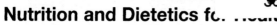
Nutrition and Dietetics for Health Care

For Churchill Livingstone:

Senior Commissioning Editor: Ninette Premdas
Project Development Manager: Mairi McCubbin
Project Manager: Joannah Duncan
Designer: Judith Wright

Nutrition and Dietetics for Health Care

Helen M. Barker BSc SRD MPH PGCE
Senior Lecturer, Dietetics, School of Health and Social Sciences,
University of Coventry, Coventry, UK

TENTH EDITION

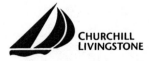

CHURCHILL
LIVINGSTONE

EDINBURGH LONDON NEW YORK OXFORD PHILADELPHIA ST LOUIS SYDNEY TORONTO 2002

CHURCHILL LIVINGSTONE
An imprint of Elsevier Limited

Tenth edition published 2002

ISBN 13: 978 0 443 07021 1
ISBN 10: 0 443 07021 0

British Library Cataloguing in Publication Data
A catalogue record for this book is available from the British Library

Library of Congress Cataloguing in Publication Data
A catalogue record for this book is available from the Library of
Congress

Note
Medical knowledge is constantly changing. As new information
becomes available, changes in treatment, procedures, equipment and
the use of drugs become necessary. The editors, contributor and the
publishers have taken care to ensure that the information given in
this text is accurate and up to date. However, readers are strongly
advised to confirm that the information, especially with regard to
drug usage, complies with the latest legislation and standards of
practice.

ELSEVIER   your source for books,
journals and multimedia
in the health sciences
www.elsevierhealth.com

Working together to grow
libraries in developing countries
www.elsevier.com | www.bookaid.org | www.sabre.org
ELSEVIER   BOOK AID International   Sabre Foundation

Transferred to Digital Printing 2010

The
publisher's
policy is to use
paper manufactured
from sustainable forests

Essential nutrient. This is a nutrient which is necessary for life and cannot be synthesised by the body; therefore it must be included in the diet.

Diet. This is the selection of foods which are normally eaten by a person or population.

Food. This is a substance that, when eaten, digested and absorbed, provides at least one nutrient.

Balanced diet. This is a diet which provides adequate amounts of all nutrients—not too much and not too little.

Malnutrition. This occurs when the diet contains an incorrect amount of one or more nutrients.

Nutritional status. This is the state of health produced by the balance between requirement and intake of nutrients.

Nutritional assessment. This is the measurement of nutritional status. It is based on anthropometric and biochemical data, and a dietary history.

Dietitian. This is a person who applies the science of nutrition to the feeding of individuals and groups, both in health and disease.

METABOLISM

This term is used to describe all the changes which are constantly taking place in the body as a result of tissue activity. The word itself means change; and, in the course of metabolism, nutrients take part in many transformations, as a result of which energy is liberated, tissue is formed, and the body functions necessary for the maintenance of life are stimulated and controlled. There are two types of metabolism.

1. *Anabolism:* complex molecules are synthesised from simpler ones—this reaction requires energy.
2. *Catabolism:* complex molecules are broken down to simpler ones and energy is released.

The type of metabolism that occurs in growth is anabolism. Catabolism occurs during starvation and illness, when the energy intake is inadequate.

FUNCTION OF NUTRIENTS IN THE BODY

A rigid classification of the functions of nutrients is impossible because their functions often overlap. A brief outline, however, is presented in Table 1.1.

MEASUREMENT OF NUTRIENTS IN FOODS

The majority of foods have been analysed, and details of their composition are available (Holland et al 1991).

The energy value of foods can be expressed as either calories or joules. In the UK the calorie is the more familiar term. It is a unit of heat. The unit used in nutrition is the kilocalorie, often incorrectly referred to as a calorie for the sake of convenience.

The calorie, however, is not recognised in the international system of units (Système International; SI), agreed in 1960, and has been replaced by the joule. The joule is a unit of energy, irrespective of the form in which that energy is manifested; for example it can denote heat, muscular energy or electrical energy. In nutrition, large amounts of energy are being considered, and the most convenient units are the kilojoule (kJ) and the megajoule (MJ), the prefix 'mega' denoting 1 million. For example, the estimated average daily energy requirement for a male aged 19–50 years who is inactive is usually expressed as 10.7 MJ rather than 10 669 kJ. One kcal is equivalent to 4.184 kJ.

Further information on units of measurement will be found in Appendix 1. The calorie and the joule are discussed in more detail in Chapter 7.

Nutritionists and dietitians need a standard against which they can compare the nutrient content of a specific diet to see whether the diet:

- contains an adequate amount of the nutrient, or
- is likely to be deficient in that nutrient, or
- contains an amount of a particular nutrient that is likely to be toxic.

Table 1.1   Main functions of nutrients

Nutrient	Function
Carbohydrate	Metabolised to produce energy 1 g of carbohydrate provides 16 kJ (3.75 kcal)
Protein	Utilised for tissue formation, growth and repair Metabolised to produce energy 1 g of protein provides 17 kJ (4.0 kcal)
Fat	A concentrated source of energy Acts as a carrier for fat-soluble vitamins Contains essential fatty acids which are important for cell-membrane formation 1 g provides 37 kJ (9 kcal)
Water	Provides the fluid medium essential for metabolic processes and the excretion of waste products
Vitamins	Act as co-factors in enzyme activity Act as antioxidants preventing damage by free radicals Prevent deficiency diseases
Minerals	Bone and teeth formation Components of enzyme systems Nerve function Maintaining cell homeostasis

1

Introduction to nutrition

LEARNING OBJECTIVES

After studying this chapter you should be:

- familiar with the terminology used in nutrition
- able to describe dietary reference values and explain how they are used.

Human nutrition is the study of the effects that any constituent of the diet has on the human. This is a rapidly expanding science which overlaps with physiology, biochemistry, psychology and sociology (see Box 1.1).

TERMINOLOGY IN NUTRITION

Nutrition may be described as the sum of the processes by which a living organism receives materials from its environment and uses them to promote its own vital activities. Such materials are known as nutrients.

Nutrients. This term is commonly applied to any substance which is digested and absorbed and used to promote body function. These nutrients include protein, fat, carbohydrate, minerals, vitamins and water.

Box 1.1 A summary of the topics included in the study of human nutrition

- The physiological and biochemical processes by which food is digested, absorbed and utilised, either to produce energy or to be converted into body tissues.
- The diseases that result from malnutrition.
- The role of diet in the development of chronic degeneractive diseases such as heart disease and cancer.
- The effects of diet upon human growth, function and intellectual development.
- The factors which influence dietary choice.

Contents

Contents

Preface

It is now accepted by all those involved in health care that good nutrition is essential for maintenance of good health, prevention of disease and recovery from illness. All health care workers have a role to play in this. They need to have a sound knowledge and a clear understanding of the principles of nutrition and how these can be applied, to ensure that their clients have the best possible diet. This book has been written to provide health care workers and students of nutrition and dietetics with clear, concise, evidence-based information that is practical in use with patients and clients.

The contents of this new edition have been expanded and more detail provided. The work has been fully referenced and further reading recommended to meet the varied needs of health care professionals.

The text is divided into three sections. The first provides the scientific basis of nutrition, which is then applied in the other two sections. The Public Health and Community Nutrition section covers dietary needs and nutritional care of all members of the community. There are specific chapters on ethnic minority groups, elderly people, people with learning disabilities and people with mental health problems. Up-to-date information is given on the dietary recommendations for children and adults, including how these can be achieved on low incomes. The chapter on factors influencing food choice will be of particular interest to all involved in health promotion. A chapter on public health nutrition has been included to meet the needs of those health care workers who are involved in improving public health by promoting good nutrition for all members of the community.

The section on therapeutic diets covers conditions that have dietary modification as an essential component of their treatment and includes a revised and enlarged chapter on malnutrition in hospital and nutrition support, which should be of particular value to all those who are trying to reduce the incidence of malnutrition in hospitals.

Coventry, 2002   Helen M. Barker

The science of nutrition

The Committee on Medical Aspects of Food Policy (COMA) report *Dietary Reference Values for Food Energy and Nutrients for the United Kingdom* (DoH 1991) was designed to provide these standards and the terms used in this report are outlined below.

DIETARY REFERENCE VALUES

This is a general term used to cover four different sets of reference values (LRNI, EAR, RNI and safe intake—see below) which have been produced by the COMA panel (see Fig. 1.1). These reference values are intended to be used to assess the adequacy of a diet for a group of individuals and to act as a guide for specific individuals. They are divided into age and sex groups. As individuals have a range of requirements, they should be used with caution to assess the diet of any individual.

Lower reference nutrient intake (LRNI)

This is the amount of the nutrient that supplies the needs of the small group of the population who have the lowest needs. Most people will require more than the LRNI of a nutrient. If the population has a dietary intake that corresponds to the LRNI, many people will be receiving a diet that is deficient in that nutrient.

Estimated average requirement (EAR)

This value is always higher than the LRNI. It is the average amount of a nutrient required by a group of people. Since it is an average, some individuals will require more than the EAR and others less.

Reference nutrient intake (RNI)

This value is always higher than the EAR and is the intake of a nutrient which fulfils the needs of 97% of the population. It exceeds the actual requirements of most individuals within a population. When the intake of a nutrient by a population is the same as the RNI, it is unlikely that a particular member of that population will have a diet deficient in that nutrient.

Safe intake

The LRNI, EAR and RNI values have been set by the panel after consulting published literature, balance studies and observed intakes. If, however, there is insufficient information to establish these levels, the panel have set a level, known as the safe level, on the basis of information available, which they felt was adequate for most people's needs but not high enough to be harmful.

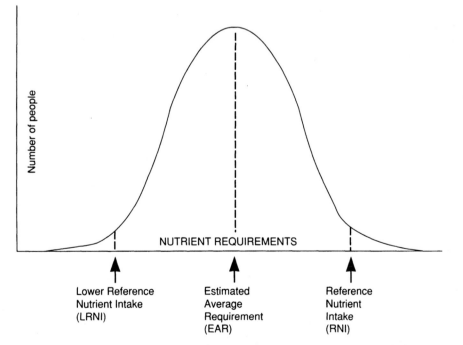

Figure 1.1 Relationship between various reference values (from Salmon 1991 with permission of HMSO).

REFERENCES

Department of Health (DoH) 1991 Dietary reference values for food energy and nutrients for the United Kingdom. Report of the Panel on Dietary Reference Values of the Committee on Medical Aspects of Food Policy (COMA). (Report on Health and Social Subjects 41) HMSO, London

Holland B, Welch A A, Unwin I D, Buss D H, Paul A A, Southgate D A T 1991 McCance and Widdowson's composition of foods, 5th Edn. Cambridge, Royal Society of Chemistry

Salmon J (for the Department of Health) 1991 Dietary reference values—a guide. HMSO, London

FURTHER READING

Directorate General Industrial Affairs 1993 Reports of the Scientific Committee for Human Nutrition Series 31. Nutrient and energy intakes for the European Community Office des Publications Officielles des Communautés Européennes

Ministry of Agriculture, Fisheries and Food 1995 Manual of Nutrition, 10th Edn. HMSO, London

USEFUL WEBSITES

www.nutrition.org.uk
The website of the British Nutrition Foundation which contains fact-sheets, work-sheets and press releases on a broad range of nutrition issues.

www.eatright.org
The website of the American Dietetic Association which contains consumer advice, nutrition information and position papers.

www.bda.uk.com
The website of the British Dietetic Association which contains position papers, press releases on topical issues and nutrition information.

USEFUL ADDRESSES

British Nutrition Foundation
High Holborn House
52–54 High Holborn
London
WC1V 6RQ
Tel: 0207 404 6504

2

Carbohydrates

LEARNING OBJECTIVES

After studying this chapter you should be able to:

- describe the chemical structure of carbohydrates
- list the different types and sources of carbohydrate in the diet
- outline how carbohydrates are digested, utilised and absorbed
- discuss the dietary reference values for carbohydrates
- describe the consequences of insufficient carbohydrate in the diet.

Carbohydrates are compounds consisting of carbon, hydrogen and oxygen. Plants have the ability to produce sugar and starch from the carbon dioxide of the air and water from the soil. Carbohydrate is the most important source of energy in the human diet. Humans obtain the carbohydrate in their diet by eating foods which have a plant origin, e.g. grains, vegetables and fruit.

Carbohydrate is oxidised in the body to give heat and energy for all forms of body activity. Carbon dioxide and water are formed as end-products and are excreted principally by the lungs and kidneys.

One gram of carbohydrate provides 16 kJ (3.75 kcal) on oxidation in the body, which is often 'rounded up' to 4 kcal.

CHEMICAL STRUCTURE OF CARBOHYDRATES

Monosaccharides

The simplest forms of carbohydrate with which we are concerned in human nutrition are the simple sugars, glucose, fructose and galactose (see Fig. 2.1). These are known as monosaccharides. The structure of the glucose molecule is shown in Figure 2.2.

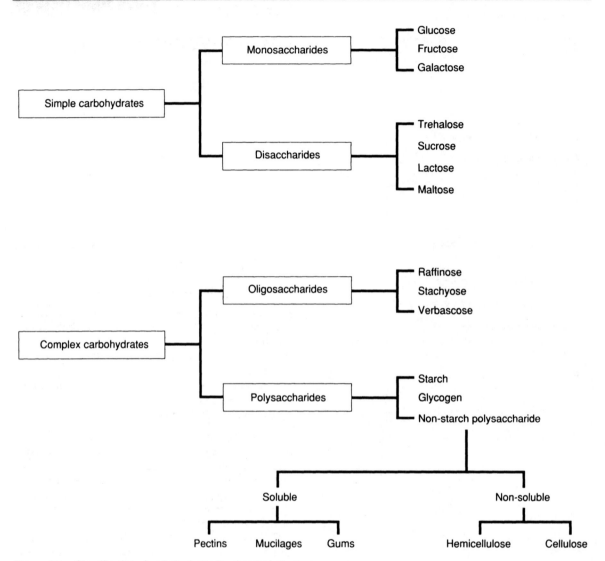

Figure 2.1 Classification of carbohydrates by chemical structure.

Dissacharides

Pairs of monosaccharides combine to form disaccharides. The disaccharides which are most important in human nutrition are sucrose, lactose and maltose. Their composition is illustrated below:

glucose + fructose → sucrose
glucose + galactose → lactose
glucose + glucose → maltose

Figure 2.3 shows the structure of the sucrose molecule.

Oligosaccharides

These are formed from 3–11 monosaccharide units joined together. The most commonly occurring dietary oligosaccharides are raffinose, stachyose and verbascose.

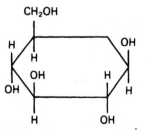

Figure 2.2 Structure of the glucose molecule.

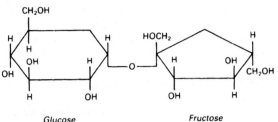

Figure 2.3 Structure of the sucrose molecule.

Polysaccharides

Polysaccharides are formed from large numbers of monosaccharides joined together.

The most important polysaccharide in human nutrition is starch, which is composed of many glucose units.

There are two types of starch: amylose and amylopectin.

Amylose consists of a straight chain of 70–350 glucose molecules. Part of an amylose chain is illustrated in Figure 2.4.

Amylopectin is a branched chain of up to 100 000 glucose molecules (Fig. 2.5).

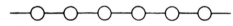

Figure 2.4 Part of an amylose chain: ○ = 1 glucose molecule.

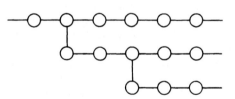

Figure 2.5 Part of an amylopectin chain: ○ = 1 glucose molecule.

DIETARY SOURCES OF CARBOHYDRATE

Naturally occurring carbohydrates

Glucose is prepared commercially from starch and is found in some fruits, notably grapes.

Fructose is found in honey and in fruits; it is sometimes called 'fruit sugar'.

Sucrose is the table sugar we are all familiar with. It is obtained from sugar beet and sugar cane and occurs in some fruits and vegetables.

Lactose is the sugar found in all mammalian milks.

Maltose is found in sprouting grain and is formed during the manufacture of beer.

Starch is the storage carbohydrate produced by plants. Considerable amounts are found in all grains, unripe fruit and certain vegetables such as potatoes, yams, plantains, peas, beans and lentils.

Galactose does not occur naturally in the diet, but is produced by the digestion of lactose.

Glycogen: animals store carbohydrate as glycogen in the liver and muscles. Meat is not a dietary source of carbohydrate because most of the glycogen is destroyed naturally prior to use.

Non-starch polysaccharides (NSP) are components of plant-cell walls. They are found in cereals, vegetables and fruit and used to be known as dietary fibre. They are not available to the human body as an energy source, as the body produces no digestive enzymes with which to break them down. They are nevertheless a valuable constituent of the diet, adding bulk to the intestinal contents, stimulating peristalsis and aiding excretion of the faeces. Other important roles of NSP are discussed in Chapter 8.

In the case of herbivorous animals, NSP are available as an energy source. This is because of the presence in the gut of bacteria which convert them to substances which can be absorbed and utilised.

The accepted method for the analysis of NSP is that of Englyst & Cummings (1988).

Synthetic carbohydrates

Food technologists have developed a range of carbohydrates which are prepared commercially and used in the place of sugars and fats in food processing and production.

Maltrodextrins: these are small oligosaccharides formed by the hydrolysis of starch. They are used to add sweetness, improve the texture and as a fat substitute in cakes and biscuits.

Polydextrose: this carbohydrate has a cream-like texture and is produced from glucose, sorbitol (an alcohol of glucose) and citric acid. Unlike maltrodextrins which are digested, absorbed and metabolised by the same mechanisms as the naturally occurring oligosaccharides, polydextrose cannot be digested by humans. Polydextrose is used as a substitute for fat in the production of reduced fat, lower calorie dairy products and in slimming products.

Corn syrup is a glucose syrup produced by hydrolysis of corn starch, which is digested normally and used to sweeten soft drinks, sauces and jams.

Invert sugar is a mixture of glucose and fructose produced by the acid hydrolysis of sucrose, which is used in the place of sucrose because of its greater sweetening power.

CARBOHYDRATE DIGESTION

The long-chain starch molecules are insoluble in water and difficult to digest. They are broken down to the shorter-chain maltose, maltotriose and α-limit dextrins. This hydrolysis occurs in the gut lumen and is brought about by the enzymes salivary α-amylase and pancreatic α-amylase.

These shorter chains are then converted to their constituent monosaccharides by a group of enzymes found on the brush border surface of the mucosal cells. This group of brush border enzymes includes:

- glucoamylase, the most important of these enzymes quantitatively
- sucrase/isomaltase which splits sucrose and α-limit dextrins into glucose
- β-galactosidase which acts on lactose.

The monosaccharides are then absorbed into the cells by an active mechanism which is partially dependent on a sodium gradient. This link between glucose and sodium absorption is of particular relevance in the preparation of rehydration solutions for diarrhoea.

Dietary disaccharides are digested rapidly by the brush border enzymes and therefore provide a more immediate source of energy than starch, which has the longer digestive process to undergo. Different carbohydrate-containing foods are digested and absorbed at different rates. This is discussed in Chapter 27, 'Diet in Diabetes Mellitus'. The rate of digestion is influenced by the food form, NSP content and type of carbohydrate present. High-amylose starches digest more quickly than high-amylopectin starches (Vinik & Jenkins 1988).

ABSORPTION AND UTILISATION OF CARBOHYDRATES

After absorption into the capillaries of the intestinal villi, the materials resulting from the digestion of carbohydrate (glucose, fructose and galactose) travel to the liver in the portal vein.

These sugars derived from dietary carbohydrate are utilised in four ways:

1. *Metabolised to produce energy.* Much of the glucose leaves the liver in the bloodstream and is conveyed around the body to be used as a fuel for the production of energy for cell activity. The brain, nervous system and red blood cells must have glucose as an energy source—no other sugar will do.

2. *Converted to glycogen.* Glycogen is synthesised from glucose in the muscles and stored to be released when it is required for the performance of muscular work. Glycogen is also synthesised by, and stored in, the liver. Liver glycogen is synthesised from glucose, galactose, fructose and the breakdown products of protein and fat.

3. *Converted to fat.* When muscles and liver are stocked with glycogen, excess carbohydrate is converted to fat, which is stored in the adipose tissues.

4. *Converted to more complex biomolecules.* Glucose is the precursor for the development of complex biomolecules, such as glycoproteins, glycolipids and proteoglycans, which are components of cell membranes, body fluids and matrix tissues.

Blood sugar level

A certain concentration of glucose is available at all times in the blood, varying between 3.5 and 10 millimoles per litre (mmol/l) in normal individuals. This blood sugar level is maintained by the liver, the glycogen stores of which are broken down into glucose and liberated into the bloodstream in this form when the level falls below approximately 4 mmol/l.

In normal circumstances, the blood sugar rarely rises above 10 mmol/l. In abnormal circumstances however (and notably in the case of diabetic people who do not metabolise carbohydrate correctly), the glucose level rises above this figure, in which case the excess will be excreted in the urine via the kidneys. The renal (or kidney) threshold for glucose is said to be 10 mmol/l.

In a small proportion of people the renal threshold is lower than normal and glucose appears in the urine when the level in the blood is not abnormally high. It is important to distinguish this benign condition from diabetes mellitus.

Hormonal control

Certain hormones play a part in the metabolism of carbohydrate.

Insulin, secreted by the β cells of the pancreatic islets, acts by assisting the passage of glucose through the cell membrane into the interior of the cell, where it is then available for metabolic activity.

Adrenaline, secreted by the adrenal medulla, stimulates the release of glucose from the breakdown of glycogen in the liver.

Glucagon, from the α cells of the pancreatic islets, also promotes release of glucose from liver glycogen.

Growth hormone, from the pituitary gland, reduces the ability of insulin to cause glucose uptake by muscle and adipose tissue, bringing about a rise in blood sugar level.

Daily intake

In UK diets, carbohydrate accounts for between 40% and 50% of the total energy intake. Figure 2.6 shows the types and sources of carbohydrate in the UK diet.

The Committee on Medical Aspects of Food Policy (COMA) report on sugars (DoH 1989) shows that breast- and bottle-fed infants obtain 40% of their energy requirement from sugars, primarily lactose. This reduces to 25–30% in pre-school children and 17–25% in older children and adolescents. This is further reduced to 18% in adults (Gregory et al 1990), of which at least half of the intake of total sugars is provided by non-milk extrinsic sugars (sucrose) that have been added to food.

Foods high in carbohydrate are plentiful, cheap, palatable, easily prepared and usually have a low fat content. Surveys show that as income levels rise in developing countries the proportion of energy in the diet derived from carbohydrate decreases and the proportion derived from fat increases.

Every culture has its staple carbohydrate food, to which small amounts of other foods are added for their protein, vitamin and minerals content to ensure a balanced diet. For example, staple carbohydrate foods in the UK are wheat (for bread) and potatoes, in the Indian sub-continent, rice or wheat (for chapattis) and in Afro-caribbean communities starchy roots and tubers. Starch may provide 80% of the energy requirement in some situations. Starchy foods contain vitamins, minerals and some protein and fat, the amounts varying with the type of food (Table 2.1).

Unfortunately, a substantial part of the carbohydrate in the Western diet is taken in the form of sucrose—sugar as it is found in the sugar bowl and in cakes and confectionery—which is almost entirely pure carbohydrate with a negligible vitamin and mineral content.

PROPERTIES AND USES OF SUGARS

An important characteristic of sugars is their sweetness. The degree of sweetness varies with different sugars. They are listed in descending order of sweetness below, fructose being the most sweet and lactose the least sweet:

- fructose
- sucrose
- glucose
- maltose
- galactose
- lactose.

All sugars are soluble in water, lactose being the least soluble.

Sucrose is used as the sweetener of choice for most domestic purposes; it is used both as a sweetener and a preservative. Sucrose is added to many manufactured foods to improve the taste, texture, appearance and shelf-life.

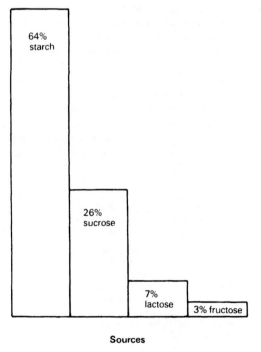

64%
starch

26%
sucrose

7%
lactose

3% fructose

Sources

Bread	Preserves	Milk	Fruit
Cereals	Confectionery	Milk products	
Potatoes	Added to		
Biscuits	drinks		
Confectionery			

Figure 2.6 Sources of carbohydrate in the UK diet.

Table 2.1 Protein, fat and carbohydrate content of some starchy foods

Food	Protein	Fat	Carbohydrate
	(g)	(g)	(g)
1 slice bread	3.0	0.6	22
1 cup boiled rice	2.5	0.4	36
1 medium boiled potato	3.5	–	50
1 portion boiled yam	1.7	–	33

Glucose is sometimes used where a high-energy intake is required, as it is easily obtained, soluble and not as sweet as sucrose, although in most therapeutic situations its use has been replaced by that of glucose polymers and maltodextrins.

Fructose is occasionally used as a sweetner instead of sucrose by diabetics and those trying to lose weight; less is used because of its more intense sweetness, so reducing the actual energy intake.

Intrinsic and extrinsic sugars

In addition to classifying by their chemical structure, nutritionists also classify sugars into two groups, intrinsic and extrinsic (DoH 1991)—see Figure 2.7.

Intrinsic sugars are sugars that are contained within the cell walls of a food, for example the fructose, glucose or sucrose which occurs naturally in a food. If this sugar is extracted from the food, it becomes an *extrinsic sugar*, for example sucrose which, once extracted from sugar beet, becomes an extrinsic rather than an intrinsic sugar.

Extrinsic sugars particularly sucrose, are frequently incorporated into other foods by adding them to drinks or using them in baking. However, this process does not reincorporate the sugar into the cells of the other foods so the sugar does not become intrinsic.

The lactose present in milk and milk products is classified as a subgroup of extrinsic sugars—*milk extrinsic sugars*. Other extrinsic sugars (mainly sucrose) are referred to as *non-milk extrinsic sugars*.

DIETARY REFERENCE VALUES FOR SUGARS

The COMA report on dietary reference values for foods does not recommend any limitation on the intake of intrinsic sugars or milk sugars. Starch, intrinsic sugars and milk sugars should provide the balance of energy which is not provided by alcohol, protein, fat and non-milk extrinsic sugars (the intake of all these should be limited) to ensure an adequate energy intake.

Sucrose, the extrinsic sugar which is quantitatively most important, should be restricted to an intake of 10% of total dietary energy intake or not exceed 60 g/day. This figure was set because of the relationship between sucrose intake and dental caries, which in practice is related to the frequency with which non-milk extrinsic sugars are eaten, rather than the quantity (i.e. the number of sugar-containing snacks, drinks and meals eaten).

The conclusions of the COMA panel on dietary sugars are summarised in Box 2.1.

DIETARY REFERENCE VALUES FOR STARCH

The basis for many healthy eating campaigns is to reduce fat consumption while maintaining energy balance by increasing carbohydrate intake, particularly the intake of starchy foods. In practice this means encouraging people to eat more bread, pasta, rice and potatoes. Gregory et al (1990) showed that the average amount of energy provided by starch in the diet of UK adults was 24%. It has been proposed by the COMA report (DoH 1991) that 39% of energy should be provided by carbohydrates (starch, intrinsic sugars and milk sugars). However, it did not state how much should be provided as starch. It did, however, state that there are no known detrimental effects of high or very high starch intakes (provided the requirements for all other nutrients are met).

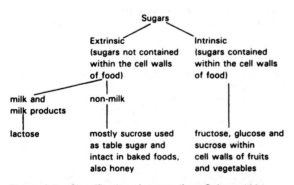

Figure 2.7 Classification of sugars (from Salmon 1991, with permission of HMSO).

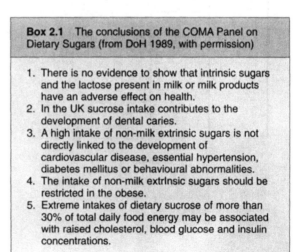

Box 2.1 The conclusions of the COMA Panel on Dietary Sugars (from DoH 1989, with permission)

1. There is no evidence to show that intrinsic sugars and the lactose present in milk or milk products have an adverse effect on health.
2. In the UK sucrose intake contributes to the development of dental caries.
3. A high intake of non-milk extrinsic sugars is not directly linked to the development of cardiovascular disease, essential hypertension, diabetes mellitus or behavioural abnormalities.
4. The intake of non-milk extrinsic sugars should be restricted in the obese.
5. Extreme intakes of dietary sucrose of more than 30% of total daily food energy may be associated with raised cholesterol, blood glucose and insulin concentrations.

INSUFFICIENT CARBOHYDRATE

1. Lack of carbohydrate in the diet results in insufficient glucose being available for production of energy, with the result that fat is used as an energy source to an extent greater than normal. During fat metabolism, substances known as ketones are produced. In the absence of sufficient carbohydrate these are produced at a rate exceeding that of their disposal, their accumulation in the body giving rise to ketoacidosis.

2. The primary function of protein is to build body tissue. However, if a lack of carbohydrate and fat occurs, protein will be diverted from this purpose and used instead to give energy. Carbohydrate is therefore said to be a protein sparer, and lack of carbohydrate can cause depletion of body tissue, as in starvation resulting from famine, or from the inability to take food during illness.

REFERENCES

Department of Health (DoH) 1989 Dietary sugars and human disease. Committee on Medical Aspects of Food Policy (COMA). Report of the panel on the dietary sugars. (Report on Health and Social Subjects 37). HMSO, London

Department of Health (DoH) 1991 Dietary reference values for food energy and nutrients for the United Kingdom. Report of the Panel on Dietary Reference Values of the Committee on Medical Aspects of Food Policy (COMA). (Report on Health and Social Subjects 41). HMSO, London

Englyst H N, Cummings J H 1988 An improved method for the measurement of dietary fiber as non-starch polysaccharides in plant foods. Journal of the Association of Analytical Chemistry 71: 808–814

Gregory J, Foster K, Tyler H, Wiseman M 1990 The dietary and nutritional survey of British adults. HMSO, London

Salmon J (for the Department of Health) 1991 Dietary reference values—a guide. HMSO, London

Vinik I A, Jenkins D J A 1988 Dietary fibre in the management of diabetes. Diabetes Care 11: 160–173

FURTHER READING

Department of Health (DoH) 1991 Dietary reference values for food energy and nutrients for the United Kingdom. Report of the Panel on Dietary Reference Values of the Committee on Medical Aspects of Food Policy (COMA). (Report on Health and Social Subjects 41). HMSO, London

Holmes S 1993 Building blocks—foods, metabolism. Nursing Times 89(21): 28–31

3

Fats

LEARNING OBJECTIVES

After studying this chapter you should be able to:

- describe the chemical structure of fats
- explain the differences between saturated and unsaturated fats
- list the types, sources and dietary reference values for fats in the diet
- outline the digestion, absorbtion, utilisation and function of fats.

STRUCTURE OF FATS

Fats, like carbohydrates, are composed of atoms of carbon, hydrogen and oxygen, but they are arranged in different patterns and proportions.

Fats are formed by the combination of glycerol with fatty acids, each unit of glycerol combining with three fatty acid units to give a triglyceride (triacylglycerol). Many different fatty acids occur. They can be divided into three types: saturated fatty acids, monounsaturated fatty acids and polyunsaturated fatty acids (Box 3.1). A triglyceride can contain three identical fatty acids or a mixture of different fatty acids.

1 molecule glycerol + 3 molecules fatty acid → 1 molecule triglyceride (fat) and water

It is the particular types and combination of fatty acids which give each type of fat its own identity and physical properties. The fats with which we are familiar, for example in butter, lard and olive oil, are mixtures of triglycerides. Examples of the fatty acids occurring in dietary fats are stearic, palmitic and oleic acids (see Box 3.1).

Hydrogenation of fatty acids

The carbon atoms in the hydrocarbon chain of the fatty acid part of the triglyceride molecule can be linked by

---

> **Box 3.1 Types of fatty acid**
>
> **Saturated**
> Palmitic (16 carbon atoms in chain) and stearic acids (18 carbon atoms in chain), which are found in lard and suet, are examples of saturated fatty acids. All the bonds in the fatty acid chain have been hydrogenated.
>
> **Monounsaturated**
> Oleic acid (18 carbon atoms in chain), which is found in many fats, particularly olive oil, is an example of a monounsaturated fatty acid. Although the carbon chain is 18 atoms long there is one double bond, so that two hydrogen atoms are missing.
>
> **Polyunsaturated**
> These contain more than one double bond, for example linoleic acid which has four hydrogen atoms missing, and linolenic acid which has six hydrogen atoms missing.

'single' or 'double' bonds. If all the bonds are single the fatty acid is called saturated; if double bonds are present (i.e. there are hydrogen atoms missing) the fatty acid is unsaturated. If only one double bond is present, the fatty acid is monounsaturated. The fatty acids of saturated fats are more stable than those of unsaturated fats. The double bonds in unsaturated fatty acids can be converted to single bonds; this process is known as hydrogenation.

Figure 3.1 shows the structures of palmitic acid, oleic acid, linoleic acid and alpha-linolenic acid.

Saturated—Palmitic acid

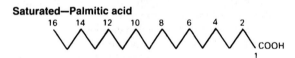

Monounsaturated—Oleic acid

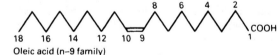

Polyunsaturated—Linoleic acid

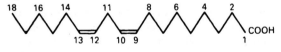

Alpha-Linolenic acid

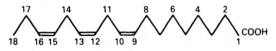

Figure 3.1 The structures of palmitic, oleic, linoleic and alpha-linolenic acids (adapted from Garrow et al 2000).

Saturated and unsaturated fats

The fatty acids present in most soft fats and oils contain less hydrogen than those in the harder fats and are therefore referred to as being unsaturated. More hydrogen can be introduced into their structure by chemical means. This process of hydrogenation alters both the chemical structure and the physical properties of the fat, making it harder and raising its melting point. Margarine is produced by the hydrogenation of oils such as palm oil, corn oil and soya oil.

Cis *and* trans *forms of fats*

If a fat contains a double bond, as in monounsaturated and polyunsaturated fat, it can exist in two isomeric forms. These are known as the *cis* form and the *trans* form. It is usual for the monounsaturated and polyunsaturated fatty acids occurring naturally to exist in the *cis* form. The exception to this is the fat present in some meats. This is because the *cis* form is converted to the *trans* form in the stomach of some ruminants. However, when polyunsaturated fats are hydrogenated to be used for margarines and in the food industry, they usually adopt the *trans* form. It has been suggested that an increased intake of *trans* fatty acids may be linked to an increased incidence of coronary heart disease (Willett et al 1993).

ESSENTIAL FATTY ACIDS

Certain polyunsaturated fatty acids are needed by the body and are known as the essential fatty acids. The essential fatty acids are linoleic and alpha-linolenic. Arachidonic, eicosapentanoic and decosahexanoic acids can all be manufactured from linoleic and alpha-linolenic acid, but if the supply of linoleic and alpha-linolenic acid is limited, they then become essential fatty acids.

Arachidonic, eicosapentanoic and decosahexanoic acids are precursors of prostaglandins, thromboxane which promotes platelet aggregation in clotting, and leukotrienes. The use of long-chain n-3 fatty acids (derived from alpha-linolenic acid) to treat the inflammatory condition rheumatoid arthritis (Geusens et al 1994), and for asthma, psoriasis and Crohn's disease (BNF 1999) has therefore been researched.

Vitamin E is important in preventing oxidation of essential fatty acids in the body, thus preserving their chemical structure.

STEROLS

Sterols are also made up of carbon, hydrogen and oxygen atoms, but arranged in a different configuration to fats. The atoms are arranged in a series of four rings with a range of side-chains. The principal sterol found in animal tissue is cholesterol. This sterol is not found in plants; over 40 sterols have been identified in plants and these are known as phytosterols. The average UK diet contains approximately 0.25 g plant sterols and 0.3 g cholesterol per day.

Cholesterol

Cholesterol is synthesised in the body and is also obtained from the diet. It occurs in association with animal tissues and, in the UK, the principal dietary sources are full-fat dairy products, fatty meat, egg yolks and offal.

Cholesterol is excreted from the body in the bile, where it is held in solution by combining with bile salts. If it is precipitated out of solution, it appears in solid form as gallstones. Hegsted et al (1965) were able to show that an increase in saturated fatty acids leads to a rise in serum cholesterol.

Phytosterols

The most abundantly occurring phytosterols are beta sitosterol, campesterol and stigmasterol. They reduce absorption of cholesterol from the intestinal lumen by competing with cholesterol for space in the micelles (Heinnemann 1991) (see Fig. 3.2). This has led to the development of polyunsaturated margarines that contain additional sterols for use in the primary prevention of ischaemic heart disease (Law 2000).

PHOSPHOLIPIDS

Essential fatty acids are part of phospholipids, which have these important functions:

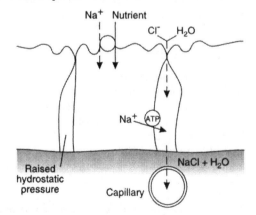

Figure 3.2 Transport of Na^+ can drive absorption of Cl^- and osmosis of water from the intestine. This is accelerated in the presence of nutrient molecules (e.g. glucose) (McGeown 1999).

- maintaining the structure and function of cell membranes
- regulating cholesterol metabolism.

Phospholipids occur in small amounts in most foods. Eggs, liver, pulses and nuts are particularly rich sources of them. The most commonly occurring phospholipid is phosphatidylcholine (lecithin), the richest dietary source of which is eggs.

The chemical structure of phospholipids enables them to act as emulsifying agents. They are important components of cell membranes and lipoproteins.

LIPOPROTEINS

Fats, cholesterol, phospholipids and fatty acids are insoluble in water, but in blood plasma they form soluble combinations with some of the plasma proteins, and in this form they are known as lipoproteins.

RANCIDITY AND SOLUBILITY OF FATS

Fats are insoluble in water, but in certain circumstances will form a suspension of minute particles known as an emulsion. This process takes place during the digestion of fats in the intestine.

Rancidity in dairy fats is due to the liberation of free fatty acids, some of which have a disagreeable odour and flavour, resulting from hydrolysis of the triglycerides by bacteria. Exposure to the oxygen of the air causes unsaturated fats in meat, fish oils and non-dairy fats to become oxidised and develop rancidity.

DIETARY SOURCES OF FATS AND ESSENTIAL FATTY ACIDS

Most vegetable and marine oils are good sources of essential fatty acids. A dietary survey of UK adults in 1990 (Gregory et al 1990) showed that they obtained their essential fatty acids from vegetables, fruit, nuts, cereal products and fat spreads.

Fats are derived from both animal and vegetable sources. Fats and oils have similar structures. Fats which are liquid below 20°C are called oils. Fish and vegetable fats are referred to as oils, as they are liquid at room temperature.

Meat fats include beef dripping, suet, mutton fat and lard (pork fat).

Dairy fats include milk and its products, cream, butter and cheese. These contain cholesterol, either in the free form or combined with glycerol to form an ester.

Eggs also contain cholesterol.

Fish oils: the tissues of some fish are rich in long-chain polyunsaturated fatty acids, of the omega-3 (n-3) series. These fish are known as fatty fish and include herring, mackerel, sardine, salmon and trout. Fish that does not accumulate fat in the tissues are known as white fish. White fish accumulate oils in their livers which are a rich source of vitamins A and D.

Vegetable fats include olive oil, coconut oil, palm oil, cotton-seed oil, corn oil and others. These do not contain cholesterol but contain plant sterols instead, which are poorly absorbed by humans.

DIGESTION AND ABSORPTION

Fat digestion starts in the stomach where it is broken up by the mechanical action of the stomach movements, while the lingual lipase partially hydrolyses some of the triglycerides to diglycerides and free fatty acids. The gastric contents then enter the duodenum where the fats are further emulsified by bile from the gall bladder and hydrolysed by the action of pancreatic lipase to form micelles. The micelles diffuse into the intestinal epithelium where they reform as triglycerides which then combine to form chylomicrons, which pass into the lacteals and then enter the portal circulation via the lymphatic system.

FUNCTIONS OF FATS

1. *Source of energy.* Fats are oxidised in the body to provide energy for tissue activity and for the maintenance of body temperature. They are a concentrated source of energy, providing 37 kJ (9 kcal) per gram, compared with 16 kJ per gram from carbohydrate and 17 kJ per gram from protein. An adequate supply of energy from carbohydrate and fat ensures that protein is available for tissue formation and repair.

2. *Incorporation into body structure.* Some fat enters the body cells and constitutes an essential part of their structure. Fat is particularly important in the structure of the brain and nervous tissue.

3. *Protection.* The deposits of fatty tissue around the vital organs hold these organs in position and protect them from injury.

4. *Insulation.* Subcutaneous fat prevents loss of heat from the body.

5. *Satiety.* The presence of fat in the chyme as it passes into the duodenum results in inhibition of gastric peristalsis and acid secretion, thus delaying the emptying time of the stomach and preventing early recurrence of hunger after a meal.

6. *Fat-soluble vitamins.* The fats of the diet provide the fat-soluble vitamins and assist in their absorption from the intestine.

7. *Energy storage.* The storage of fat in the adipose tissue enables the body to store energy for a prolonged period of time.

BODY-FAT STORES

The chief stores of fatty tissue are under the skin and around the abdominal organs; these are sometimes referred to as the fat depots. Large amounts of fat can be stored in this way. These fat stores are not inert, but are continually being interchanged with the fats circulating in the bloodstream, and being mobilised for use as fuel.

The metabolism of an unusually large proportion of fat may give rise to ketosis (p. 13). This can occur when the diet has a very low carbohydrate content, for example in some slimming regimes, and is a feature of diabetes mellitus where carbohydrate metabolism is impaired through lack of insulin.

Fats have a higher energy value, weight for weight, than carbohydrate, protein or alcohol. They contribute an important part of the energy content of the diet and improve its palatability.

In the UK individual fat intakes range between 80 and 160 g daily. It is not known whether any definite amount of fat is necessary for the maintenance of health, other than to provide an adequate supply of essential fatty acids. Eating more energy than the body needs, whether it is as fat, carbohydrate or protein, leads to deposition of fat in the adipose tissues and contributes to the development of obesity.

DIETARY REFERENCE VALUES

The dietary reference values for fat are expressed as a percentage of the total energy intake.

The dietary reference value for total fat intake is that 35% of energy should be provided by fat. This figure is derived by adding up the individual reference values for the different types of fatty acids and adjusting the amount to take account of the weight of glycerol in fat. The dietary reference values for fatty acids are listed in Table 3.1.

The recommendations of the panel in relation to heart disease are discussed in Chapter 22.

Table 3.1 Dietary reference values for fatty acids and total fat

Fatty acids	Population average intake as % of energy consumed (excluding that provided by alcohol)
Saturated fatty acids	11
Cis-monounsaturated fatty acids	13
Cis-polyunsaturated fatty acids (these should not exceed 10% of total energy)	65
Trans fatty acids	2
Total fatty acids	**32.5**

When adjusted for the weight of glycerol, the 32.5% becomes 35%
In practical terms: 35% of the energy in a 2500 kcal diet is provided by 97 g fat; 35% of the energy in a 1900 kcal diet is provided by 74 g fat.

REFERENCES

British Nutrition Foundation (BNF) 1999. n-3 Fatty acids and health—A briefing paper. British Nutrition Foundation, London

Garrow JS, James WPT, Ralph A 2000 Human nutrition and dietetics, 10th Edn. Churchill Livingstone, Edinburgh

Geusens P, Wouters C, Nijs J, Jiang Y, Dequeker J 1994 Long-term effect of omega-3 fatty acid supplementation on active rheumatoid arthritis. Arthritis and Rheumatism 37(6): 824–829

Gregory J, Foster K, Tyler H, Wiseman M 1990 The dietary and nutritional survey of British adults. HMSO, London

Hegsted D M, McGandy R B, Myers M L, Stare F J 1965 Quantitative effects of dietary fat on serum cholesterol in man. American Journal of Clinical Nutrition 17: 281–295

Heinnemann T, Kullack-ublick A, Pietruck B, Von Bergmann K 1991 Mechanisms of action of plant sterols on inhibition of cholesterol absorption. European Journal of Clinical Pharmacology 40 (Suppl. 1): 59–635

Law M 2000 Plant sterol and stanol margarines and health. British Medical Journal 320: 861–864

McGeown JG 1999 Physiology. Churchill Livingstone, Edinburgh

Willett W C, Stampfer M J, Manson J E et al 1993 Intake of *trans* fatty acids and risk of coronary heart disease among women. Lancet 341: 581–585

FURTHER READING

Coultate T P 1984 Food—the chemistry of its components. The Royal Society of Chemistry, London

Department of Health (DoH) 1991 Dietary reference values for food, energy and nutrients for the United Kingdom. Report of the Panel on Dietary Reference Values of the Committee on Medical Aspects of Food Policy (COMA). (Report on Health and Social Subjects 41). HMSO, London

4

Proteins

LEARNING OBJECTIVES

After studying this chapter you should be able to:
- describe the chemical structure of proteins
- discuss the role of essential amino acids
- explain the concept of nitrogen balance
- outline the digestion, absorption, utilisation and function of proteins
- explain the causes and consequences of dietary protein deficiency.

STRUCTURE OF PROTEINS

Every living cell has protein as one of its principal constituents. In structure, proteins resemble chains, consisting of amino acids linked together. Animals can synthesise proteins from amino acids but are unable to synthesise amino acids de novo. Plants are able to synthesise amino acids from carbon dioxide, water and nitrogen-containing compounds from the soil. Thus, humans obtain protein only by eating plants or other animals.

Amino acids are composed of carbon, hydrogen, oxygen and occasionally sulphur (see Fig 4.1).

Chains of amino acids are formed when the amino group of one amino acid links with the acid group of another amino acid. Two amino acids link together to form a dipeptide. A polypeptide is formed when many amino acids link together.

Very large protein molecules contain many thousands of amino acids, whereas small proteins, such as insulin, contain less than 100. In some cases, mineral elements such as sulphur, phosphorus, iodine and iron are also present.

The proteins of the diet are the body's only source of nitrogen. Structurally, proteins are divided into two types depending on the shape of the molecule:

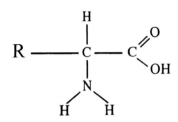

Figure 4.1   General structure of an amino acid (Garrow et al 2000).

- *fibrous*, where the chain remains in its extended form, and
- *globular*, where the chain is folded to form an irregularly shaped bulky molecule.

There are thousands of different plant and animal proteins. All are hydrolysed to amino acids in varying proportions. Examples of proteins found in food include:

- myosin—in meat
- albumin—in eggs
- casein—in milk
- vitellin—in eggs
- gluten—in wheat.

The amino acid content and sequence is specific to the protein and shows a species variation. Thus, the myosin in beef has a different amino acid sequence to the myosin in lamb.

ESSENTIAL AMINO ACIDS

The human body requires amino acids in order to make the specific proteins required by its many specialised tissues. Some amino acids can be made by converting one into another. This occurs in the liver by a process known as transamination. Those amino acids which the body is either unable to make, or unable to make in sufficient quantities, are called essential amino acids and are listed in Box 4.1. Histidine is an essential amino acid for children.

Cystine and tyrosine are semi-essential amino acids. Semi-essential amino acids are produced by the body from essential amino acids. Cystine can be synthesised from methionine, and tyrosine from phenylalanine, if these amino acids are present in the diet in adequate amounts. Glycine, arginine, proline, glutamic acid, aspartic acid, serine and alanine can be synthesised by the body from other carbon-and nitrogen-containing substances.

A more detailed description of the characteristics of individual amino acids can be found in *Human Nutrition and Dietetics* (Garrow et al 2000).

Biological value of proteins

If the diet contains adequate supplies of all the essential amino acids, proteins can be synthesised. If, however, it contains an inadequate amount of one of these amino acids, synthesis cannot occur. Protein foods which contain all the essential amino acids in the proportions required to support growth and/or maintain nutritional status are said to have a high biological value. Examples of foods with a high biological value are human breast-milk, eggs and meat.

Limiting amino acids

Protein foods from plant sources tend to have a lower biological value than animal protein foods. The essential amino acids that they lack, or only supply in small amounts, are called the limiting amino acids. Not all foods have the same limiting amino acid (see Table 4.1).

This is very important in assessing the adequacy of dietary protein supplies.

Supplementation of amino acids

The lack of an essential amino acid in a food can be overcome by eating, at the same time, another protein food which contains that amino acid.

For example, a meal containing wheat as the only protein source lacks lysine, and so has a low biological value, as does a meal of soya beans only for, although beans are a rich source of lysine, they contain very little methionine.

However, a meal which contains both soya beans and wheat has adequate supplies of both lysine and methionine. This fact is of great importance to strict vegetarians who derive their protein entirely from vegetable sources. They need to eat not only adequate amounts

Table 4.1   Examples of limiting amino acids in foods

Food	Limiting amino acid
Wheat	Lysine
Soya beans	Methionine
Maize	Tryptophan

but also a variety of protein-containing foods to ensure a sufficiency of the essential amino acids. A mixture of low biological value proteins will complement each other to provide a diet with a wide range of essential amino acids, thus improving its biological value.

In many parts of the world the staple diet consists largely, or entirely, of foods of vegetable origin, containing only low biological value proteins. Efforts are at present being made to increase the nutritive value of these diets by the addition of foods which can be produced locally, and which supply the essential amino acids lacking in those already consumed. Some products which have proved of value in this respect are groundnuts (peanuts), soya beans and cotton-seed. In a mixed diet, such as that normally eaten in the UK, the protein is derived from foods of both high and low biological values. Approximate protein content for some food portions are given in Table 4.2.

FUNCTIONS OF PROTEINS

Proteins are essential constituents of all body tissues:

1. They replace the protein lost during normal metabolism and normal wear and tear. Protein is lost in the formation of hair and nails, and as dead cells from the surface of skin and the alimentary tract. It is also lost in digestive secretions.

2. They produce new tissue. New tissue is formed during periods of growth, recovery from injury, pregnancy and lactation.

3. They are needed in the manufacture of new proteins which perform specific functions in the body—enzymes, hormones and haemoglobin.

4. They can be used as an energy source.

NITROGEN BALANCE

It is known that 1 g of nitrogen is contained in approximately 6.25 g of protein, the exact figure depending upon the nature and source of the protein. High biological value proteins are digested to give more nitrogen than lower biological value proteins. It is thus possible to calculate the nitrogen value of the diet from its protein content. A person is said to be in nitrogen balance when the intake of nitrogen in the diet is equal to the output in urine and faeces and from the skin.

Positive nitrogen balance. Nitrogen intake exceeds nitrogen loss, so it can be assumed that new tissue is being formed, e.g. growth, tissue repair.

Negative nitrogen balance. Nitrogen loss exceeds nitrogen intake, so it can be assumed that tissue is being broken down to provide energy, e.g. during starvation. The negative nitrogen balance which occurs after injury or surgery is discussed in Chapter 23.

Nitrogen balance studies are sometimes performed in order to obtain information about protein requirements, or to assist in the diagnosis of disease, or to assess the adequacy of a particular protein intake.

PROTEIN TURNOVER

The proteins of the body exist in a dynamic state, this means that they are constantly undergoing a process of breakdown and synthesis from amino acids. This is known as protein turnover and is illustrated schematically in Figure 4.2.

Table 4.2 Protein content of food portions

Portion	Protein content (g)
50 g egg (1 egg)	6
30 g cheese	6
50 g cottage cheese	7
200 ml milk (1 glass)	6
60 g fish, cooked	12
50 g meat, cooked	12
30 g cereal (e.g. flour, oatmeal, rice, semolina, cornflakes)	2
100 g (3 tablespoons) cabbage or carrot, boiled	1
180 g potato, boiled (1 medium size)	3
50 g butter beans, boiled (2 tablespoons)	5
100 g baked beans in tomato sauce (2 tablespoons)	5
200 g vegetable soup, canned	3
1 slice toast and a serving of baked beans in tomato sauce	8
1 slice bread spread with 2 teaspoons peanut butter	6

These figures are approximate and for the purpose of comparison only. For more precise information on the composition of specific foods, see *McCance and Widdowson's Composition of Foods* (Holland et al 1991).

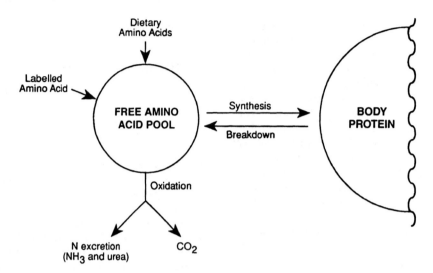

Figure 4.2 Protein turnover: simple representation of whole-body protein and amino acid metabolism (Garrow et al 2000).

Digestion, absorption and disposal

Proteins are hydrolysed to amino acids and dipeptides and tripeptides by digestion.

1. Digestion starts in the stomach, where the combination of an acid pH and the proteolytic enzyme pepsin hydrolyses the proteins to oligopeptides, which enter the duodenum.

2. These oligopeptides are further hydrolysed by the proteolytic enzymes trypsin, chymotrypsin and carboxypeptidase to di-and tripeptides and amino acids. Proteolytic enzymes are secreted in an inactive form that is then activated preventing autodigestion of the gastrointestinal tract.

The amino acids and peptides produced enter the intestinal cells and from there have three fates:

1. They enter the body's circulating amino acid pool, from which they are built into the structural proteins and specific enzymes which are needed by each cell.

2. They are converted to other amino acids.

3. They are oxidised to produce energy; in some cases the amino acids are converted to glucose first. The urea formed in this process is excreted by the kidneys.

Daily intake

The Committee on Medical Aspects of Food Policy (COMA), reporting in 1991 (DoH 1991), recommended average daily intakes of protein for the UK. It will be seen from Table 4.3 that for adults the RNI is 55.5 g/day for men and 45 g/day for women, with an increase for pregnant and lactating women. These figures allow for the fact that only about 90% of the protein in food is digested and, of this, only about 70% is incorporated into body tissue. In general, a higher percentage of the protein in animal material is digested than in plant material.

In their deliberations the members of the panel considered, firstly, minimum protein requirements. They found it necessary, however, to recommend intakes higher than the minimum in order to allow for a palatable diet. They also considered other important nutrients such as B-complex vitamins, which are found in

Table 4.3 Reference nutrient intakes (RNI) for protein

Age	RNI (g/day)	
0–3 months	12.5	
4–6 months	12.7	
7–9 months	13.7	
10–12 months	14.9	
1–3 years	14.5	
4–6 years	19.5	
7–10 years	28.3	
	Male	Female
11–14 years	42.1	41.2
15–18 years	55.2	45.4
19–49 years	55.5	45.0
50+ years	53.3	46.5
Pregnancy		51.0
Lactating up to 6 months		56.0
6 months +		53.0

association with protein in foods. The final figures are therefore intended to be used as a guide in the planning and assessment of diets, rather than a prescription for actual protein intake. Calculation of nitrogen requirement for a specific individual is discussed in Chapter 23.

It is advisable that some protein should be derived from foods of animal origin—milk, eggs, cheese, fish and meat—which are best able to supply the essential amino acids. It should be remembered also that the value of these foods is partly determined by the relatively high contribution they make towards the intake of other essential nutrients.

Table 4.2 gives the approximate protein content of some average food portions. High protein intakes have been linked to reduced kidney function in the elderly (Brenner et al 1982) and it has been recommended that the daily protein intake for adults should not exceed twice the RNI. Amino acid dietary supplements should be used with extreme caution; the COMA report (DoH 1991) recommends that dietary amino acids should be taken in a balanced mixture. There is little published information about the possible toxic effects of amino acid supplements.

INSUFFICIENT PROTEIN INTAKE

It is most unusual in the UK to meet with obvious signs of protein deficiency resulting from a grossly defective diet, but it is not known to what extent minor deficiencies may arise, and may be responsible for ill-health and impaired development. Marginal intakes should be avoided, especially in times of increased need such as growth, pregnancy, lactation, and during recovery from injury, when insufficient protein can impair wound healing and increase susceptibility to infection.

Situations where protein deficiency can develop as a result of illness include:

1. If the energy requirement is increased, and this is not met by the provision of extra dietary energy, the use of protein for energy production may result in a lack of protein for growth and replacement. This may be aggravated by the withdrawal of protein from the body tissues to help meet energy needs, e.g. in fevers or hyperthyroidism.

2. Trauma such as burns, fractures and surgery is followed by a period when breakdown of body protein exceeds intake, resulting in a period of negative nitrogen balance.

3. Deficiency may also result from failure to absorb or utilise dietary protein, as occurs in some disorders affecting the gastrointestinal tract, and when the liver is diseased.

4. Protein deficiency may be the result of excessive loss of protein from the body; for example:
   a. as occurs in some kidney disorders
   b. as a result of haemorrhage
   c. in the fluid which exudes from burns.

Protein energy malnutrition (PEM)

Protein energy malnutrition is the general term used to describe the spectrum of illnesses caused by an inadequate diet deficient in protein, and often in energy too, that occurs mainly in developing countries. There are two extreme forms:

- *kwashiorkor* due to a dietary deficiency of protein
- *marasmus* due to dietary deficiencies of both protein and energy.

In practice, the clinical picture is usually mixed and is often complicated by other specific vitamin and mineral deficiencies, for example vitamin A and iron. The treatment and prevention of these conditions is discussed by Truswell in 'Malnutrition in Developing Countries' in the *ABC of Nutrition* (1999).

Kwashiorkor

In rural areas, this is the form of PEM that predominates. It develops during early childhood when, after prolonged breast-feeding, the child is weaned onto a diet based on a starchy staple food, such as cassava or plantain porridge, which has a low protein content. This often occurs when the next baby is born, so the older child no longer receives breast-milk. Although he/she is able to eat sufficient to satisfy his/her energy requirements, his/her food does not contain enough protein.

Children with kwashiorkor are sometimes normal weight for their height. Oedema develops because synthesis of plasma albumin is reduced—this oedema may mask the physical signs of muscle wasting. A fatty liver develops because the synthesis of lipoproteins for lipid transport is reduced and lipids accumulate in the liver. Children whose diet is deficient in protein are unable to synthesise sufficient new body proteins. This results in retardation of growth, increased susceptibility to infection and slow recovery from injury and infection.

Some physiological adaptation to a low protein intake does occur, but any condition which increases protein requirement, e.g. injury or infection, can precipitate severe kwashiorkor. The clinical signs are:

- growth retardation
- oedema

- muscle wasting
- liver enlargement
- skin and hair pigmentation changes.

Kwashiorkor is likely to be accompanied by deficiencies of retinol, iron, folate, magnesium and potassium.

Marasmus

Unlike kwashiorkor, this is more common in urban areas, where its incidence is increasing, particularly among those who have recently moved from rural areas. Marasmus develops when the diet lacks sufficient energy and protein. It is sometimes referred to as childhood starvation and is most commonly caused by incorrect bottle-feeding or early weaning. The milk is over-diluted and so provides an inadequate diet containing both too little energy and too little protein.

Gastroenteritis is common in developing countries and may precipitate marasmus by increasing intestinal losses and nutritional requirements, and also because it is often treated with starvation by parents.

The clinical signs of marasmus are:

- muscle wasting
- loss of subcutaneous fat layer
- growth retardation.

PEM also occurs in adults, though it is generally less severe because the relative protein requirement is lower. It results in small stature and low weight, high disease prevalence, a shorter life-expectancy and low birth-weight in the babies of marasmic mothers.

PEM is a major problem that confronts developing countries. It is likely that there are 7–10 less severe cases for every severe case. The problem can be overcome by the following public health measures:

Growth monitoring. It may be more appropriate to measure mid-upper-arm circumference than weigh the child. These records show when the child's weight and growth begin to drop and PEM is developing. It is easier to treat at this stage than in the more advanced state.

Breast-feeding should be encouraged. Bottle-feeding is unsatisfactory because of both its cost, and the need for sterilisation and clean water. The nutritional advantages of breast-feeding are discussed in Chapter 15. It must be remembered that the nutritional requirements of the mother are increased while she is breast-feeding. A combination of poor maternal diet and prolonged breast-feeding can cause kwashiorkor in infants.

Nutritional supplements are needed for vulnerable groups. Children and pregnant and lactating women whose nutritional needs are not met by their diet are vulnerable and should be the priority groups in feeding programmes.

Nutrition education is essential. This must be specific to the community and is most successfully carried out in maternal and child health centres, where mothers can learn not only of the need for an adequate diet but also how to provide it.

Improved sanitary conditions and provision of clean water will reduce the incidence of infectious disease, particularly gastroenteritis.

Immunisation prevents the extra metabolic demands of infection and increases survival rate because resistance to infection is reduced by malnutrition.

Oral rehydration of those children with gastroenteritis is needed to prevent the marasmic cycle.

REFERENCES

Brenner B M, Meyer T W, Hostetter T H 1982 Dietary protein intake and the progressive nature of kidney disease: the role of hemodynamically mediated glomerular injury in the pathogenesis of progressive glomerular sclerosis in aging, renal ablation, and intrinsic renal disease. New England Journal of Medicine 307: 652–659

Department of Health (DoH) 1991 Dietary reference values for food energy and nutrients for the United Kingdom. Report of the Panel on Dietary Reference Values of the Committee on Medical Aspects of Food Policy (COMA) (Report on Health and Social Subjects 41). HMSO, London

Garrow J S, James W P T, Ralph A 2000 Human nutrition and dietetics, 10th Edn. Churchill Livingstone, Edinburgh

Holland B, Welch A A, Unwin I D, Buss D H, Paul A A, Southgate D A T 1991 McCance and Widdowson's composition of foods, 5th Edn. Royal Society of Chemistry, Cambridge

Truswell A S 1999 ABC of nutrition, 2nd Edn. British Medical Journal, London

FURTHER READING

UNICEF 2000 The state of the world's children. Oxford University Press, Oxford

Wiseman M J, Hunt R, Goodwin A, Gross J L, Keen H, Viberti G 1987 Dietary composition and renal function in healthy subjects. Nephron 46: 37–42

World Health Organization 1985 Energy and protein requirements. Report of a joint FAO/WHO/UNU meeting (WHO Technical Report Series 724). World Health Organization, Geneva

5

Minerals, trace elements and water

LEARNING OBJECTIVES

After studying this chapter you should be able to:

- describe the importance of minerals and trace elements in the diet
- list the dietary sources, reference nutrient intakes (RNIs) and functions of minerals and trace elements
- describe the consequences of an inadequate or excessive intake of minerals and trace elements
- explain the importance of fluid in the diet and the importance of its contribution to the maintenance of fluid balance.

Minerals and trace elements are inorganic substances that are essential for the normal function and development of body cells and systems. They make up approximately 3% of the total body-weight. The dietary intake of minerals and trace elements comes from those present in food and water; this is usually in the form of mineral salts or incorporated into tissue.

The minerals and trace elements that are essential for human health are listed in Box 5.1.

Table 5.1 summarises the RNIs, dietary sources and effects of inadequate and excessive intakes of minerals and trace elements.

Functions of minerals in the body include:

1. Formation and maintenance of strength and rigidity of bones and teeth
2. Regulation of fluid balance
3. Regulation of acid/base balance
4. Components of enzymes and hormones and, as such, essential for energy metabolism and functioning of the immune system
5. Transmission of action potential along nerves
6. Contraction of muscle fibres.

Table 5.1 Reference nutrient intakes, sources and effects of incorrect intakes

UK RNI/day	Dietary sources	Functions	Deficiency symptoms	Toxicity symptoms
Calcium 700 mg	Dairy products	Bone and teeth formation Muscle contraction Nerve transmission Blood clotting	Rickets Osteoporosis Convulsion Stunted growth	—
Phosphorus 550 mg Dairy products Meat and fish Wholegrain cereal		Bone and teeth formation Acid–base balance	Deminerilisation of bone	Low blood calcium levels
Iron 8.7 mg male 14.8 mg female	Meat Dried fruit, green vegetables Fortified cereals	Component of haemoglobin	Pallor Tiredness Breathlessness Reduced resistance to infection	Cirrhosis of liver
Iodine 140 µg	Seafish and shellfish Milk Some vegetables Iodised salt	Component of thyroid hormones Controls metabolic rate	Enlarged thyroid Foetal abnormality Retarded growth	Hyperthyroid
Flourine 50 µg	Seafood Tea Drinking water	Helps prevent caries	Increased frequency of dental caries	Tooth mottling Skeletal changes
Sodium 1600 mg	Cheese Preserved foods Pre-prepared foods Added to cooking	Acid-base and fluid balance Nerve transmission Muscle contraction	Muscular fatigue Nausea Reduced appetite	Hypertension Vomiting
Potassium 3500 mg	Fruit Vegetables	Acid–base and fluid balance Nerve transmission Muscle contraction	Muscle weakness Confusion Cardiac arrest	Irregular heart rate
Magnesium 300 mg	Wholegrain cereals Green vegetables Nuts	Protein and DNA synthesis Bone development	Neuro muscular dysfunction	Hypertension
Copper 1.2 mg	Meat Shellfish Vegetables	Enzyme function Ion absorption	Reduced resistance to infection	—
Zinc 9.5 mg	Meat Eggs Pulses Wholegrain cereals	Enzyme function Immune system	Skin lesions Growth failure Reduced immunity	Diarrhoea Nausea

CALCIUM

Of all the minerals in the body, calcium occurs in the greatest amount. The body of a well-nourished adult contains 1–1.5 kg calcium, 99% of which is found in the bones and teeth in the form of hydroxyapetite. The functions of calcium in the body are listed in Box 5.2.

Absorption and utilisation

Where the type of diet normally consumed by western peoples is concerned, it has been estimated that only 20–30% of the calcium intake is absorbed from the alimentary tract. However, if the intake is lower than 250 mg/day then 70% of the intake will be absorbed.

Box 5.1 Essential minerals and trace elements

Minerals	Trace elements	
Calcium	Iron	Manganese
Phosphorus	Fluoride	Chromium
Potassium	Copper	Selenium
Sodium	Zinc	Molybdenum
Chlorine	Iodine	
Magnesium	Cobalt	

Box 5.2 Functions of calcium

- Deposits of calcium in the original soft matrix give bones their necessary rigidity.
- In the case of teeth, calcium contributes to hardness and resistance to decay.
- The small amount of calcium remaining in the tissue fluids plays a part in controlling the action of heart and skeletal muscle and the excitability of nerves.
- Calcium also has a role in the clotting of blood.

Absorption occurs predominantly in the jejunum but also in the ileum and colon.

Calcium is absorbed both by simple passive diffusion across the gut cell wall and by active transport. The absorption of calcium is affected by ageing, renal efficiency, hormone balance (see Chapter 6), intestinal integrity and diet. The active transport mechanism predominates when the dietary intake of calcium is low and requires the active metabolite of vitamin D, calcitriol. Hegsted (1963) has shown that there is an increased efficiency in the absorption of calcium during pregnancy.

Dietary factors that increase calcium absorption are the amino acids lysine and arginine, fat, vitamin D and lactose. Those which decrease absorption are cocoa, soya beans, spinach, wheat bran and wholemeal cereals.

Amino acids have a favourable effect on calcium absorption because soluble salts which can be easily absorbed are formed between calcium and the amino acid.

Wholemeal cereal products and some fruits and vegetables reduce calcium absorption. This happens because the phytic acid in wholegrain cereals and the oxalic acid occurring in some vegetables and fruit combine with calcium to form insoluble salts which cannot be absorbed from the gut. Yeast contains the enzyme phytase which destroys phytic acid, so wholemeal bread in the diet does not reduce calcium absorp-

tion but the phytate present in wheat bran, taken as a dietary supplement, will. Diets containing a lot of wholegrain cereal are only likely to cause calcium deficiency if the cereal is eaten in an unleavened form, such as chapattis.

Dietary sources

Milk has a high content of available calcium, is palatable, inexpensive and a staple food in many societies. Cheese also has a high calcium content. Two-thirds of the calcium content of the UK diet is provided by dairy produce. Flour, with the exception of wholemeal, is fortified with calcium, with the result that bread and similar foods made from fortified flour are of value as a source of this mineral (Box 5.3). In the UK, most of the calcium of the diet comes from these foods. Other foods containing useful supplementary amounts are eggs, fish such as salmon and sardines (of which the small bones are eaten), cabbage and broccoli. Dried milk is a concentrated source of calcium. A significant amount may be obtained from hard water, which can contain up to 50 mg per litre.

Dietary requirement

Calcium is lost in the urine, faeces, skin, hair and nails. Dietary calcium is required to make good these losses. The calcium present in bile and pancreatic secretions may be reabsorbed in the ileum and colon.

Additional amounts of calcium are needed:

- for growth throughout childhood and adolescence
- during pregnancy to meet the requirements of the foetus
- during lactation for secretion in the milk, which supplies the calcium needed by the growing infant.

Growth. Reference nutrient intakes of calcium at different ages are given in Table 5.2. The RNI of a 6-year-old child can be met easily by including half a pint of milk and a yoghurt or portion of cheese in the daily diet (see Box 5.2).

Box 5.3 Calcium content of some dairy products and white bread

- 500 ml milk contains approximately 500 mg calcium.
- 30 g cheddar cheese contains 240 mg calcium.
- 125 g pot low-fat yoghurt contains 200 mg calcium
- Two thick slices white bread contain 74 mg calcium.

Table 5.2 Reference nutrient intakes for calcium (from DoH 1991, with permission)

Age	RNI (mg/day)	
0–12 months	525	
1–3 years	350	
4–6 years	450	
7–10 years	550	
	Male	Female
11–18 years	1000	800
19+ years	700	700

Pregnancy. No extra calcium is required in the diet during pregnancy because of the increase in calcium absorption (Heaney et al 1971). However, Chan et al (1987) have suggested that the intake of calcium for pregnant adolescents should be increased, because the adolescent will have a high calcium requirement herself, to which the needs of the developing foetus are added.

Lactation. During lactation, there is an additional requirement of 550 mg of calcium per day. This can easily be met as most lactating women increase their food intake, and all should be encouraged to increase their fluid intake. The absorption of calcium from breast-milk is more efficient than from infant formula milks.

Calcium intake and osteoporosis

Peak bone mass (PBM) is reached by the age of 35; most of it is achieved during the growth period. There are wide variations in PBM. It is influenced by gender, genetic, hormonal and dietary factors.

Once PBM has been reached, a loss of cortical bone occurs within a few years. This occurs at a rate of 0.35% per year in males and in females prior to the menopause. This rate increases in females for 5 years after the menopause. Nordin and Heaney (1990a, b) have proposed that the increase in incidence of osteoporosis and associated fractures in elderly women is due to a dietary deficiency of calcium. However, osteoporosis results from an atrophy of the bone and loss of all components, not just calcium specifically. This post-menopausal bone loss can be prevented by oestrogen replacement. Calcium supplementation without the addition of oestrogens does not achieve this.

High intakes of calcium are not toxic for healthy individuals because of the body's homeostatic mechanism which controls both the amount absorbed from food and the amount excreted in the urine. The Committee on Medical Aspects of Food Policy (COMA) panel (DoH 1991) remained unconvinced of the value of high calcium intake in preventing osteoporosis, but because such an intake is not toxic, proposes that an increase in calcium intake for people at risk of osteoporosis may be prudent.

The COMA recommendations were intended for healthy individuals. The National Osteoporosis Society recommends an increased calcium intake for those at risk of osteoporosis (NOS 1999). Their recommendations are 1000 mg calcium per day for women aged over 45 years taking hormone replacement therapy, 1500 mg calcium per day for women aged over 45 years and men aged over 60 years. These figures are based on the NHI Consensus Statement (NHI 1994).

Calcium deficiency

Calcium may be lacking in the body if absorption is impaired, as in the malabsorption syndrome (see Chapter 25) or as a result of a lack of vitamin D. A diet low in available calcium may also be a contributing factor. Gregory (2000) identified a low intake of calcium in girls aged 15–18 years. This was associated with a low intake of milk and would be of particular significance for pregnant teenagers.

Deficiency of calcium in the body gives rise to the development of rickets in childhood and osteomalacia in adult life. These conditions are discussed further in the section on vitamin D (Chapter 6).

PHOSPHORUS

Phosphorus is the mineral which occurs in the second largest amount in the body. It occurs both as organic phosphates such as adenosine mono-, di-and triphosphates and creatine phosphate, and as inorganic phosphates which occur in the bone matrix and extracellular fluid. Its functions are listed in Box 5.4.

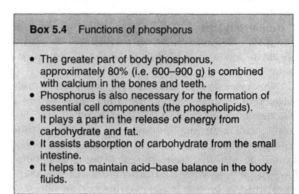

Box 5.4 Functions of phosphorus

- The greater part of body phosphorus, approximately 80% (i.e. 600–900 g) is combined with calcium in the bones and teeth.
- Phosphorus is also necessary for the formation of essential cell components (the phospholipids).
- It plays a part in the release of energy from carbohydrate and fat.
- It assists absorption of carbohydrate from the small intestine.
- It helps to maintain acid–base balance in the body fluids.

Absorption

As in the case of calcium absorption, which is regulated by parathyroid hormone, absorption of phosphorus depends upon the formation of soluble salts. Marshall et al (1976) have shown that it is normal for about 60% of dietary phosphorus intake to be absorbed. Excessive use of antacids containing magnesium and aluminium can limit phosphorus absorption by the formation of insoluble salts.

Dietary sources

Phosphorus is widely distributed in foods. In general, meat, fish, milk, cheese, eggs and cereals contain more phosphorus than vegetables and fruits. It is also present in many food additives.

Dietary requirement

Most foods which are rich sources of calcium are also rich sources of phosphorus. The diet should have a ratio of 1 mmol phosphorus to 1 mmol calcium, reflecting the normal bodily concentrations. Therefore the RNI for phosphorus has been set as the same as that of calcium in mmol. When the calcium intake differs from the RNI, the phosphorus intake should be the same as the calcium intake. This is particularly important for infants (DoH 1991). It is usual for serum phosphate and calcium levels to show an inverse relationship. It is therefore important to measure both serum levels to check this, not just to evaluate serum calcium levels.

Phosphorus deficiency

Dietary deficiency is unlikely to occur. The foods upon which we depend for much of our calcium have a high phosphorus content, and it may be said that dietary adequacy of calcium ensures also a sufficiency of phosphorus. However, deficiency can occur in alcoholics, patients with renal disease, patients receiving total parenteral nutrition and patients with malabsorption syndrome.

IRON

The functions of iron in the body are given in Box 5.5.

Iron stores

0.5–1 g of iron is stored as ferritin and haemosiderin in the liver, spleen and bone marrow. These stores are mobilised when requirement for iron exceeds the amount absorbed from the diet. The plasma ferritin

---

Box 5.5 Functions of iron

- Iron is necessary for the formation of haemoglobin, a constituent of the red blood cells. Haemoglobin is responsible for the transport of oxygen and carbon dioxide between the lungs and the tissues and is the pigment which gives the blood its red colour.
- Iron is found in the muscle pigment myoglobin.
- It is also an important constituent of many enzyme systems.

---

concentration is a guide to the level of iron stores. If the plasma ferritin level is less than 12 µg/l it can be assumed that the iron stores have become depleted.

The total iron content of the body is quite small, and in the case of a man of average size is estimated to be about 4 g.

Absorption

Not all the iron in the diet is absorbed. FAO (1988) suggest that in industrialised countries, where the diet contains adequate amounts of meat and ascorbic acid, it is usual for only 15% of dietary iron to be absorbed.

Iron absorption occurs in the duodenum and jejunum, where the ferrous form of iron is bound to the transport protein transferrin which enters the mucosal cell by endocytosis. Figure 5.1 shows the process by which iron forms the Fe^{2+} –transferrin complex and is transported from the gut lumen into the plasma.

Dietary sources

The relative availability to the body of the iron present in foods differs depending on the type of iron and other components of the diet. These are shown in Box 5.6.

Two types of iron are found in foods:

- meat and meat products contain haem iron (i.e. the iron in haemoglobin)
- fruit and vegetables contain iron as ferric complexes.

The iron contents of some foods in each category are listed in Box 5.7 (see page 37).

Dietary requirement

Iron is needed in the diet:

- to make good the very small amount which is constantly lost from the body, principally in the urine

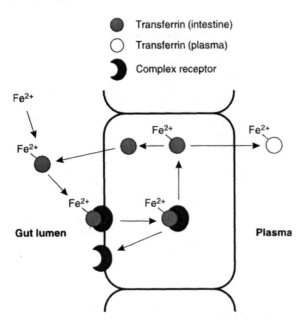

● Transferrin (intestine)
○ Transferrin (plasma)
◗ Complex receptor

Figure 5.1 Outline of iron absorption mechanisms in the upper small intestine (McGeown 1999).

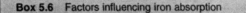

Box 5.6 Factors influencing iron absorption

- Gastric secretions. Gastric enzymes and hydrochloric acid convert iron in the ferric form to the better absorbed ferrous form.
- Total diet. The presence of ascorbic acid in the diet enhances iron absorption. Phytates present in wholegrain cereals, oxolates present in rhubarb and spinach and the iron-binding phenolic compounds present in tea, calcium and soy protein all inhibit iron absorption.

- to replace loss due to menstruation
- for the formation of additional haemoglobin in pregnancy, childhood and adolescence
- in lactation for secretion in the milk
- to make good loss of iron due to bleeding.

Infants and children need iron for growth and to develop their own iron stores.

Men and post-menopausal women are estimated to lose 0.86 mg iron/day and their iron intake needs to replace it.

Reference nutrient intake

The RNIs for iron at different ages are listed in Table 5.3. These are difficult to set because of the range of levels of absorption from foods and the range of individual requirements.

Groups with increased iron needs

Menstruating women. Hallberg et al (1966) showed that although menstrual loss for individual women from period to period was relatively constant, there was a great variation between women. The RNI of 14.8 mg/day will not meet the requirements of approximately 10% of menstruating women and these women should receive an iron supplement.

Pregnancy and lactation. Those women who start their pregnancy with good iron stores do not require iron supplements. Their increased needs are met by increased absorption, cessation of menstrual losses and mobilisation of their iron stores. The amount of iron secreted into breast-milk is offset in part by lactational amenorrhoea.

Blood donors. Those who give blood regularly at intervals of not less than 6 months are able to replace their stores. Donors of child-bearing age or who give blood more regularly may need supplements.

Iron deficiency

Groups of the population who may suffer from iron deficiency are those with:

- increased needs
  — infants and toddlers (Chapter 15)
  — adolescents (Chapter 15)
  — pregnant women
- high losses
  — menstruating women
- poor or reduced absorption
  — elderly people (Chapter 17)
  — vegetarians (Chapter 14).

Table 5.3 Reference nutrient intakes for iron (from Salmon 1991, with permission of HMSO)

Age	RNI (mg/day)	
0–3 months	1.7	
4–6 months	4.3	
7–12 months	7.8	
1–3 years	6.9	
4–6 years	6.1	
7–10 years	8.7	
	Male	Female
11–18 years	11.3	14.8
19–49 years	8.7	14.8
50+ years	8.7	8.7

These groups are discussed in greater detail in the chapters indicated.

High iron intakes

Haemochromatosis is an inherited condition in which iron absorption is inappropriately high and results in an accumulation of iron in the tissues—a diet low in iron is not sufficient to prevent this.

Iron poisoning does occur in children and adults—a dose of 200–300 mg/kg body-weight is lethal for children.

IODINE

The trace element iodine is a constituent of thyroxine (T_4) and triiodothyronine (T_3), the hormones which are secreted by the thyroid gland. These hormones control the rate of tissue activity, metabolic rate and integrity of connective tissue. They are also necessary for the development of the foetal nervous system during the first trimester of pregnancy. They are therefore vital for normal physical and mental development. A deficiency in the mother's diet during early pregnancy results in cretinism, a syndrome of mental retardation and dwarfism.

Dietary sources

Iodine is present in very small amounts in many foods. The best sources are vegetables and sea fish.

In the UK, cow's milk is a major source of iodine in the diet. This has not always been the case, but changing practice in animal husbandry has led to an increase in its content (Wenlock 1987).

The iodine content of agricultural produce depends upon the amount of iodine in the soil in the district where the food was produced, rather than on the nature of the food itself. Soils vary greatly in iodine content, some containing very little.

Goitrogens

Some foods have been found to contain substances which interfere with the uptake of iodine by the thyroid gland. These substances are known as goitrogens.

- Cabbage and turnip contain goitrogenic cyanoglucosides.
- Cassava, maize, sweet potato and lima beans also contain goitrogens.
- There is evidence to suggest that water may have goitrogenic properties when contaminated with faeces.

- Calcium, fluoride, manganese and magnesium ions present in hard water are also goitrogenic.

Reference nutrient intake

The RNIs for iodine at different ages are given in Table 5.4. No increase is required during pregnancy and lactation.

Iodine deficiency

Iodine deficiency is prevalent in communities where dietary intake is low, or insufficient to counteract the effect of goitrogenic factors operating in that particular area.

Although the dietary intake of iodine exceeds requirements in most European countries, iodine deficiency is still an important global public health issue, usually occurring in isolated, inland, rural communities which depend on local produce. If the soil iodine content is low, then the iodine content of the vegetables will also be low. This, in combination with a diet containing goitrogens, leads to endemic goitre leading to preventable physical and mental disability. Goitre can be eradicated by a range of public health measures, such as the provision of salt iodised with potassium iodate, iodised oil injections and iodising the water supply.

Goitre

If sufficient iodine is not available for formation of thyroxine and triiodothyronine, the thyroid gland enlarges in an effort to maintain its normal output of the hormones, and gives rise to a swelling of the neck. This condition is known as endemic goitre. The word 'endemic' means 'commonly found in certain populations'.

Excess iodine intake can also cause goitre.

Table 5.4   Reference nutrient intakes for iodine (from Salmon 1991, with permission of HMSO)

Age	RNI (μg/day)
0–3 months (formula fed)	50
4–12 months	60
1–3 years	70
4–6 years	100
7–10 years	110
11–14 years	130
15+ years	140

FLUORINE

The body contains traces of fluorine, principally in the teeth and the skeleton, where it is present as the salt calcium fluorapatite. However, it has no known essential function in humans. This mineral is present in water, which, although containing only minute amounts, is the chief dietary source. Traces are also present in many foods. In the UK up to 70% of fluoride is provided by tea.

Interest in fluorine where human nutrition is concerned centres around its association with the prevention of dental caries. It has been shown that in districts where fluorine is present in water to the extent of 1 part per million, teeth are more resistant to decay than in districts where the water contains smaller amounts. To bring about this effect, the fluorine must be available while calcification is taking place, rather than after the teeth have already matured. If the fluorine content of the water is in excess of this amount, permanent chalk-white mottling appears on the teeth in a proportion of cases. Higher concentrations result in an increase in the proportion of cases of mottling and in the mottling taking on a permanent brown discoloration. This has raised the question of whether or not public water supplies that are deficient in fluorine should have this mineral added to the level required for maximum prevention of dental caries, but not high enough to cause discoloration (see Chapter 16).

Studies in the USA have shown that children living in areas where the drinking water contains 1 part per million or more of fluorine show an incidence of dental caries up to 60% less than in areas where the water is deficient in this mineral. It has also been shown that a comparable effect may be obtained by artificial fluoridation of water supplies which are naturally low in fluorine content. Trials carried out in this country have furnished similar evidence of the benefits of the protective level of fluorine in drinking water.

The role of fluorine in dental health is further discussed in Chapter 16.

SODIUM

Physiological functions

In the body sodium is found principally in the blood plasma and the fluid surrounding the tissues. It plays an important part in the production of the osmotic pressure which regulates fluid exchanges between the cells and the surrounding tissue fluid, and is vital for the transmission of impulses in nerves, for muscle contraction and for active transport mechanisms, such as the absorption of sugars from the gut.

Table 5.5 Reference nutrient intakes for sodium (from Salmon 1991, with permission of HMSO)

Age	RNI (mg/day)
0–3 months	210
4–6 months	280
7–9 months	320
10–12 months	350
1–3 years	500
4–6 years	700
7–10 years	1200
11+ years	1600

Sodium is also important for acid–base regulation; by combining with chloride and bicarbonate ions it helps to maintain the balance between anions and cations.

Dietary sources

Most of the sodium of the diet comes from sodium chloride (common salt), which is used as a condiment in cooking and at the table, and for the preservation of such foods as cheese, ham, bacon, fish and vegetables. Sodium also occurs as a natural constituent of foods. On the whole, milk, cheese, eggs, meat and fish have a higher sodium content than fruits, vegetables and cereals. At least 80% of the salt in the UK diet comes from processed foods.

Dietary requirement

Sufficient sodium is present in foods to ensure an adequacy of this mineral, and the body can adjust itself to wide variations in intake by excreting any excess in the urine. In certain diseases, however, sodium is retained in the body in excessive amounts, and in these circumstances it may be necessary to restrict dietary intake.

Sodium is excreted principally in urine and in sweat. Normally, the sodium content of the body is maintained by the kidneys at an almost constant level. Changes in the sodium concentration in the extracellular fluid (ECF) are compensated for by changes in the ECF volume. So if the ECF sodium concentration increases, more water is retained in the ECF to keep a constant concentration. The absorption of sodium and water are under the complex hormonal control of aldosterone and ACTH. Changes in ECF volume are detected by pressure sensors in the circulation, which stimulate changes in sodium and water absorption in the kidneys. This process is discussed more fully in Lee et al (1996).

Reference nutrient intake

The RNIs for sodium at different ages are listed in Table 5.5. It is important that infants do not receive too much sodium because their immature kidneys cannot compensate for it, so they rapidly become hypernatraemic.

Sodium deficiency

When sweating is very profuse, as occurs in hot climates, sodium depletion can occur. This gives rise to symptoms which include excessive fatigue and muscle cramps. These symptoms are also experienced by people whose occupations involve working in extremely hot surroundings. The condition may be remedied, or its occurrence prevented, by an increased salt intake.

In temperate climates, such as that of the UK, sodium depletion due to excessive sweating is only likely to occur either as an occupational hazard or due to unusual weather conditions, or due to increase of physical activity.

Although the sodium intake should be adequate to compensate for these increased losses, extra salt will be needed initially. Adaptation to the increased loss occurs over a few days and more dilute sweat is produced.

Other groups which may suffer from sodium deficiency are those whose losses are excessive because of prolonged vomiting or diarrhoea, exudate from tissue damage such as burns, or those with poor kidney function. In the elderly, where the ability to concentrate urine has reduced, sodium deficiency can lead to confusion.

Dietary salt and hypertension

There is much conflicting evidence about the links between hypertension and dietary sodium intake. Law et al (1991) have been able to show a consistent link between salt intake and rise in blood pressure. High alcohol intake, smoking and obesity also contribute to a rise in blood pressure with age. As the link between hypertension and cardiovascular disease is well documented, it is sensible to reduce salt intake. This is recommended in the *Health of the Nation* report (DoH 1992).

Approximately 10% of the population may have a genetic predisposition to developing raised blood pressure on moderate sodium intakes. This group of the population may be particularly successful at lowering their blood pressure by reducing their sodium intake.

OTHER MINERALS

Potassium

Potassium is present principally in body cells. Its action complements that of sodium. Normally, the kidneys play an important part in regulating the potassium content of the body. Excessive retention occurs in association with some kidney disorders and also in Addison's disease, and may cause cardiac arrest. Deficiency can result from prolonged vomiting or diarrhoea, or as a result of oral diuretic therapy, and causes muscle paralysis.

Over 90% of dietary potassium is absorbed in the proximal small intestine. Fruit and vegetables are the major contributors of potassium to the diet, bananas and fruit juices being particularly rich sources. Coffee is also a good source. Increasing the dietary potassium intake has been shown to reduce blood pressure in normotensive and hypertensive individuals (Matlou et al 1986). The increase in fruit and vegetable consumption and the resulting increase in potassium intake recommended in the *Health of the Nation* report (DoH 1992) may contribute to the reduction of hypertension.

The RNIs for potassium are given in Table 5.6.

Table 5.6 Reference nutrient intakes for potassium (from Salmon 1991, with permission of HMSO)

Age	RNI (mg/day)
0–3 months	800
4–6 months	850
7–12 months	700
1–3 years	800
4–6 years	1100
7–10 years	2000
11–14 years	3100
15+ years	3500

Magnesium

Magnesium has many important roles. It is necessary for skeletal development and for maintaining the electrical potential across the cell membranes of nerves and muscles.

Dietary sources of magnesium are hard water, cereals, green vegetables, meat and animal products. The magnesium available from meat and animal products is less than that from plant products, because animal products contain calcium, protein and phosphate, all of which make the magnesium less available for absorption.

Absorption of magnesium from the small intestine is efficient. This efficiency is reduced if the intake is excessive, in which case magnesium passes through the intestine unabsorbed and has a laxative effect. It is also excreted by the kidneys.

Magnesium deficiency can occur accompanying starvation, malabsorption syndromes, acute pancreatitis, alcoholism and prolonged diarrhoea or vomiting. It is usually accompanied by low blood calcium levels. The symptoms of the deficiency are progressive muscle weakness, failure to thrive, neuromuscular dysfunction, tachycardia and ventricular fibrillation. It has also been known to occur following surgical removal of parathyroid glands and in conjunction with prolonged use of diuretics.

Copper

Copper is a component of many of the enzyme systems of the body. The best dietary sources are cereals, cereal products and nuts.

Copper deficiency is associated with many clinical symptoms including defects in hair pigmentation, increased susceptibility to respiratory infections and a reduced immune response. The raised plasma cholesterol shown by Klevay et al (1984) to accompany experimental copper depletion has led to interest in the link between lack of dietary copper and coronary heart disease.

Copper has been found to be necessary along with iron to promote recovery from anaemia in malnourished infants in impoverished communities, where feeding has depended upon cow's milk and cereals rather than upon breast-milk or infant formulae and cereals. Deficiency has occurred during rehabilitation from kwashiorkor and marasmus, if the food supplement used has been low in copper (cow's milk has a low copper content and so, when used, may precipitate the deficiency).

Copper is also necessary for normal red blood cell development, blood clotting and phospholipid synthesis.

Zinc

There is approximately 2 g of zinc in the adult human, about 60% of which is in skeletal muscle and 30% in bone. Zinc is an essential part of many enzymes, including those in all the major metabolic pathways.

Zinc is essential for the synthesis of lean tissue, so is needed for wound healing. However, zinc has only been shown to be beneficial for wound healing in people who are zinc-deficient. Zinc deficiency may also contribute to reduced cellular immunity.

High intakes of zinc, in excess of 2 g, can cause nausea and vomiting. Long-term ingestion of high intakes can lead to copper deficiency.

Deficiency of zinc can cause symptoms which include growth failure and impaired healing of wounds. Factors predisposing to deficiency include:

- diets lacking in zinc in a form readily available to the body, for example those containing wholegrain cereals which can interfere with zinc absorption
- infestation with parasites causing chronic blood-loss
- excessive sweating due to high environmental temperature
- malabsorption of food
- surgery
- burns.

Dietary sources of zinc are seafood, meats, eggs, whole cereals and pulses. Simple dietary deficiency appears to be uncommon in western communities. The first case of zinc deficiency was identified in 1958 in the Middle East where the diet consisted of unleavened bread, beans and clay. There is an increasing amount of interest in the role of zinc in appetite control. Patients with anorexia nervosa often have a low serum zinc level.

Cobalt

Cobalt is the constituent of vitamin B_{12} that is necessary for normal development of red blood cells. It is found in meats, milk products and seafoods.

Chloride

Chloride is important because it balances the sodium and potassium in the cells and in the ECF. Depletion can result from prolonged vomiting, but inadequate intake is not likely to occur.

In the UK the major dietary source of chloride is salt. Currently the dietary intake exceeds requirements.

Selenium

Selenium is part of one of the enzymes which protects intracellular structures from damage by oxidation. This antioxidant property has led to suggestions that it may be protective against the development of some forms of cancer. Cereals, meat and fish are the best sources of selenium in the diet.

Molybdenum

Molybdenum is essential for some of the enzymes involved in DNA metabolism. Dietary sources of molybdenum are milk, pulses, liver, kidney and cereals. High dietary intakes may reduce the absorption of copper from the diet.

Manganese

Manganese is a component of some enzymes and activates others, so has many roles. It occurs in small amounts in many foods. The major dietary source of manganese in the UK is tea. When excessive amounts of the element are consumed, absorption is very low and excess is excreted by the kidneys, making this one of the least toxic of all elements.

Chromium

Chromium increases the action of insulin and plays a part in lipid metabolism. Dietary sources are meat, wholegrain cereals, pulses, nuts and yeast.

Aluminium

Aluminium is found in all plants and animals, the concentration depending upon the soil in which the vegetables, cereals or animal-feed crops grew and the amount present in the water. It does not appear to have any function.

Sulphur

Although involved in many metabolic processes, there is no dietary requirement for sulphur because it can be derived from the amino acids cysteine and methionine.

Box 5.7   Dietary sources of iron

Meat and meat products:

- Lean meat—an average portion contains 6 mg iron
- Eggs—1 egg contains 1.8 mg iron

Sources suitable for vegetarians:

- Bread—thick slice contains 0.7 mg iron
- Green-leafed vegetables—average portion contains 1.5 mg iron
- Pulses—150 g baked beans contains 3 mg iron
- Dried fruit—portion of prunes contains 0.8 mg iron
- Fortified breakfast cereals—average portion contains 0.3 mg iron

---

Other minerals are present, some in trace amounts, in human tissues. Some of these are essential, but in many cases their function is poorly understood. As they are not likely to be lacking in a balanced diet, and as no deficiency states have been reported, they do not require consideration from a nutritional point of view.

- Arsenic, antimony, cadmium, bromine, boron, caesium, germanium, lead, lithium, mercury, silver, strontium and tin have not yet been shown to be essential micronutrients.
- Nickel, silicon and vanadium have been shown to be essential micronutrients for humans.

WATER

Water constitutes about 65–70% of the total bodyweight and is the medium in which almost every body process takes place. When one considers some of the many ways in which it promotes the functions of the body, its importance becomes apparent.

- Water is the basis of intracellular and extracellular fluids and is a constituent of all the body's secretions and excretions.
- The products of digestion are absorbed into the body in a fluid medium and distributed in blood and lymph.
- The chemical reactions involved in metabolism also require a fluid medium.
- The waste products are conveyed in the bloodstream to the kidneys and the lungs for excretion.
- Sufficient water is required to ensure an adequate urine flow and to facilitate the passage of the faeces along the colon so that constipation does not occur.
- The joints are bathed in a lubricating fluid which prevents friction when movement takes place.
- Body temperature is largely controlled by evaporation of moisture from the skin and the lungs.

A constant supply of water is essential. Thus people who undergo long fasts can live on their body reserves of protein, fat, carbohydrate and other nutrients for several weeks—provided water is available. If water were withheld they would die after a few days.

Figure 5.2 shows the fluid compartments within the body and the relative volumes occupied by intracellular fluid, extracellular fluid and plasma.

Sources

A large part of the water required by the body is supplied by milk, tea, water and other beverages, and such foods as fruit and vegetables.

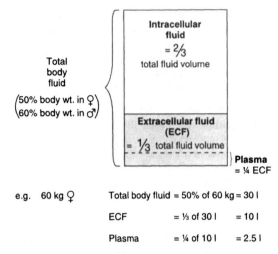

e.g. 60 kg ♀   Total body fluid = 50% of 60 kg = 30 l

                ECF   = ⅓ of 30 l   = 10 l

                Plasma   = ¼ of 10 l   = 2.5 l

Figure 5.2 Fluid compartments within the body showing the relative volumes occupied by intracellular fluid, extracellular fluid and plasma (part of the extracellular space) (McGeown 1999).

Water is a constituent of most foods, even though they may be solid in consistency:

- bread contains approximately 35% water
- fish 65%
- meat 50–70%
- vegetables and fruits 80–90%.

When carbohydrates, fats and proteins are metabolised, water is produced. This water is known as metabolic water. It is of particular importance to certain forms of animal life. Hibernating animals depend during their dormant period on water produced as a result of metabolism.

Water balance

Water is lost from the body in urine, faeces, sweat and expired air. The sensation of thirst normally ensures an adequate intake. The regulatory mechanisms in the kidneys result in a variable volume of urine being secreted—consequently a balance is maintained between intake and output of water.

Requirement

An average adult living in a temperate climate requires approximately 2500 ml of water daily. The actual amount that is ingested depends both on climate and habit:

- drinks provide 1000–2500 ml
- food provides 1000–1500 ml
- metabolism provides 200–400 ml.

Requirements vary according to the amount lost in sweat, and more water is required by people who exercise vigorously, or who work in hot surroundings. As we have already seen, loss of a large volume of sweat necessitates the replacement of salt as well as water.

In addition to occurring when fluid intake is inadequate, water depletion can occur in conditions such as prolonged vomiting and diarrhoea, haemorrhage, extensive burns and in uncontrolled diabetes mellitus. The term 'dehydration' means loss of water, but is often used as implying a loss of certain mineral elements also, particularly sodium. Loss of up to 5% of body-weight by dehydration results in thirst and discomfort, loss of 6–10% results in dizziness, absence of saliva and inability to walk, loss of 11–12% results in delirium, swollen tongue, inability to swallow and shrivelled skin.

REFERENCES

Chan G M, McMurray M, Westover K, Engelbert-Fenton K, Thomas M R 1987 Effects of increased dietary calcium intake upon calcium and bone mineral status in lactating adolescent and adult women. American Journal of Clinical Nutrition 46: 319–323

Department of Health (DoH) 1991 Dietary reference values for food energy and nutrients for the United Kingdom. Report of the Panel on Dietary Reference Values of the Committee on Medical Aspects of Food Policy (COMA) (Report on Health and Social Subjects 41). HMSO, London

Department of Health (DoH) 1992 The Health of the Nation: a strategy for health in England. HMSO, London

Food and Agriculture Organisation (FAO) 1988 Requirements of vitamin A, iron, folate and B_{12}. Report of a joint FAO/WHO consultation (Food and

Nutrition Series 23). Food and Agriculture Organisation, Rome

Gregory J 2000 National Diet and Nutrition Survey: young people aged 4 to 18 years. HMSO, London

Hallberg L, Hogdahl A-M, Nilsson L, Rybo G 1966 Menstrual blood-loss—a population study. Acta Obstetrica Gynaecologica Scandanavica 45: 320–351

Heaney R P, Skillman T G 1971 Calcium metabolism in normal human pregnancy. Journal of Clinical Endocrine Metabolism 33: 661–670

Hegsted D M 1963 Symposium on human calcium requirements. Journal of the American Medical Association 185: 588–593

Klevay L M, Inman L, Johnson L K et al 1984 Increased cholesterol in plasma in a young man during experimental copper depletion. Metabolism 33: 1112–1118

Law M R, Frost C D, Wald N J 1991 By how much does dietary salt reduction lower blood pressure? British Medical Journal 302: 811–824

Lee C A B, Barrett C A, Ignatavicius D D 1996 Fluids and electrolytes. A practical approach, 4th Edn. F.A. Davis, Philadelphia

McGeown 1999 Physiology. Churchill Livingstone, UK

Marshall D H, Nordin B E C, Speed R 1976 Calcium, phosphorus and magnesium requirement. Proceedings of the Nutrition Society 35: 163–173

Matlou S M, Isles C G, Higgs A et al 1986 Potassium supplementation in Blacks with mild to moderate essential hypertension. Journal of Hypertension 4: 61–64

National Osteoporosis Society (NOS) 1999 Diet and Bone Health. National Osteoporosis Society, Bath

National Health Institutes (NHI) 1994 Consensus Statement. Optimal Calcium Intake 12(4): 1–31

Nordin B E, Heaney R P 1990a Calcium supplementation of the diet: justified by present evidence. British Medical Journal 300 (6731): 1056-60

Nordin B E, Heaney R P 1990b Calcium supplementation of the diet. British Medical Journal 301 (6743): 120

Salmon J (for the Department of Health) 1991 Dietary reference values—a guide. HMSO, London

Wenlock R W 1987 Changing patterns of dietary iodine intake in Britain. In: dietary iodine and other aetiological factors in hyperthyroidism. Conference report (MRC Scientific Report 9). MRC Environmental Epidemiology Unit, Southampton

FURTHER READING

British Nutrition Foundation 2001 Selenium and Health. British Nutrition Foundation, London

Delange F 2000 The role of iodine in brain development. Proceedings of the Nutrition Society 59: 75–79

Garrow J S, James W P T, Ralph A 2000 Human nutrition and dietetics, 10th Edn. Churchill Livingstone, Edinburgh

USEFUL ADDRESSES

The National Osteoporosis Society
P O Box
Radstock
Bath BA3 3YB
Website: www.nos.org.uk

The National Dairy Council Website: www.milk.co.uk

6

Vitamins

LEARNING OBJECTIVES

After studying this chapter you should be able to:

- discuss the differences between fat soluble and water soluble vitamins
- describe the structure, function and dietary sources of vitamins
- list the dietary reference values for vitamins
- explain the consequences of inadequate and excessive vitamin intakes.

INTRODUCTION

The term vitamin is a shortened form of vitalamine. This term was first used in 1911 by Casimir Funk to describe a substance that he isolated from rice polishings that both cured and prevented beriberi in chickens.

One of the earliest records of the cure of a vitamin deficiency disorder, although it was not recognised as such then, was in an Egyptian medical treatise of 1500 BC, where eating roast ox liver was recommended as a treatment for night-blindness. During the 18th century, Lind (1753) cured sailors with scurvy using citrus fruit juice, and, during the 19th century, beriberi was cured in Japanese sailors by adding extra meat and dried milk to their daily rice ration. It was not, however, realised that a specific deficiency was causing the disease and that the food cured this deficiency. At this time, the only known nutrients were protein, fat, carbohydrate, minerals and water.

Vitamins are organic substances or groups of related substances which have specific biochemical functions in the body. They are essential for normal metabolism and are provided by the diet. The body can manufacture some vitamins but must have adequate amounts of the precursor, e.g. tryptophan for niacin products.

Structure and function of vitamins

Vitamins have different specific chemical structures and physiological functions. Generally, they act by promoting a specific chemical reaction or group of reactions in a metabolic process. If the vitamin is lacking, the metabolic process cannot proceed, the symptoms of the disease develop and the body develops specific deficiency symptoms.

When vitamins were first isolated they were identified by a letter of the alphabet. Once their chemical composition was understood, they were given an appropriate name; for example, vitamin C became ascorbic acid.

Sometimes the vitamin can only be obtained directly from food, for example ascorbic acid. In other instances foods also contain a very closely related substance known as the pro-vitamin or vitamin precursor, which can be converted into the vitamin in the body, for example vitamin A is produced from β-carotene.

Vitamin D is unusual in that diet is not its only source. The precursor is manufactured in the body and converted in the skin to the vitamin under the influence of sunlight.

Some vitamins are formed in the intestine by bacteria, and part of the body's requirement is met in this way. Vitamin K and some of the B-group vitamins are produced in the intestine as a result of this bacterial action. In some cases, however, there is doubt as to how much of the vitamin formed in this way is absorbed from the digestive tract.

Classification of vitamins

Vitamins may be classified as either fat-soluble or water-soluble:

- Fat-soluble vitamins:
  — vitamin A
  — vitamin D
  — vitamin E
  — vitamin K
- Water-soluble vitamins:
  — vitamins of the B group
  — vitamin C.

Large doses of fat-soluble vitamins are harmful because they cannot be excreted and are stored in the body. Water-soluble vitamins are excreted in the urine so large doses are not usually harmful, although in some situations they can be.

Vitamin requirements

The exact amount of each vitamin needed for optimum health is not known and shows individual variation. The Committee on Medical Aspects of Food Policy (COMA) has made certain recommendations about vitamin intake which, it considers, would meet the requirements of average healthy persons (DoH 1991a). These reference values are explained in Chapter 1 and reproduced in Appendix 2.

VITAMIN A (RETINOL)
Functions

1. *Night vision.* Vitamin A is essential for the formation of the retinal pigment rhodopsin. It is this pigment that enables the eye to see in dim light. Rhodopsin decomposes in the presence of bright light. It is regenerated and requires vitamin A for its regeneration.
2. *Healthy epithelial tissue.* Vitamin A is necessary for maintaining the integrity of epithelial tissue and mucous membranes.
3. *Normal development of teeth and bones.*
4. *Functioning of the immune system.*

Sources

The carotenoid group of plant pigments can be converted to vitamin A. Although there are about 100 pigments in this group, the most commonly occurring is β-carotene, which is split, by an enzyme that occurs naturally in the mucosa of the small intestine, to yield two molecules of retinol. This conversion can also occur in the liver. In the UK diet, about 30% of the vitamin A intake is provided by carotenoids, mostly β-carotenes.

β-carotene is the precursor of vitamin A; it is a yellow pigment which occurs in many plants, particularly those with yellow, red or dark green colouring. Humans obtain the vitamin partly from foods of animal origin in which it has already been formed, and partly from the carotene present in vegetables, fruits and some animal products (Box 6.1).

Vitamin content of source foods

This varies greatly with the diet of the animal concerned. For example, if cows are grazing on grass in summer and their diet is high in the plant pigment carotene, the vitamin content of milk and its products is at its highest.

Effect of cooking and storage of foods

Vitamin A and carotene are not destroyed by most methods of cooking. However, some losses occur at

Box 6.1 Dietary sources of carotenoids and of preformed vitamin A

Carotenes
Foods rich in carotene include:

- cabbage and lettuce, especially the dark-green leaves
- spinach
- tomatoes
- carrots
- peaches
- apricots
- prunes
- pumpkins
- mangoes

Preformed vitamin A
The best sources of the already formed vitamin are:

- liver
- kidney
- egg yolk
- milk
- butter
- cheese
- cream
- oily fish such as herrings, sardines and salmon
- vitamin-fortified margarine
- cod and halibut liver oils

Table 6.1 Carotene contents of food portions

Food	β-carotene (μg)
Portion of cooked carrots	4536
1 raw tomato	544
Portion of cooked broccoli	428

carotene (Colditz et al 1985). In the UK it is recommended that the intake of fruit and vegetables is increased to protect against the development of some cancers (DoH 1998). Table 6.1 gives the carotene content of some foods.

Effects of deficiency

Night-blindness

The first sign of vitamin A deficiency is impaired ability of the eye to adapt to vision in a dim light. This is known as poor dark adaptation, or night-blindness.

Retinol in the diet or produced from β-carotene is absorbed from the intestine and, as it is fat-soluble, is transported to the liver in chylomicrons. Any vitamin A not needed immediately is stored in the liver. The liver of a well-nourished person in the UK contains about 400 μg retinol (Huque & Truswell 1979), sufficient to last for at least 6 months. The liver is very efficient at mobilising its retinol stores to ensure an adequate circulating level of retinol. This means that levels of circulating retinol are not a good indicator of the vitamin A status of a person who is suspected of having a vitamin A deficiency. It is only during the later phases of deficiency that circulating levels drop. At this time, clinical symptoms of the deficiency are also present.

Deficiency occurs in developing countries where there is a shortage of foods containing β-carotene and occasionally in more affluent countries where it may be associated with malabsorption or chronic biliary obstruction.

Deterioration of mucous membranes

A more serious deficiency results in deterioration of mucous membranes, which become dried and hardened, or keratinised. The resultant accumulation of dead cells encourages local infections, for example of the respiratory tract. In some cases, the skin becomes dried and the ducts are blocked with dead cells, giving rise to a roughened appearance. These infections can cause death in malnourished children.

high temperatures, for example during frying. As vitamin A is destroyed by light, dried forms of fruit such as dried apricots or prunes have a lower content than the fresh form.

Dietary requirement

Although one molecule of β-carotene is cleaved to provide two molecules of retinol, the absorption of β-carotene by the gut is not very efficient. As a result of this, 6 μg dietary β-carotene is considered to be equivalent to 1 μg dietary retinol (WHO 1967). Dietary reference values for vitamin A are expressed as μg retinol equivalent per day. This is a total from the sum of retinol and dietary β-carotene.

The reference nutrient intakes for children and adults are listed in Appendix 2.

Different diets will obviously contain vitamin A from different sources, and there are as yet no recommendations for the proportions of vitamin A that should be provided by preformed retinol and β-carotene. However, a prospective study of elderly people in Massachusetts showed that a decreased risk of all cancers was associated with increased consumption of green and yellow vegetables, i.e. those rich in β-

Xerophthalmia

This is also common among children where the diet is deficient in retinol. The conjunctiva becomes keratinised, giving rise to xerophthalmia, sometimes known as dry eye, and a softening of the cornea—keratomalacia—may take place, resulting in infection, ulceration of the cornea and permanent blindness. This corneal damage was estimated to cause 500 000 new cases of blindness a year in children in Southeast Asia.

Poor growth

Retinol is important for both proliferation and differentiation of cells, so in a deficiency state, growth will be retarded (see Box 6.2).

Prevention of deficiency

The COMA report recommended that vitamin drops be available for children up to the age of 5 years (DHSS 1988). The recommended dose of 5 drops contains 200 µg vitamin A, which is the lower reference nutrient intake (LRNI) (see p. 5).

In developing countries a dose of 60 mg every 6 months is recommended to prevent deficiency developing. The usual pharmacological form used is retinol palmitate.

Vitamin A and pregnancy

The dietary reference values for retinol during pregnancy recommend an extra 100 µg. However, because of the teratogenic effects of retinol, pregnant women are advised not to take vitamin A supplements and avoid foods that are very rich sources of it, such as liver.

Vitamin A excess

Large intakes of β-carotene are not harmful but can lead to a yellow/orange appearance of the skin, particularly the palms. Large intakes of retinol are harmful and can cause liver and bone damage, hair loss, double vision, headaches and vomiting. Regular intakes should not exceed 7500 µg/day for adult women and 9000 µg/day in adult men (DoH 1991a). Children are more sensitive to increased retinol intake and the daily intake in infants should not exceed 90 µg.

VITAMIN D
Formation

There are two main forms of vitamin D, both of which are sterols. Cholecalciferol (vitamin D_3) is formed by the action of sunlight on 7-dehydrocholesterol, which occurs naturally in the skin of humans and other animals.

Ergocalciferol (vitamin D_2) is formed by the action of sunlight on ergosterol, which occurs naturally in plants and fungi. This form of the vitamin is prepared commercially and used in medicinal preparations and for the fortification of such foods as margarine. It is known as vitamin D_2 or ergocalciferol.

Functions

Vitamin D is needed for the absorption of calcium from the small intestine and the calcification of the skeleton.

Cholecalciferol is not the active form of vitamin D. Cholecalciferol is hydroxylated by the liver to 25-hydroxycholecalciferol (25-OHD_3), which is further hydroxylated in the kidneys to 1,25-dihydroxycholecalciferol ($1,25$-$(OH_2)D_3$), also known as calcitriol. It is the calcitriol which is the active form. Its prime function is to act as a hormone by stimulating the production of the transport protein necessary for calcium transport across the epithelium of the small intestine. Vitamin D acts with parathyroid hormone to release calcium from bone into the circulation to maintain calcium homeostasis, facilitate phosphate absorption and increase bone formation (see Fig. 6.1).

The level of 25-OHD_3 in the plasma is a good measure of vitamin D status. The normal range is 25–75 nmol/l.

Box 6.2 Vitamin A

Sources
- Formed in human tissues from plant pigment β-carotene
- Formed in tissues of food-producing animals and found in milk, eggs, liver and other foods

Functions
- Integrity of epithelial tissue
- Dark adaptation
- Normal growth

Deficiency
- Night-blindness
- Mucous membrane infections
- Growth retardation

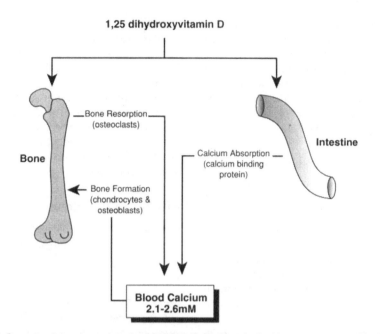

1,25 dihydroxyvitamin D

Bone

Bone Resorption
(osteoclasts)

Bone Formation
(chondrocytes &
osteoblasts)

Calcium Absorption
(calcium binding
protein)

Intestine

**Blood Calcium
2.1-2.6mM**

Figure 6.1 1,25(OH)$_2$D$_3$ and calcium homeostasis. 1,25(OH)$_2$D$_3$ is the principal hormone responsible for calcium absorption from the intestine where it stimulates the production of an intracellular calcium-binding protein. 1,25(OH)$_2$D$_3$ also affects bone metabolism, stimulating both resorption and formation (Garrow et al 2000).

Sources

Non-dietary

The major source of vitamin D for most of the population of the UK is the vitamin D formed in the body as a result of ultraviolet irradiation of the skin (DoH 1991a).

There is considerable variation in vitamin D status among the population of healthy individuals. This is due to the differing amounts of time spent outside and the differing intensity of solar radiation (McLaughlin et al 1974).

The intensity of solar radiation in the UK varies with latitude, time of year, time of day and climatic conditions. In the UK, ultraviolet radiation of the right wavelength for cholecalciferol conversion (290–310 nm) only occurs during the 7-month period of April to October. The radiation is most effective between 11 a.m. and 3 p.m., and complete cloud cover reduces its effect by 50%.

Dietary

Vitamin D is present in foods of animal origin in which it has already been formed; it is found in eggs, butter and oily fish such as herrings, sardines and salmon. Cod and halibut liver oils are particularly rich sources.

It is also prepared artificially by irradiation of a plant sterol and used in medicinal preparations and vitaminised foods; margarine is artificially fortified with the vitamin. It might be expected that milk and cheese would be good sources of vitamin D, but in fact they contain only small amounts. Infant formula milks and fortified infant cereal foods are in many cases almost the only components of the diet of infants that contain vitamin D.

Fortification of dairy produce and margarine with vitamins A and D

This process was started as a preventive measure when margarine was used as a substitute for butter.

Margarine was developed as a substitute for butter in the 19th century. Its use in the 20th century is widespread. In the UK during the Second World War, legislation was passed to ensure that margarine was fortified with retinol and vitamin D, those vitamins which occur naturally in butter. This measure was intended to ensure that changing from butter to margarine in the diet did not result in a dietary deficiency. This statute means that margarine must contain 700 µg retinol and 8 µg vitamin D/100 g.

Vitamins A and D are both removed with the fat from milk during the skimming process. Many products made from skimmed milk have vitamins A and D added. This fortification process was reviewed by the COMA panel (DoH 1991b) and it was agreed to continue the fortification process because margarine provides a good source of vitamin D for those members of the population whose skin is not exposed to sufficient sunlight, for example people with reduced mobility, who live in institutions or who, because of their culture, choose not to expose their skin.

Effect of cooking, storage and preservation

Vitamin D in food is not affected by storage, preservation or cooking of food.

Dietary reference values for vitamin D

In the UK, the average dietary intake of vitamin D is 3 µg and the range is 0.5–8 µg/day. However, there is no dietary reference value for adults living a normal lifestyle because they manufacture an adequate supply.

For those people who do not go out in the sun, in particular older people, an intake of 10 µg/day is recommended (DoH 1991a). This should be supplied by including fortified margarine, oily fish and eggs in the diet. Supplements will be necessary for those housebound people who have poor diets and those with poor appetites. Compston (1998) suggests that the elderly and other populations at high risk of vitamin D deficiency should be routinely supplemented with 800 iu (20 µg) vitamin per day, and that this would reduce incidence of osteoporotic fractures in the elderly. An intake of 10 µg/day is also recommended for pregnant and lactating women. Some of this will be supplied by sunshine but supplements may be required to ensure an adequate intake.

In Scotland, where there is less of the necessary ultraviolet radiation, there is a higher incidence of hypocalcaemia and a defect of dental enamel (both related to vitamin D deficiency) in the infants of women who have not received vitamin D supplements (Cockburn et al 1980), but this does not occur in infants in the South of England.

Very little information is available on which to base an estimation of vitamin D requirements. It is possible that for adults no dietary intake is necessary, provided there is adequate exposure to sunlight. This is not always the case in the UK. Children and adolescents during the winter may also lack adequate vitamin D. Those who are partially or totally housebound certainly require a dietary source, or alternatively a supplement of the vitamin. The reference nutrient intake (RNI) for the housebound is 10 µg/day (see Appendix 2).

Children aged 0–6 months have an RNI of 8.5 µg/day; from 6 months to 3 years it is 7.0 µg/day; and after the age of 4 years they do not have a requirement for vitamin D providing their skin is exposed to sun.

This intake is initially provided by breast-milk, fortified infant milks, infant foods and infant vitamin drops which provide 7 µg/day (DHSS 1988). In infants it is important to ensure that overdose does not occur. However, once weaning is established and fewer fortified foods are being used, it is important to maintain an adequate intake.

Effects of deficiency

Deficiency of vitamin D leads to rickets in young children and osteomalacia in adults.

Rickets

Rickets is known to have occurred frequently in the UK for some hundreds of years. It was particularly prevalent among the poor of large cities, who could not afford to feed their children adequately and who did not benefit from the effect of sunlight because of their poor social conditions and the prevalence of cloud and smoke.

Since the discovery in the 1920s of vitamin D and its antirachitic effect, much has been done to improve this situation. Improved standards of living, education in nutrition, the routine administration of vitamin concentrates to infants and pregnant and nursing mothers, and the addition of vitamin D to margarine and to the infant formula milks and cereal foods used in infant feeding, have combined to make rickets uncommon among children in the UK but not eradicated, particularly in infants who are exclusively breast-fed (Train et al 1995).

In rickets the calcification of the skeleton is impaired. The bones remain stunted and soft and the weight of the child and the pull of the muscles give rise to deformities such as bow legs, narrowing of the pelvis, curvature of the spine and undue prominence of the sternum, which is known as pigeon chest.

Other symptoms include:

- the delayed development of teeth
- the child is restless and excessive perspiration occurs, especially around the head
- there is impaired muscle tone, giving rise to a pot-bellied appearance
- gastrointestinal upsets also occur.

Children are particularly vulnerable to a deficiency between the ages of 6 months and 3 years when calcium is being deposited in their bones and the amount of sunshine available to them is limited. There is an increased likelihood of Asian children living in northern latitudes developing rickets and this is discussed in Chapter 18.

Osteomalacia

Osteomalacia in adults corresponds to rickets in children. It is a generalised bone disorder which occurs when mineralisation is impaired leading to the accumulation of unmineralised matrix in the skeleton. Osteomalacia can be diagnosed histologically and it is usually accompanied by a plasma 25-OHD_3 level of below 10 nmol/l. In some countries it is a complication of pregnancy, occurring when the increased vitamin D requirements to meet the needs of the mother and the foetus are not met, when the skeleton of the mother becomes demineralised. Bone deformities and fractures occur, and deformity of the pelvis may make normal delivery of the child impossible.

Incidence of rickets and osteomalacia

Vitamin D is present in foods of the normal diet in comparatively small amounts that vary with the extent to which the source animal has been exposed to sunlight; naturally occurring foods cannot therefore be depended upon as a source of supply. The action of the ultraviolet rays of sunlight cannot be depended upon either as they are impeded by cloud, atmospheric dust, window glass and clothing.

Low vitamin D intake probably contributes to the development of osteomalacia, which has been reported among elderly women in the UK. Recently, osteomalacia has been encountered among immigrants from India and Pakistan. Osteomalacia in its most serious form occurs in some eastern countries, where the diet is lacking in calcium and vitamin D and where there is very little sunshine. It occurs also in women who are never exposed to the sun, for example among those whose style of dress shields them from the sun.

In both rickets and osteomalacia, a low blood calcium level may give rise to a form of muscle spasm known as tetany.

The incidence of osteomalacia in older people is discussed in Chapter 17.

VITAMIN E (TOCOPHEROL)
Functions

Vitamin E has been shown to be essential for some animal species. Most of the experimental work has been done on rats, in which deficiency of this vitamin causes failure of reproduction. The function of vitamin E in the human body is not fully understood. It has an important role in protecting membrane lipids from oxidative damage and so is important in the prevention of cancers and cardiovascular disease and maintaining the integrity of cell membranes. Deficiency is unknown under normal conditions.

Sources

Vitamin E is a fat-soluble vitamin which is found in all cell membranes. There are eight compounds which have vitamin E activity. These can be divided into two groups of compounds, the tocopherols and the less potent tocotrienols.

This vitamin is widely distributed in foods. Wheatgerm and wheatgerm oil are particularly rich sources. It is also present in the germinating part of other seeds and in green leafy vegetables like broccoli and spinach. Other foods such as eggs and butter contain smaller amounts.

Dietary reference values for vitamin E

The requirement for vitamin E depends on the amount of polyunsaturated fatty acids (PUFA) in the diet. Vitamin E acts as an antioxidant, so the greater the PUFA content of the diet the greater will be the need for vitamin E. As the PUFA content of the diet is very varied, the COMA panel felt unable to give a specific RNI for vitamin E, but rather set levels of safe intakes. The safe levels of intake have been set as more than 3 mg/day for women and 4 mg/day for men. The safe intake set for infants is based on the vitamin E content of breast-milk. Infant formulae should provide at least 0.3 mg/100 ml and at least 0.4 mg/g PUFA.

Effects of deficiency

As dietary sources of vitamin E are varied it is unusual for children and adults to suffer from a deficiency. As a fat-soluble vitamin, absorption of vitamin E relies on normal digestion and absorption of dietary fat. Deficiency can occur in children or adults who are unable to absorb or utilise vitamin E adequately, for example patients with malabsorption syndrome, cystic fibrosis or abetalipoproteinaemia. These patients have a low plasma tocopherol and mild haemolytic anaemia.

Vitamin E status is measured as the serum tocopherol: cholesterol ratio. This is because serum levels are increased when serum lipids are raised. This is due to the tocopherols passing out of the cell membranes into the circulation, so giving a raised serum tocopherol value.

The lowest satisfactory serum tocopherol:cholesterol ratio is 2.25 µmol/mmol.

Vitamin E deficiency can occur in premature infants, where it shows as a specific syndrome with the symptoms of haemolytic anaemia, thrombocytosis, and oedema. Most infant formulae for pre-term babies now contain vitamin E.

High intakes

Vitamin E influences normal immune function but there is as yet no evidence to show that increasing vitamin E intake improves immune response. High intakes have been associated with the prevention of ischaemic heart disease and cancer but the evidence is still inconclusive (DoH 1991a). Large doses do not appear to be harmful. An intake of up to 3200 mg/day has been shown to be safe (Bendich & Machlin 1988).

VITAMIN K

Functions

Vitamin K, identified as the 'koagulatious vitamin' by Dam in 1935, is known as the anti-haemorrhagic vitamin, because it maintains the blood's normal levels of prothrombin and other factors necessary for blood clotting.

Sources

Vitamin K occurs in three chemical forms.

Phylloquinone. Most of our dietary intake comes from this form, which occurs in green leafy vegetables and to a lesser extent in a wide range of foods including fruits, cereal, meat, dairy produce and vegetable oils.

Menaquinones. These are produced by bacteria, particularly those found in the gut.

Menadione. This is a synthetic water-soluble form which is rarely used because it can cause jaundice (DoH 1991a).

Dietary reference values (DRVs) for vitamin K

Vitamin K requirement is believed to be very small and easily met by bacterial synthesis and dietary intake. There is too little information to provide accurate DRVs for vitamin K but the COMA report (DoH 1991a) states that intakes of 1 µg/kg body-weight per day are safe and seem to be adequate. To prevent haemorrhagic disease of the newborn, which is discussed below, many paediatricians recommend that newborn babies receive a single 1 mg dose of vitamin K.

Effects of deficiency

When deficiency of vitamin K is observed, it is usually due to a failure of absorption of the vitamin from the alimentary tract, often accompanying impaired fat absorption, e.g. in disease of the small bowel.

Haemorrhagic disease of the newborn, a rare life-threatening condition, develops in the first few days of life when it is thought to be caused by the low dietary intake of vitamin K, and the fact that the bacteria responsible for synthesis of this vitamin have not yet become established in the intestine. This low dietary intake means that the activity of vitamin-K-dependent clotting factors is reduced and bleeding can occur. Large doses of the naturally occurring vitamin K, phylloquinone, have now been shown to be harmful.

ABSORPTION OF FAT-SOLUBLE VITAMINS

Absorption of the fat-soluble vitamins is associated with the simultaneous absorption of fat and is assisted by the emulsifying action of bile. A deficiency of fat-soluble vitamins can occur when excessive amounts of fat escape digestion and absorption and are excreted in the faeces. Such disturbances have been known to induce rickets and osteomalacia.

In obstructive jaundice, when bile is prevented from entering the duodenum, poor absorption of vitamin K can result in serious haemorrhage during surgery to remove the obstruction. The administration of the vitamin by injection before the surgery eliminates this risk.

Fat-soluble vitamins are also soluble in mineral oils, which, when consumed, are not absorbed to any important extent. Thus, when liquid paraffin is used as a laxative, fat-soluble vitamins may be carried by it, in solution, into the faeces and so excreted, leading to vitamin deficiency.

VITAMINS OF THE B COMPLEX

INTRODUCTION

The first vitamin B identified was shown to cure the disease beriberi, and was later found to be associated in foods with another factor effective in curing pellagra. The anti-beriberi factor was called vitamin B_1, and the anti-pellagra factor vitamin B_2. Later, vitamin B_2 itself was shown to contain the anti-pellagra vitamin nicotinic acid, and riboflavin. Other dietary factors have since been assigned to the B group, among which are vitamin B_{12}, folic acid and vitamin B_6 or pyridoxine.

THIAMIN (VITAMIN B_1)

Functions

Thiamin constitutes part of an enzyme system concerned in the metabolism of carbohydrates, alcohol and fat. It is necessary for the metabolism of pyruvic acid, a substance which is produced during the breakdown of glycogen in the muscles to yield energy.

Sources

Thiamin is found in small amounts in many foods. The best sources are the germinating parts of cereals and other plants.

Wholemeal flour and bread are of importance as sources of thiamin. Unfortified white flour and bread made from unfortified white flour contain relatively little thiamin, as it is removed with the germ and bran during milling of the wheat. In the UK, however, white flour is artificially fortified with this vitamin as are many breakfast cereals and baby foods. This ensures that these foods are good sources of the vitamin.

Yeast extracts are also good sources of thiamin. Other moderately good sources are milk, eggs, liver, kidney, pork and pulses.

Effect of cooking

Thiamin is soluble in water, so some loss occurs when cooking water is discarded. It is destroyed by alkalis and by very high temperatures. Some of the thiamin present in bread is destroyed by toasting. This is only significant if all bread eaten is toasted and the diet is very limited in the range of foods eaten.

Dietary requirements

Thiamin requirements are related to energy intake as this vitamin is essential for energy metabolism.

The RNI is 0.4 mg/1000 kcal for most individuals (Table 6.2) and should not be reduced below 0.4 mg/day for people on a very low calorie intake. It is not necessary to increase this figure during pregnancy and lactation; the increase in energy intake that occurs is from a wide range of sources, so a proportionate increase in thiamin will occur (Oldham et al 1950).

Table 6.2 Reference nutrient intakes for thiamin

Age	RNI (mg/1000 kcal)
0–12 months	0.3
1–10 years	0.4
11–50 years males and females	0.4

Effects of deficiency

The body only contains 30 mg of thiamin, approximately 30 times the normal daily requirement. Thiamin deficiency develops quickly once the body store has been utilised. It can develop after 1 month on a diet containing little thiamin. There are two deficiency diseases caused by lack of thiamin; beriberi and Wernicke–Korsakoff syndrome. These diseases do not usually occur together and it is unclear why deficient individuals develop beriberi instead of Wernicke–Korsakoff syndrome or vice-versa.

Beriberi

Lack of thiamin is believed to be the principal cause of this disease, which occurs among people whose staple food is polished rice. The peripheral nerves are affected, resulting in a condition referred to as polyneuritis. The legs and feet, particularly, are involved and there is pain, weakness, degeneration of the muscles and inability to perform coordinated movements. This is known as dry beriberi.

In some cases, fluid accumulates in the tissues (oedema) and the resultant swelling can obscure the wasting of muscle. Heart function may be impaired and death can occur from heart failure. This form of the disease is known as wet beriberi.

Infantile beriberi with cardiovascular symptoms occurs in breast-fed infants if the diet of the mother is grossly deficient in thiamin. If the vitamin is provided in time, these changes are reversed and little permanent injury remains.

It is believed that, although thiamin deficiency is the principal cause of beriberi, a lack of other dietary factors, particularly other vitamins of the B complex, plays a part in bringing about the condition. As well as a diet deficient in thiamin, beriberi can be caused by a diet containing a lot of antithiamin compounds. These contain the enzyme that destroys thiamin, thiaminase, which is found in raw fish and raw shellfish.

Other compounds which have an antithiamin activity, and so can cause beriberi, are found in betel nuts, tealeaf extracts, fermented tea and coffee. Treatment involves providing a diet adequate in all essential nutrients, with supplements of the vitamins of the B group, emphasis being placed on thiamin.

In the past, beriberi has been the cause of much disease and death. It was particularly prevalent among men who were at sea for long periods of time and unable to obtain fresh foods. Beriberi still occurs where highly refined rice is the staple food and very little fresh food is eaten, it is also seen occasionally in alcoholics.

Wernicke–Korsakoff syndrome

This condition is sometimes seen in people who have undergone a long period of fasting or who suffer from persistent vomiting, such as in hyperemesis gravidarum, but it is most commonly seen among alcoholics whose energy sources are high in carbohydrate and alcohol but contain no thiamin.

The symptoms of this syndrome include poor memory, confusion, apathy, nystagmus and ataxia and it has been suggested that thiamin deficiency may contribute to the development of confusional states among elderly people in institutional care (Older & Dickerson 1982).

High doses of thiamin are toxic, causing headache, irritability, insomnia, rapid pulse and weakness and can cause death. A chronic intake of more than 3 g/day has been shown to be toxic.

RIBOFLAVIN (VITAMIN B₂)

Functions

Riboflavin is a constituent of a number of enzymes concerned in oxidation and reduction processes in body tissues.

Sources

Riboflavin is found in many foods. The most valuable dietary source is milk (500 ml supplies half of the recommended daily intake for an average person). Other valuable sources are egg yolk, liver, kidney and heart. Some proprietary breakfast cereals and cereal foods for infants are fortified with riboflavin. Meat, fish, vegetables and wholegrain cereals contain small amounts. Yeast has a high riboflavin content, as does yeast extract.

Effects of cooking, storage and preservation

This vitamin is not affected greatly by the cooking, drying, canning or freezing of foods. It is sensitive to light, and much of the riboflavin in milk is destroyed after several hours' exposure to sunlight. This fact is important for people who rely on doorstep deliveries of milk. The riboflavin content of foods is reduced by the addition of alkalis such as baking soda, but not to the same extent as occurs in the case of thiamin.

Dietary reference values for riboflavin

Although riboflavin has an essential role in the release of energy from carbohydrates, fats and proteins, the riboflavin requirement only correlates with the energy intake for sedentary people, not for those who are more active. So RNIs for riboflavin are expressed as a daily intake rather than per 1000 kcal (Table 6.3).

An increased intake during pregnancy and lactation is needed to meet the requirements of the developing foetus and to ensure that the breast-milk contains sufficient riboflavin. Phenothiazines—a group of drugs used to treat some psychoses—increase the riboflavin requirement.

Effects of deficiency

The liver of a healthy individual contains enough riboflavin, as coenzymes, to last 3 months. The effects of riboflavin deficiency are apparent in the skin, particularly that of the face, and also in the eyes. The effects include:

* inflammation of the lips and tongue
* a waxy skin eruption around the nose and lips
* cracks at the corners of the mouth
* the cornea of the eye is infiltrated by small blood vessels, producing a bloodshot appearance
* the eyes are painful and sensitive to light.

Table 6.3   Reference nutrient intakes for riboflavin

Age	RNI (mg/day)	
0–12 months	0.4	
1–3 years	0.6	
4–6 years	0.8	
7–10 years	1.0	
	Males	Females
11–14 years	1.2	1.1
15–18 years	1.3	1.1
19–50+ years	1.3	1.1
Pregnancy		+0.3
Lactation		+0.5

These symptoms are found not only in association with riboflavin deficiency but are known to accompany other disorders and dietary deficiencies.

Deficiency of riboflavin is believed to be rare in the UK because of the contribution milk makes to the diet. However, the National Diet and Nutrition survey of young people aged 4–18 years (Gregory 2000) showed low riboflavin, folate and thiamin levels in some young people, along with an increased intake of soft and carbonated drinks. In other areas when deficiency occurs it is usually associated with deficiency of thiamin, nicotinic acid and other factors as well.

Large doses of riboflavin do not appear to be toxic. Large amounts are not absorbed from the small intestine because of the vitamin's poor solubility.

NIACIN (VITAMIN B₃)

Niacin is the name given to two related compounds: nicotinamide and nicotinic acid. They are part of the coenzymes nicotinamide adenine dinucleotide (NAD) and nicotinamide adenine dinucleotide phosphate (NADP), which are involved in the oxidative release of energy.

Functions

Nicotinic acid, like riboflavin, is a component of enzyme systems concerned in oxidation and reduction processes in body tissues.

Sources

Wholegrain cereals and wholemeal bread, meat, liver, kidney, fish and pulse vegetables are all natural sources of this vitamin. It appears, however, that not all of the nicotinic acid occurring in cereals can be absorbed by the body.

In the preparation of refined flours, nicotinic acid is progressively removed during milling. However, in the UK, flours other than wholemeal (white and brown flours, see Chapter 9) are artificially fortified with the vitamin in an available form, with the result that flour products are an important source of nicotinic acid. Some proprietary breakfast cereals and cereal foods for infants are fortified with this vitamin. Yeast has a high nicotinic acid content.

The essential amino acid tryptophan found in many protein foods can be converted to nicotinic acid in the body and is thus a precursor of the vitamin. The normal conversion is for 60 mg tryptophan to be converted to 1 mg nicotinic acid. This process is more efficient in pregnant women.

Reference nutrient intakes for niacin

RNIs are expressed as mg niacin equivalent/1000 kcal. 1 mg niacin equivalent is 1 mg dietary nicotinic acid or nicotinamide or 60 mg tryptophan.

With the exception of lactating women, both sexes and all ages have an RNI of 6.6 mg niacin equivalent/1000 kcal (Salmon 1991).

Lactating women require an extra 2.3 mg/day; a lactating woman with an energy intake of 2800 kcal would have an RNI of 17.5 mg niacin equivalent.

Effects of deficiency

Deficiency of nicotinic acid is usually accompanied by deficiency of several vitamins of the B group. Other dietary factors may be lacking also. In the initial stages there is loss of weight and appetite, accompanied by general ill-health. Prolonged deficiency gives rise to a condition known as pellagra:

- Reddish-brown pigmented areas appear on the skin, especially on areas which are exposed, such as the neck, face and hands. They occur equally on both sides of the body, giving a symmetrical appearance.
- There is inflammation of the gastrointestinal tract, resulting in diarrhoea.
- Mental changes include:
  — irritability
  — anxiety
  — depression, progressing in severe cases to hallucinations and dementia.

Dermatitis, diarrhoea and dementia have become known as the three Ds of pellagra.

Symptoms resulting from a deficiency of other factors such as thiamin and riboflavin also occur. This condition responds to a balanced diet with supplements of the missing factors.

Pellagra is predominantly a disease of maize-eating peoples. Maize is not a good dietary source of nicotinic acid; it also has a low tryptophan content. Pellagra is still seen in some countries, including India, central Asia and parts of Africa.

VITAMIN B₆
Functions

This vitamin is a mixture of the compounds pyridoxine, pyridoxal and pyridoxamine, and their phosphates. They act as cofactors for a large number of enzymes which catalyse amino acid reactions, so are very important for protein metabolism.

Sources

Vitamin B_6 occurs in a wide range of foods including liver, wholegrain cereals, meat, fish, bananas and pulses. The B_6 present in some vegetables may be in an unavailable form. Deficiency of B_6 is rare because this nutrient is found in such a wide variety of foods.

Reference nutrient intakes for vitamin B_6

Vitamin B_6 is essential for protein metabolism, so the RNIs are calculated in $\mu g/g$ protein (Table 6.4). An increased amount is not required during pregnancy and lactation, other than the increase that would accompany the normal increase in energy and protein requirements.

Effects of deficiency

Because of its widespread distribution in food, deficiency of vitamin B_6 is rare. However, if deficiency does occur, it is more likely to do so, and develop more quickly, when the diet has a high protein content (Canham et al 1969).

The best-known documented cases of vitamin B_6 deficiency occurred during the 1950s, when an infant formula which contained insufficient vitamin B_6 was available (Bessey et al 1957). The symptoms of convulsions and metabolic abnormalities were corrected by treatment with vitamin B_6.

The plasma level of pyridoxal phosphate drops in pregnant women. This appears to be a normal response and does not require vitamin B_6 supplementation.

Pharmacological use of vitamin B_6

Vitamin B_6 is used in the treatment of a range of disorders: homocystinuria, hyperoxaluria, and radiation sickness. It is also used to treat some of the side-effects of contraceptive steroids and for premenstrual tension (PMT) (Bender 1987). However, oral contraceptives do not increase vitamin B_6 requirements.

Sensory neuropathy was shown to develop in patients taking high doses of vitamin B_6 (Dalton & Dalton 1987). Because of the interest in self-medication for premenstrual syndrome, it has been recommended that vitamin B_6 should be available in tablets containing no more than 50 mg (Truswell 1999). Wyatt et al (1999) have published a systematic review evaluating the efficacy of vitamin B_6 in the treatment of premenstrual syndrome, which suggested that doses of B_6 of up to 100mg/day were likely to be beneficial in treating premenstrual symptoms and premenstrual depression.

VITAMIN B_{12} (CYANOCOBALAMIN)

Functions

Vitamin B_{12} is necessary for normal protein metabolism as it has a role, with folic acid, in the metabolism of some amino acids. It is also necessary for the production of the myelin sheath around nerves.

Sources

Meat and offal are the best dietary sources of vitamin B_{12}, but milk, cheese and eggs also contain valuable amounts. Vitamin B_{12} is not found in vegetables, so this means vegans and vegetarians may have a diet that is deficient in vitamin B_{12}. Vitamin B_{12} is also synthesised by bacteria and found in some seaweeds. It is supplements from these sources that will be acceptable to vegetarians.

The reference nutrient intakes for vitamin B_{12} at different ages are given in Table 6.5.

Effects of deficiency

In order for Vitamin B_{12} to be effective, it has to be absorbed from the diet. It is absorbed in the terminal ileum, but before this can happen the vitamin must bind to salivary haptocorrin and then to a protein produced by the parietal cells of the stomach. This protein is known as intrinsic factor.

A deficiency of vitamin B_{12} usually results from lack of the intrinsic factor necessary for its absorption,

Table 6.4 Reference nutrient intakes for vitamin B_6 (from Salmon 1991, with permission of HMSO)

Age	RNI ($\mu g/g$ protein)
0–6 months	8
7–9 months	10
10–12 months	13
From 1 year	15

Table 6.5 Reference nutrient intakes for vitamin B_{12} (from Salmon 1991, with permission of HMSO)

Age	RNI ($\mu g/day$)
0–6 months	0.3
7–12 months	0.4
1–3 years	0.5
4–6 years	0.8
7–10 years	1.0
11–14 years	1.2
15+ years	1.5

rather than inadequate dietary intake. This may be seen in persons in whom gastric secretion is impaired, or intestinal absorption reduced, so it can occur following gastric and ileal surgery. As the body contains a large store of vitamin B_{12} in the liver, deficiency will take a long time to develop.

The symptoms of deficiency are a megaloblastic anaemia and neurological symptoms.

Large doses of vitamin B_{12} have not been shown to be toxic to humans (see Table 6.6).

FOLIC ACID (FOLATE)

Sources

Folic acid is widely distributed in foods in a variety of forms which are chemically related and are known collectively as folate. Green vegetables, pulses, yeast extract and wholemeal bread are particularly rich sources.

The folate content of foods decreases the longer the foods are kept and the forms in the food change slowly to those that are less available. It is not a stable vitamin and considerable losses occur during cooking, particularly if vegetables are cooked for a long time.

Requirement

Requirement is increased during pregnancy. The megaloblastic anaemia which is sometimes observed in this condition, and which responds to treatment with folic acid, is due in part to defective diet. Folate deficiency sometimes occurs in premature babies, in association with the malabsorption syndrome, and in elderly persons living on poor diets. Dietary deficiency of folic acid, giving rise to anaemia, occurs in tropical countries.

Reference nutrient intakes for folate

Table 6.7 lists RNIs for folate in different age-groups. The role of supplementation of the diet with folate

Table 6.7 Reference nutrient intakes for folate (from Salmon 1991, with permission of DoH)

Age	RNI (µg/day)
0–1 year	50
1–3 years	70
4–6 years	100
7–10 years	150
11–50+ years	200
Pregnant women	+100
Lactating women	+60

during the preconceptual period in the prevention of neural tube defects is discussed in Chapter 14.

Effects of deficiency

Folate deficiency can develop quickly because the body does not have large stores; the lower limit of normal serum folate concentration is 3 mg/ml. Deficiency develops when diet is generally poor, as in the elderly, or when requirements are increased during pregnancy or when the folate in the diet is not absorbed properly.

Before it can be absorbed, folate in the food must be hydrolysed by an enzyme in the intestine; deficiency may occur when the small intestine is diseased, such as in coeliac disease, and when malabsorption occurs. Deficiency can also develop in alcoholic patients being treated with anticonvulsants, as these substances interfere with folate metabolism.

The symptom of deficiency is megaloblastic anaemia and, in children, growth may be stunted.

PANTOTHENIC ACID

This nutrient is essential for energy production and is widely distributed in plant and animal tissues. It therefore occurs in a wide range of foodstuffs.

Deficiency has only been shown to occur in humans when they are fed an artificial pantothenic-acid-free

Table 6.6 Vitamin B complex

	Sources	Functions	Deficiency
Thiamin Riboflavin Nicotinic acid	Fresh unprocessed foods and wholegrain cereals	Components of enzyme systems concerned in oxidation of foodstuffs	Beriberi Skin lesions Corneal vascularisation Pellagra
Vitamin B_{12} Folic acid		Red blood cell formation	Pernicious anaemia Nutritional megaloblastic anaemia

diet. The COMA report (DoH 1991a) therefore considers that the current UK diet containing 3–7 mg/day is adequate, but does not give an RNI.

No toxic effects have been shown from large doses.

BIOTIN

This nutrient is important in lipogenesis, gluconeogenesis and branched-chain amino acid catabolism. It is synthesised by the gut flora and found in a wide range of foods. Deficiency, the symptoms of which include anorexia, depression, hallucinations and desquamating dermatitis, has been shown to occur in patients on an inadequate regime of total parenteral nutrition and experimentally in subjects who have eaten large quantities of raw egg white (which contains the glycoprotein avidin, which binds with biotin making it unavailable).

ASCORBIC ACID (VITAMIN C)

Functions

Ascorbic acid has three important functions, which are well proven:

- prevention of scurvy
- aiding wound healing
- assisting the absorption of non-haem iron (Hunt et al 1990).

It has also been suggested that large doses of this vitamin are beneficial for a range of conditions, including improving immune function, physical working capacity, male fertility, lipid metabolism and resistance to stress. These claims are as yet not completely proven.

There is increasing interest in the role of ascorbic acid as an antioxidant in the prevention of the development of malignant disease. Interest has been around the link between it and the prevention of the formation of nitrosamines; this is discussed further in Chapter 11.

Vitamin C and wound healing

Ascorbic acid is necessary for the reduction of the amino acid proline to hydroxyproline. Hydroxyproline is essential for the formation of collagen (Fig. 6.2). It is inadequate collagen formation that is the biochemical basis for the development of scurvy (see below).

The requirement for vitamin C is increased after trauma and surgery, when the rate of collagen synthesis is increased. Adequate ascorbic acid is essential in the diet for the prevention and treatment of pressure sores (Taylor et al 1974). This is particularly relevant for the care of elderly patients who may already have a low store of ascorbic acid prior to the accident or fall which has led to their admission to hospital.

Sources

Ascorbic acid is found principally in fresh fruits and vegetables.

Good sources are oranges, grapefruit, lemons, tomatoes and leafy vegetables such as cabbage, broccoli, cauliflower and spinach (Table 6.8). Blackcurrants, gooseberries, raspberries and strawberries contain considerable amounts of ascorbic acid, but their season is short. Other fruits contain small amounts.

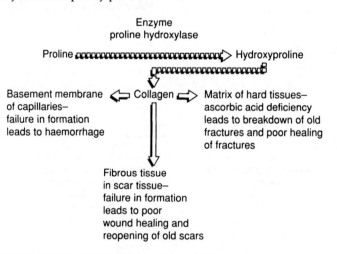

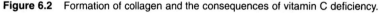

Figure 6.2 Formation of collagen and the consequences of vitamin C deficiency.

Table 6.8 Vitamin C content of food portions

Food	Vitamin C (mg)
1 large boiled potato	3.6
1 portion Brussels sprouts	54.0
1 small orange	57.0
1 tomato	14.5

Table 6.9 Reference nutrient intakes for vitamin C

Age	RNI (mg/day)
0–12 months	25
1–10 years	30
11–14 years	35
15+ years	40
Pregnant women	50
Lactating women	70

Potatoes and turnips have a comparatively small ascorbic acid content, but, as staple foods, they constitute a very important dietary source. This is especially so for people who cannot afford the more expensive fruits and vegetables, or who are living on a diet which contains very little fruit or vegetables.

Milk has a low ascorbic acid content and this is still further reduced by pasteurisation.

Conservation of ascorbic acid in foods

Storage, preparation and cooking of foods can result in much loss of ascorbic acid, because the vitamin is soluble in water and easily oxidised and so destroyed. This oxidation occurs more rapidly in the presence of alkalis, and when exposed to heat or light.

The ascorbic acid content of foods is much reduced during storage:

• New potatoes have a higher content of ascorbic acid than old ones which have been stored during the winter.
• Wilted vegetables contain less than fresh ones.
• The enzyme ascorbic acid oxidase occurs in many fruits and vegetables. It increases the rate of oxidation of ascorbic acid. This enzyme is brought into contact with the vitamin by bruising, shredding and grating. Food should be prepared and cooked carefully to minimise vitamin loss. This is discussed further in Chapter 9.

Reference nutrient intakes for vitamin C

There is considerable international variation in the RNIs for ascorbic acid. This is because they have been calculated in different ways. The UK dietary reference values for ascorbic acid (Table 6.9) have been based on the amount of the vitamin needed to prevent scurvy developing and on vitamin C turnover studies, not on the amount required for total tissue saturation.

This difference has occurred because most animals are able to synthesise ascorbic acid and so have tissues that are saturated with it. Humankind does not synthesise this vitamin, so some authorities feel that our dietary intake should be sufficient to ensure tissue saturation like other animals.

Ascorbic acid status is measured either as leukocyte vitamin C level or plasma vitamin C level. The leukocyte level parallels the level found in most tissues and organs. It is usual to accept a level of 15 $\mu g/10^8$ cells as a sign of deficiency. The plasma ascorbic acid concentration reflects recent dietary intake and a value of less than 11 $\mu mol/l$ indicates a biochemical depletion of ascorbic acid which should occur in all tissues.

Ascorbic acid and smoking Smokers have an increased requirement for vitamin C. However, increasing vitamin C intake does not eliminate the health problems caused by smoking. Smith & Hodges (1987) have proposed that the dietary intake of smokers should be increased by 80 mg/day.

Vitamin C and the elderly This important topic is discussed in Chapter 17.

Effects of deficiency

Scurvy

Scurvy is probably the most well known deficiency disease and one of the first to be scientifically proven to be caused by diet. This disease, which was common among 18th-century sailors, was shown by James Lind (1753) to be both prevented and cured by the addition of citrus fruit to the diet. This work was very important for the wellbeing of the British Navy at that time.

Prolonged deficiency of vitamin C results in scurvy. This condition is characterised by multiple haemorrhages. It is usually accompanied by:

• swollen, bleeding and inflamed gums—the gums remain unaffected if no teeth are present
• spontaneous haemorrhages under the skin, which are apparent as small red dots or patches, or as extensive areas of bruising
• haemorrhages into the joints, under periosteal membranes and into the muscles
• degenerative changes in the bones.

Anaemia is also frequently present.

In infancy, scurvy is characterised by painful, swollen joints. The limbs are tender and the child cries when being handled. Bone degeneration may give rise to deformities resembling those seen in rickets. Spontaneous haemorrhages can also occur.

Scurvy responds readily to an improved diet which contains additional ascorbic acid.

Incidence. Scurvy is known to have been the cause of disease and death for some hundreds of years. It has been of frequent occurrence in the UK and other northern European countries. Early navigators, at sea for long periods of time, lost large numbers of men through death from scurvy. Armies have suffered its effects; Florence Nightingale reported a high incidence among the British troops during the war in the Crimea.

Today scurvy is no longer encountered on this scale, but may be seen occasionally in persons eating very restricted diets, for example elderly people living alone and unable to cater adequately for themselves. Infants, especially if artificially fed, are liable to develop scurvy if they are not given a dietary source or supplement of ascorbic acid, particularly if the introduction of mixed feeding is delayed. Varying degrees of ascorbic acid deficiency have been observed in the past in people living in institutions and also those on badly planned gastric diets, which lacked fruit and vegetables.

Fain et al (1998) have identified an increased incidence of scurvy among cancer patients because of the high incidence of malnutrition caused by cachexia and poor dietary intake.

Large doses of vitamin C

As so many claims have been made for the value of increasing vitamin C intake, it is not surprising that many people take supplements, particularly during winter. Large doses are excreted via the kidneys. However, the possible risks of a very high intake include diarrhoea and increased risk of oxalate stones in the kidney. Also, because the body adapts to this high intake, a sudden return to a more 'normal' intake may result in scurvy developing.

Vitamin C and the common cold

Many people are convinced that an increased vitamin C intake improves their resistance to stress and to the common cold. Many studies have been conducted to clarify these points and they have been reviewed by Hemila (1992). This review shows that, while large doses of vitamin C decreased the duration and severity of symptoms, they did not prevent the infection.

REFERENCES

Bender D A 1987 Oestrogens and vitamin B_6: actions and interactions. World Review of Nutrition and Dietetics 51: 140–188

Bendich A, Machlin L J 1988 Safety of oral intake of vitamin E. American Journal of Clinical Nutrition 48: 612–619

Bessey O A, Adam D J D, Hansen A E 1957 Intake of vitamin B_6 and infantile convulsions: a first approximation of requirements of pyridoxine in infants. Paediatrica 20: 33–44

Canham J E, Baker E M, Harding R S, Sauberlich H E, Plough I C 1969 Dietary protein; its relationship to vitamin B_6 requirements and function. Annals of the New York Academy of Science 166: 16–29

Cockburn F, Belton N R, Purvis R J et al 1980 Maternal vitamin D intake and mineral metabolism in mothers and their newborn infants. British Medical Journal 281: 11–14

Colditz G A, Branch L G, Lipnick K J 1985 Increased green and yellow vegetable intake and lowered cancer deaths in an elderly population. American Journal of Clinical Nutrition 41: 32–36

Compston J E 1998 Vitamin D deficiency: time for action. British Medical Journal 317: 1466–1467

Dalton K, Dalton M J T 1987 Characteristics of pyridoxine overdose neuropathy syndrome. Acta Neurologica Scandanavica 76: 8–11

Department of Health (DoH) 1991a Dietary reference values for food energy and nutrients for the United Kingdom. Report of the Panel on Dietary Reference Values of the Committee on Medical Aspects of Food Policy (COMA). (Report on Health and Social Subjects 41). HMSO, London

Department of Health (DoH) 1991b The fortification of yellow fats with vitamins A and D. (Report on Health and Social Subjects 40). HMSO, London

Department of Health (DoH) 1998 Nutritional aspects of the development of cancer. Report of the Working Group on Diet and Cancer of the Committee on Medical Aspects of Food and Nutritional Policy. (Report on Health and Social Subjects 48). HMSO, London

Department of Health and Social Security (DHSS) 1988 Present day practice in infant feeding: third report. (Reports on Health and Social Subjects 32). HMSO, London

Fain O, Mathieu E, Thomas M 1998 Scurvy in patients with cancer. British Medical Journal 316: 1661–1662

Garrow J S, James W P T, Ralph A 2000 Human nutrition and dietetics, 10th Edn. Churchill Livingstone, Edinburgh

Gregory J 2000 National Diet and Nutrition Survey: young people aged 4–18 years. HMSO, London

Hemila H 1992 Vitamin C and the common cold. British Journal of Nutrition 62: 3–16

Huque T, Truswell A S 1979 Retinol contents from human livers from autopsies in London. Proceedings of the Nutrition Society 38: 41A

Hunt J R, Mullen L M, Lykken G I, Gallagher S K, Nielson F H 1990 Ascorbic acid: effect on ongoing iron absorption and status in iron-depleted young women. American Journal of Clinical Nutrition 51: 649–655

Lind J 1753 A treatise of the scurvy. Reprinted 1953: Edinburgh University Press, Edinburgh

McLaughlin M, Fairney A, Lester E, Raggatt P R, Brown D J, Wills M R 1974 Seasonal variations in serum 25-hydroxycholecalciferol in healthy people. Lancet i: 536–537

Older M J W, Dickerson J W T 1982 Thiamine and the elderly orthopaedic patient. Age and Ageing 11: 101–107

Oldham H, Sheft B B, Porter T 1950 Thiamine and riboflavin intakes and excretions during pregnancy. Journal of Nutrition 66: 173–188

Salmon J (for the Department of Health) 1991 Dietary reference values—a guide. HMSO, London

Smith J L, Hodges R E 1987 Serum levels of vitamin C in relation to dietary and supplemental intake of vitamin C in smokers and non-smokers. Annals of the New York Academy of Science 498: 144–152

Taylor T W, Rimmer S, Dais B, Butcher J, Dymock I W 1974 Ascorbic acid supplementation in the treatment of pressure sores. Lancet ii: 544–546

Train J J A, Yates R W, Sury M R J 1995 Lesson of the week: hypocalcaemic stridor and infantile nutritional rickets. British Medical Journal 310: 48–49

Truswell A S 1999 ABC of nutrition, 3rd Edn. British Medical Journal, London

World Health Organization (WHO) 1967 Requirements of vitamin A, thiamine, riboflavine and niacin. (WHO Technical Report Series 362). World Health Organization, Geneva

Wyatt K M, Dimmock P W, Jones P W, O'Brien PMS 1999 Efficacy of vitamin B_6 in the treatment of premenstrual syndrome: systematic review. British Medical Journal 318: 1371–1381

FURTHER READING

Basu T K, Dickerson J W T 1996 Vitamins in Health and Disease. CAB International, Guildford

Hughes D A 1999 Effects of carotenoids on human immune function. Proceedings of the Nutrition Society 58(3): 713–718

Semba R D 1999 Vitamin A and immunity to viral, bacterial and protozoan infections. Proceedings of the Nutrition Society 58(3): 719–727

7

Energy

LEARNING OBJECTIVES

After studying this chapter you should be able to:

- explain how energy intake and expenditure are measured
- describe the dietary reference values for energy intake
- discuss the factors which influence the energy requirement of an individual
- define basal metabolic rate.

ENERGY REQUIREMENT

Energy is required for the following processes:

1. *Growth and maintenance of body tissues.* The body requires energy for the activity which takes place in cells when tissues are formed from simpler components.
2. *Maintenance of body temperature.*
3. *Involuntary muscle movement.* Such movements as the beating of the heart, movements of the gastrointestinal tract and the movements of the muscles involved in respiration all require the expenditure of energy.
4. *Voluntary muscle movement.* Energy is needed for all voluntary activity such as the performance of work, walking and playing sport.

SOURCES OF ENERGY

Energy is obtained from the oxidation of the carbohydrates, fats, proteins and alcohol of the diet. The amount of energy resulting from the oxidation of carbohydrates, fats and proteins can be measured in the laboratory and, as a result of experiment, we know that in the body:

- 1 g carbohydrate supplies 16 kJ (4 kcal) approximately
- 1 g fat supplies 37 kJ (9 kcal) approximately
- 1 g protein supplies 17 kJ (4 kcal) approximately
- 1 g alcohol supplies 29 kJ (7 kcal) approximately.

Energy is essential to maintain life. Carbohydrate is the most efficiently metabolised source of energy. However, if there is an inadequate supply of carbohydrate, fat and protein will be metabolised. The metabolism of stored fat in adipose tissue as an energy source is the basis of weight-reducing diets. The use of body proteins as an energy source when energy requirements are particularly high, as during fever or after trauma, causes rapid weight loss and malnutrition.

The amount of carbohydrate, fat and protein used for energy production at a given time depends upon the rate at which tissue activity or metabolism is taking place, and a convenient way of measuring metabolism is to measure the energy produced as a result of the oxidation of food.

Units of energy

In the international system of units agreed in 1960, to which the UK subscribed, the calorie has been replaced by the joule. This is a unit of energy irrespective of the form in which it appears. For example it can denote heat, electrical energy, or mechanical energy. 4.184 joules (4.2 J) are equivalent to 1 calorie.

When considering comparatively small amounts of energy, as in average portions of individual foods, the kilojoule (kJ) is convenient. For larger amounts of energy, for example total daily requirement, the megajoule (MJ), which is equivalent to 1000 kJ, is preferable.

MEASUREMENT OF ENERGY CONSUMPTION

Calorimetry

The measurement of heat is known as calorimetry, and the energy production of an individual may be measured in either of two ways—direct calorimetry or indirect calorimetry.

Direct calorimetry. The person concerned is put into a specially insulated room where the heat given off by the body is collected by pipes of circulating water and is then measured. Any mechanical work performed by the person is also measured, expressed in terms of joules and added to the heat production to give the total energy expenditure. This method is very accurate, and is suitable for lengthy experiments, but the apparatus is expensive and elaborate.

Indirect calorimetry. This is a simpler method based on the fact that carbon dioxide is produced when food is oxidised. In this case the amount of oxygen taken in and the amount of carbon dioxide breathed out in a given time are measured, and from this it is possible to calculate the amount of food which has been oxidised and the amount of energy produced.

Doubly labelled water techniques

This method provides a way of measuring total energy expenditure (which includes basal metabolism, energy cost of physical activity, thermogenesis and energy cost of growth and repair of tissue) without confining individuals to a machine or laboratory or monitoring their food intake, and provides valuable additional information about energy requirements.

Technical difficulties in the procedure and assumptions that have to be made during the calculations mean that this method is not perfect. The subject drinks water labelled with the isotopes ^{2}H and ^{18}O. These isotopes distribute themselves throughout the body water, and the level in the body water is measured daily from the amount of the isotopes in a single daily sample of urine. The amount of carbon dioxide produced by an individual can be calculated from the rate of disappearance of the isotopes from the body and from this the rate of energy expenditure can be calculated.

Basal metabolism

Basal metabolism may be defined as the amount of energy required to carry out the basic processes of life such as cellular activity, heartbeat and respiration.

Measurement of basal metabolic rate (BMR)

This is measured by a form of indirect calorimetry when the person is completely at rest, comfortably warm and at least 12 hours since his or her last meal. This means that digestive and metabolic activity is reduced to the minimum and gives a way of providing standardised measurements while the energy used for digestive and metabolic functions is at the minimum. These standardised measurements have been used to compare energy consumption for different individuals in different physiological conditions and in different states of health. When related to lean body mass, figures for BMR are remarkably constant, although they differ with age and sex. Variation in the BMR occurs in certain pathological conditions and BMR determinations are sometimes of value in the diagnosis of disease.

In many situations it is easier to measure resting metabolic rate (RMR) instead of the BMR. This is measured under similar circumstances to BMR, but is measured first thing in the morning after an overnight fast and after the individual has rested for 30 minutes. This measurement, although not as good as the BMR, is still useful.

Total energy expenditure

In order to carry out the activities of everyday life such as walking, going up and down stairs, doing housework, working, or any form of activity, further energy is required in addition to that needed for basal metabolism. The total energy expenditure (TEE) for many activities has been measured by indirect calorimetry.

The uses of energy have already been discussed at the beginning of the chapter. Jequier (1984) has suggested that the normal distribution of TEE is 73% on BMR, 12% on activity and 15% on thermogenesis (see Table 7.1). However, this is not constant.

Specific dynamic action of food

Food has the effect of stimulating the metabolic rate while it is being metabolised, thus causing increased energy expenditure. This is known as the specific dynamic action of food, and varies with the type of food eaten. In a mixed diet, it amounts to an increased expenditure of energy equal to about 10% of the basal requirement. When accurate determination of energy requirement is being carried out, this must be taken into consideration.

Factors affecting energy requirement

We have already seen that basal requirement is affected by the size of the individual, that it is greater in men than in women, and that the total energy expenditure

Table 7.1 Factors affecting normal distribution of total energy requirement

% total energy expended on:	Increases with:	Decreases with:
BMR	Thyroid activity Protein synthesis Lean body mass	Age
Activity	Physical activity Occupation and hobbies	
Thermogenesis	Cold exposure Food consumption Stress	

depends upon the degree of muscular activity which is taking place. Various other factors should also be considered.

1. *Age*. In children, the BMR is higher per unit of surface area than in adults. BMR is lower in old age.

2. *Environmental temperature*. Metabolism is increased in cold climates, resulting in increased heat production which helps to maintain body temperature.

3. *Disease*. In fevers, the metabolic rate is increased by approximately 8% for every 0.5°C rise in temperature. Certain endocrine disorders affect BMR, for example hyperthyroidism raises it and hypothyroidism lowers it.

4. *Pregnancy*. BMR is increased during pregnancy and lactation.

5. *Energy intake*. In prolonged under-nutrition, the body compensates for the inadequate energy intake by a reduction in the metabolic rate.

Effect of excess energy intake

If the diet eaten by an individual supplies more energy than required, the excess food is used to make fat, which can be stored in the body in large amounts. This is the basis of the development of obesity.

DIETARY REFERENCE VALUES FOR ENERGY INTAKE

As has already been explained in Chapter 1, the reference nutrient intake (RNI) for a particular nutrient is sufficient to ensure that 97% of the population has enough, or more than enough, of that nutrient. An energy intake that exceeds energy consumption leads to the development of obesity. For this reason estimated average requirement (EAR) is used as a guide for assessing the energy requirement rather than the RNI. If the RNI were used, many people would obviously be receiving an amount of energy which exceeded their needs and so become obese, with all the associated health risks.

Estimated average requirements for energy

Children

The energy needs of children have been set by the panel to allow for growth and are therefore related to age and sex (see Appendix 3).

Adults

The EAR for adults is obtained by multiplying their BMR by a factor known as the physical activity level (PAL). The PAL ranges from 1.4–1.9 and takes into account lifestyle as well as occupation. Table 7.2 shows the physical activity levels for adults.

Table 7.2 Summary of physical activity levels (PAL) of adults (from DoH 1991, with permission)

PAL	Activity level
1.4	Very little physical activity during leisure time or at work This factor is the one that should be used for most people in the UK
Women 1.6 Men 1.7	Moderate levels of physical activity during leisure time and at work
Women 1.7 Men 1.9	High levels of physical activity during leisure time and at work

Table 7.3 Additional estimated average requirements for energy for lactating women (from Salmon 1991, with permission of HMSO)

Stage of breast-feeding	Additional EAR (MJ/day)	kcal/day
Up to 1 month	450 (1.9)	
1–2 months	530 (2.2)	
2–3 months	570 (2.4)	
	Group 1	Group 2
3–6 months	480 (2.0)	570 (2.4)
More than 6 months	240 (1.0)	550 (2.3)

Group 1 mothers: those whose breast-milk supplies all or most of the infant's food, for the first 3 months
Group 2 mothers: those whose breast-milk supplies all of the infant's energy and nutrient needs for 6 months or more

Table 7.4 Energy contents of some foods that are high in fat

Food	% fat	kcal/100 g
Cheddar cheese	33.5	406
Butter	82	740
Pastry	32.2	527

Table 7.5 Energy contents of some foods that are high in water

Food	% fat	% water	kcal/100 g
Apple	0	84.3	46
Orange	0	86	35

Pregnant and lactating women

During a normal pregnancy, as well as the formation of the foetus, placenta and increased mass of the uterus, an adipose tissue store of 2–2.4 kg is deposited to be used as a source of energy during lactation. The COMA panel recommend that the EAR should be increased by 200 kcal/day for women during the last trimester of pregnancy. The EAR does not increase before this because of their reduction in activity. However, this is not appropriate for women who do not reduce their activity or were underweight at the start of pregnancy; they will require extra energy during the earlier months.

The increased energy requirement during lactation depends on how long the baby is breast-fed and how soon weaning is introduced. The figures in Table 7.3 show the additional estimated average requirements for breast-feeding mothers.

Elderly people

Many people increase their activity levels after retirement (Patrick et al 1986). However, once they reach the age of 75, they are likely to reduce their physical activity. The BMR also declines with age. This is due to a decline in the amount of lean tissue and also the increased energy cost of physical activity, which occurs because of the reduced efficiency of movement (Bassey & Terry 1986). When considering these points, the panel has decided that the EARs for those aged 60 years and over should be calculated from their BMR and a PAL of 1.5. These values are in Appendix 4.

Energy balance is addressed in Chapter 21.

DIETARY SOURCES OF ENERGY

All foods provide the diet with some energy. The actual energy content depends on how much fat, protein, carbohydrate, water and alcohol the food contains (see p. 60); water provides no energy.

As a general rule, those foods with a high fat content have a high energy content (see examples in Table 7.4).

Conversely, those with a high water content, such as fruit, have a low energy content (see examples in Table 7.5).

When assessing the nutritional importance of a food, it is not only the energy that it provides that should be considered, but also its contribution to the overall nutritional status (i.e. its vitamin content) and its place in a healthy diet, (i.e. its fat content). These topics have been discussed in previous chapters and will be discussed further in Chapter 14.

Energy value of a diet

This can be calculated either by weighing and recording everything an individual eats or by asking an individual to recall what he or she ate in a preceding period. For further information see Chapter 10. However, these methods are not always reliable, particularly the recall method (Bingham 1987). For more information on the validation of dietary assessment see Nelson (1997).

REFERENCES

Bassey E J, Terry A M 1986 The oxygen cost of walking in the elderly. Journal of Physiology 373: 42P

Bingham S 1987 The dietary assessment of individuals; methods, accuracy, new techniques and recommendations. Nutrition Abstracts Review 57: 705–742

Department of Health (DoH) 1991 Dietary reference values for food energy and nutrients for the United Kingdom. Report of the Panel on Dietary Reference Values of the Committee on Medical Aspects of Food Policy (COMA). (Report on Health and Social Subjects 41). HMSO, London

Jequier E 1984 Energy expenditure in obesity clinics. Endocrinology and Metabolism 13: 563–577

Nelson M 1987 The validation of dietary assessment. In: Margetts BM, Nelson M. Design concepts in nutritional epidemiology. Oxford University Press, Oxford

Patrick J M, Bassey E J, Irving J M, Blecher A, Fentem P H 1986 Objective measurements of customary physical activity in elderly men and women before and after retirement. Quarterly Journal of Experimental Physiology 71: 47–58

Salmon J (for the Department of Health) 1991 Dietary reference values—a guide. HMSO, London

FURTHER READING

Paul A A, Black A E, Evans J, Cole T J, Whitehead R G 1988 Breast-milk intake and growth in infants from 2 to 10 months. Journal of Human Nutrition and Dietetics 1: 437–450

Prentice A M, Prentice A 1988 Energy costs of lactation. Annual Review of Nutrition 8: 63–79

8

Non-starch polysaccharides (dietary fibre)

LEARNING OBJECTIVES

After studying this chapter you should have a clearer understanding of:

- the different types of non-starch polysaccharides (NSP)
- the role of NSP in maintaining health
- the links between NSP intake and cardiovascular disease, cancer, diabetes and diseases of the gastrointestinal tract
- the possible adverse effects of a high NSP intake.

> Soon none but the poor and ignorant will use white bread; brown bread is not a luxury but a necessity for every family.

This statement was published in a pamphlet which was widely circulated by Thomas Allinson. It was part of his campaign to persuade the Victorians to adopt a healthier way of life. His campaign was successful in some circles. In 1847, Queen Victoria responded to it by changing to wholemeal bread and encouraged her Court to do the same. In spite of this auspicious start, the presence of fibre in foods and the importance of fibre in the diet was ignored for the next century. During that period, the terms roughage and fibre were assumed to be synonymous. Fibre was considered to be usefully included in the diet only as a treatment for constipation. The ideal diet was supposed to be one which contained highly refined foods and was completely digested. It was only the robust whose digestive tract could survive the onslaught of roughage!

In the last 30 years, clinical scientists have shown that non-starch polysaccharides, NSP (fibre), are an essential component of a well-balanced diet. They have many functions and not all of them are completely understood. The term 'NSP' has replaced the term 'dietary fibre'.

CHEMICAL COMPOSITION OF NSP

A wide variety of non-starch polysaccharides are found in the plant kingdom. NSP of many different types and in differing amounts are found in all plant structures. They are in the cell walls and within the cells of roots, leaves, stems, seeds and fruits.

NSP can be divided into two types: water-soluble NSP and insoluble NSP. Cellulose is insoluble, whereas the other types of NSP are soluble or partly soluble.

Insoluble NSP

Cellulose is a glucose polysaccharide and is the most common type of NSP; the long tough fibrous strands give plants their form and rigidity. Leafy vegetables are a rich source of cellulose, as are pulses and rhubarb.

Lignin is the type of NSP that gives wood its characteristic form, structure and strength. The amount of lignin in a tree varies between 10% and 50%, depending on the species and maturity of the tree. It is unimportant in the human diet.

Soluble NSP

Pectins, plant gums and mucilages have a similar composition to cellulose but contain other sugars. They are all non-cellulose polysaccharides but have different functions in plants.

Pectins are complex mixtures of polysaccharides which combine with water to form a gel. It is their presence in fruit that enables fruits to hold so much water, e.g. an orange is 85% water. Fruit and vegetables are good sources of pectins.

Plant gums are produced by plants to cover and protect the site of an injury, e.g. the gum on a fir tree. The most common dietary plant gum is gum arabic, which is used as a food additive.

Mucilages are found mixed with the endosperm in the seeds of some plants. The mucilages are able to hold water, which prevents seeds from drying out while dormant.

ANALYSIS OF NSP IN FOOD

The NSP removed from cereals during milling has been used as animal feed for hundreds of years. The first method of analysis of dietary fibre was used to check that sawdust had not been added to animal feed. The value for NSP content obtained by the old chemical analytical methods was called the crude fibre con-

tent. This term was used because it became known that, during analysis, a lot of pectin, gums and mucilages and some of the cellulose were destroyed, leaving mainly lignin to be measured. This explains why recent food tables show the dietary fibre content of the western diet to be three times the previously measured (crude fibre) value.

Definition of NSP. The term dietary fibre was used to describe plant material that is not digested by the enzymes of the human digestive tract. However, this term was an imprecise guide, because the dietary fibre left undigested varied with analytical methods and individuals. The COMA report (DoH 1991) recommended that to avoid confusion the term 'NSP' should be used and the technique used to measure them should be that of Englyst & Cummings (1988) or a comparable method.

Roughage is an old-fashioned term which does not describe NSP adequately and should not be used. It suggests that NSP is an inert substance whose only function is to provide the gastrointestinal tract with a harsh, scratchy, bulking agent. This is not so; NSP is a complex mixture of substances which have a wide range of effects on the gastrointestinal tract. Most of the NSP is removed from a carbohydrate food when it is refined.

EFFECTS OF NSP (Fig. 8.1)

Mouth. Unrefined foods are coarse and bulky, so they need to be chewed for longer than refined foods. The extra chewing stimulates increased salivation. Both the increased chewing and the salivation help to keep the teeth and gums healthy and may also contribute to an increased feeling of satiety.

Stomach. In general, unrefined foods stay in the stomach for longer than the refined forms of the same foods. This slowing of gastric emptying means that people feel fuller after a meal and so eat slightly less. It also means that food enters the small intestine more slowly, so digestion and absorption by the small intestine is slowed down.

Small intestine. Different types of NSP have different effects on the function of the small intestine. The types of NSP whose actions are best understood are the pectins, gums and mucilages. They increase the viscosity of the small intestine contents and slow the rate of absorption of the products of digestion. Though absorption is complete, it continues further down the small intestine than when NSP is absent (Holt et al 1979).

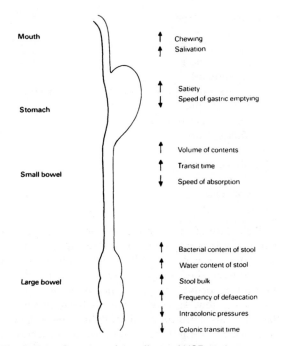

Mouth	↑ Chewing
	↑ Salivation
	↑ Satiety
Stomach	↓ Speed of gastric emptying
	↑ Volume of contents
	↑ Transit time
Small bowel	↓ Speed of absorption
	↑ Bacterial content of stool
	↑ Water content of stool
Large bowel	↑ Stool bulk
	↑ Frequency of defaecation
	↓ Intracolonic pressures
	↓ Colonic transit time

Figure 8.1 Summary of the effects of NSP on the gastrointestinal tract.

Small intestine transit time is altered by most types of NSP, though whether it increases or decreases depends largely on the type of NSP. All, except the particulate forms of NSP such as bran, slow small intestinal transit.

Large intestine. It is here that NSP has important and undisputed effects. Stephens & Cummings (1980) showed that an increase in NSP intake led to an

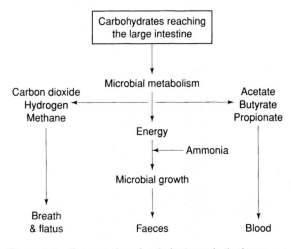

Figure 8.2 Fermentation of carbohydrates in the large intestine (Garrow et al 2000).

increase in faecal mass. Although NSP is not broken down by the enzymes and secretions of the small intestine, little is excreted in the faeces unchanged. Most is fermented by bacteria in the caecum and colon. The products of bacterial degradation are the gases carbon dioxide, hydrogen and methane and the short-chain fatty acids acetate, butyrate and propionate (Fig. 8.2). These and the water-holding property of the remaining fragments together result in a bulkier stool.

The consequences of a soft bulky stool are:

- reduced colonic transit time
- lower intracolonic pressures
- increased frequency of defaecation.

This is why increasing the NSP content of the diet prevents constipation.

NSP IN THE DIET

The NSP content of a diet depends on the amount and type of plant material eaten.

The average intake of NSP in the UK for adults is 11.2 g/day for men and 12.5 g/day for women (Bingham et al 1990); about 50% of this is from vegetable sources and 40% from cereals. There is a wide variation. Intakes as high as 25 g/day and as low as 5 g/day were recorded in this study. Vegetarians, who have a high intake of fruit and vegetables and usually eat wholegrain cereals, have an average intake of 30 g/day.

The type of NSP, as well as the amount eaten, changes with changes in the agriculature and affluence of the population. In the UK the amount of NSP from cereal sources in the diet has halved in the last 100 years. This has not been accompanied by a halving in total NSP intake, as more fruit and vegetables are now eaten. The NSP content of a selection of foods is listed in Table 8.1.

Wheat bran

The most commonly known form of NSP is wheat bran, illustrated in Figure 8.3. It is available from

Table 8.1 NSP content of a selection of food portions (Holland et al 1991)

Food portion	NSP (g)
1 thick slice white bread	0.6
1 thick slice wholemeal bread	2.6
2 Weetabix	3.9
1 medium portion branflakes	5.2
1 small orange	1.8
1 medium portion baked beans	5.0

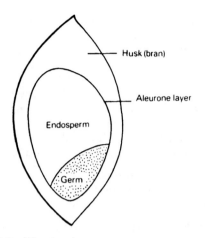

Figure 8.3 Wheat grain.

chemists, grocers and health food shops. Many claims about the beneficial effects of bran have been made. Not all of them are true. It is far better to treat constipation with a diet high in NSP-rich foods and unrefined cereals rather than to add bran to foods.

During the milling process, 11–16% of the wheat grain is removed as bran. As well as the outer husk of the grain, the aleurone layer and wheatgerm are removed. The flour produced in this way has a whiter appearance and keeps for longer, but is without its fibre and most of its B vitamins, which are present in the wheatgerm and aleurone layer.

During the Second World War, there was a shortage of wheat in the UK and less bran was removed from wheat during the production of flour. This meant that more flour could be produced from the same amount of wheat. The use of this high-fibre flour by the entire population almost doubled the intake of NSP.

THE FIBRE HYPOTHESIS

This was formulated in the 1970s by Burkitt & Trowell (Burkitt 1969). Both of these men were doctors who had been working in East Africa for over 20 years. They observed that many of the degenerative diseases which were common in the UK were rare in Africa. They also noted that the rural Africans passed frequent bulky stools. In their hypothesis they related both of these observations to the type of diet eaten by the rural Africans and proposed, 'that dietary fibre protects against a wide range of diseases'. The diseases which they suggested, on epidemiological evidence, were related to a low dietary fibre (NSP) intake are listed below. The list is divided into three groups:

- Colonic disorders:
  — constipation
  — diverticular disease
  — colonic cancer
  — appendicitis
- Disorders which are secondary to colonic disorders:
  — hiatus hernia
  — deep venous thrombosis
  — atherosclerosis
  — pulmonary embolism
- Metabolic disorders:
  — obesity
  — diabetes
  — gallstones.

As these diseases are chronic and slow to develop, it is impossible to prove that their development is due to a diet deficient in NSP alone. Epidemiological studies have shown that in areas where there is a high intake of NSP, the incidence of some of these diseases is low. However, it must be remembered that there are a multitude of differences between the lifestyles of a rural African and a western executive, and that NSP intake is only one of them. The considerable differences between the traditional diet of the rural African and that eaten in a developed country are summarised in Figure 8.4. The NSP intake of the rural African was five to six times that of the western businessman.

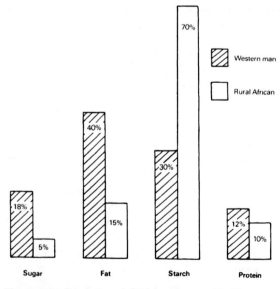

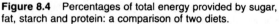

Figure 8.4 Percentages of total energy provided by sugar, fat, starch and protein: a comparison of two diets.

NSP AND DISEASE

Colonic disorders

Constipation. No-one disputes the necessity of an adequate intake of NSP for normal colonic function and the prevention of constipation. The effectiveness of different foods in increasing faecal weight and bulk depends on the type and amount of fibre they contain. For example, 50 g of wheat bran, which contains 44% NSP and 8% water, will double faecal weight, while 1550 g of eating apples, which contain 2% NSP and 84% water, are needed to have the same effect. The use of wheat bran for the treatment of constipation is discussed in Chapter 24, 'Diet in Disorders of the Gastrointestinal Tract'. A WHO (1990) report identified the importance of NSP in the prevention of constipation.

Diverticular disease. It has been suggested that diverticula form as a result of the high intracolonic pressures which occur in response to the constipation caused by diets low in NSP. Diets with a high NSP content are used successfully to treat diverticular disease. This was first reported by Painter (1971). The increased faecal volume and softer stool consistency lowers intracolonic pressures, giving symptomatic relief and reducing the frequency of episodes of diverticular inflammation (diverticulitis). Lower intracolonic pressures also probably reduce the tendency to form more diverticula.

Colonic cancer. Epidemiological evidence links the intake of NSP with the incidence of colonic cancer and it has been suggested that a NSP-rich diet may be protective against colonic cancer. The proposed mechanisms are:

- NSP binds potential carcinogens and removes them from the colon.
- The increased faecal bulk dilutes the concentration of carcinogens present.
- The reduced transit time reduces the length of time that the colon is exposed to carcinogens.

However, diets that are low in fat and sugar and diets that are high in NSP also contain more fruit and vegetables, so the link between colon cancer and NSP is still not established.

Secondary disorders

Cardiovascular disease. The link between heart disease and NSP intake is still unclear. The addition of some types of NSP, but not all types, will alter lipid metabolism and there is a lower incidence of coronary heart disease among rural African populations. This has been reviewed by Anderson et al (1990).

Hiatus hernia, haemorrhoids and varicose veins. The high intra-abdominal pressures which develop during straining to evacuate constipated stools may contribute to the development of these disorders. A high-NSP diet resulting in softer stools reduces straining and thus problems associated with these conditions. These disorders may also develop less commonly in those on a high-NSP diet.

Metabolic disorders

Obesity. During the last 40 years the amount of body fat in the adult population of the UK has increased by 10%. Many changes in lifestyle have occurred, all of which contribute to this increase. The increased consumption of fat and sugar is a more important cause of obesity than the decrease in NSP consumption. Many claims have been made about the value of dietary NSP as an aid to weight-reduction. The addition of extra NSP to the diet increases the amount of energy, or dietary calories, excreted in the faeces. This loss is only slight and of negligible value to slimmers.

The inclusion of unrefined foods in a calorie-controlled diet has two advantages:

- they are tough and bulky so they take longer to eat
- as the food stays in the stomach longer, it prolongs the feeling of fullness after a meal.

Table 8.2 shows the different times taken to eat apples in three different forms. The use of refined NSP products such as guar gum as slimming aids has been proposed, but although overall energy intake may be reduced initially, adaptation occurs and the energy intake returns to the original level.

Diabetes mellitus. In regions where the diet is based on unrefined starchy foods, the incidence of this disease is low. When people migrate from these regions to areas where the diet is rich in refined sugary foods, the incidence of diabetes increases, particularly the non-insulin-dependent type (Type 2), along with the incidence of obesity and dental caries.

The effect of NSP on slowing absorption has already been mentioned. Those which have the greatest influence on carbohydrate absorption are the viscous types (Jenkins et al 1981). These occur naturally in legumes.

Table 8.2 The times taken to eat six apples in three different forms

Form	Time in minutes
Whole apples	17
Apple puree	6
Apple juice	2

Diets containing large amounts of legumes and diets containing the viscous type of NSP, guar gum, have been used to treat diabetes by slowing carbohydrate absorption, with varying degrees of success. Interest in this was stimulated by the study of Goulder et al (1978) which showed the effect of adding NSP to the meals of diabetics on their rise in blood glucose levels. The role of NSP in the treatment of diabetes is discussed in Chapter 27.

Gallstones. Some NSP binds bile acids. This means that the bile acids are excreted with the NSP in the stool instead of being reabsorbed and recirculated in the enterohepatic circulation. By preventing the bile from becoming supersaturated, this may prevent the formation of gallstones.

The disadvantages of NSP in the diet

Mineral deficiencies. The minerals calcium, magnesium, zinc, phosphorus and iron in the diet become partly bound to NSP. Since the diet normally contains these minerals in excess, the body is able to adapt, by absorbing more. Deficiency of these minerals will occur if the dietary intake is limited and nutritional status and body stores are already poor. For example, the addition of bran to the diets of some elderly people may precipitate osteomalacia in those with a low calcium and vitamin D intake, particularly if they are housebound.

Insufficient energy intake. NSP-rich foods are bulky and take longer to eat than more refined foods. Children and those with poor appetites may not fulfil their dietary energy requirements if they have a large NSP intake.

Wind (flatulence). Most people experience the symptoms of abdominal distention, discomfort and wind after increasing their intake of NSP. This is due to the production of gas in the caecum and colon. Bacterial enzymes metabolise the NSP in the caecum and colon and produce the gases methane, hydrogen and carbon dioxide. The amount of gas produced depends on the type of NSP eaten and the bacterial flora present. The NSP and unabsorbable sugars found in peas and beans, for example, cause more wind than does wheat bran. The large bowel and its bacteria gradually adapt to the increased dietary intake and the problem of wind usually lessens, but never disappears.

DIETARY REFERENCE VALUES FOR NSP

The COMA panel (DoH 1991) proposed an average adult NSP intake of 18 g/day and that the intake should not exceed 32 g/day. They recommend that the intake for children should be proportionately lower.

REFERENCES

Anderson J W, Deakins D A, Bridges S R 1990 Soluble fibre; hypocholesterolemic effects and proposed mechanisms. In: Kritchevsky D et al (eds) Dietary fiber—chemistry, physiology and health effects. Plenum Press, New York: pp 339–347

Bingham S A, Pett S, Day K C 1990 Non-starch polysaccharide intake of a representative sample of British adults. Journal of Human Nutrition and Dietetics 3: 333–337

Burkitt D P 1969 Related disease—related cause. Lancet 2: 1229–1231 Department of Health (DoH) 1991 Dietary reference values for food energy and nutrients for the United Kingdom. Report of the Panel on Dietary Reference Values of the Committee on Medical Aspects of Food Policy (COMA). (Report on Health and Social Subjects 41), HMSO, London

Englyst H N, Cummings J H 1988 An improved method for the measurement of dietary fiber as non-starch polysaccharides in plant foods. Journal of the Association of Analytical Chemistry 71: 808–814

Garrow J S, James W P T, Ralph A 2000 Human nutrition and dietetics, 10th Edn. Churchill Livingstone, Edinburgh

Goulder T J, Alberti K G, Jenkins D J A 1978 Effect of added fibre on the glucose and metabolic response to mixed meals in normal and diabetic subjects. Diabetes Care 1: 351–355

Holland B, Welch A A, Unwin I D, Buss D H, Paul A A, Southgate D A T 1991 McCance and Widdowson's composition of foods, 5th Edn. Royal Society of Chemistry, Cambridge

Holt S, Heading R C, Carter D C, Prescott L F, Hothill P 1979 Effect of gel fibre on gastric emptying and absorption of glucose and paracetamol. Lancet 2: 636–639

Jenkins D J A, Wolever T M S, Taylor R H 1981 Dietary fibre, fibre analogues and glucose transport: importance of viscosity. American Journal of Clinical Nutrition 34: 362–366

Painter N S 1971 Treatment of diverticular disease. British Medical Journal 2: 156

Stephens A M, Cummings J H 1980 Mechanism of action of dietary fibre in the human colon. Nature 284: 283–284

World Health Organization 1990 Diet, nutrition, and the prevention of chronic diseases. Report of a WHO Study Group. (WHO Technical Report Series 797). World Health Organization, Geneva

9

An introduction to food science

LEARNING OBJECTIVES

After studying this chapter you should have a clearer understanding of:

- the chemical composition and structure of foods
- the commonly used methods of food preparation and preservation
- the use of food additives
- food labelling.

People do not eat nutrients, they eat food. In order to have a good understanding of the influence of diet on health and what the components of a healthy diet are, it is necessary to have some understanding of food science. This is particularly important in a time when our eating habits are changing and many new foods are on the market. This chapter outlines the nutrients present in particular groups of food and explains how some foods are processed to make commonly eaten foods, such as cheese.

Cooking foods often makes them more appetising and palatable, and easier and safer to eat. For example, raw meat looks unattractive, is unpalatable and difficult to chew, but when it is properly cooked all these properties are changed. In an instance such as this, cooking is beneficial. However, the reverse of this is poor cooking, which can make food unappetising, at worst inedible, and destroy many valuable nutrients.

Nutrient values are frequently reduced by poor cooking methods. This is particularly the case with vegetables and fruit, the chief nutrient to suffer in this way being vitamin C. For example, it was shown in a study on the nutrient content of meals for the elderly that up to 90% of the vitamin C content of a 'meal on wheels' could be destroyed before it was eaten. This was in part due to cooking but also due to the period of time that the meal was kept warm (Stanton 1971).

CEREALS

Most cultures have a cereal as the staple food of their diet, to which small amounts of other foods are added. Cereals such as wheat, oats, rice, rye, barley, millet, sorghum and maize are important sources of the nutrients listed in Box 9.1.

Flour and bread

Extraction rate

The staple cereal food of western people is wheat, which is converted to flour by milling. Extraction rate is the term used to indicate the proportion of the wheat grain which is retained in the flour.

In the case of flour made from the whole of the wheat grain, the extraction rate is 100%. In the preparation of flours of lower extraction rates, varying amounts of the outer layers of the grain and the germ or embryo are excluded. These parts between them contain some of the most valuable nutrients in the grain, including most of the thiamin and iron (found principally in the germ), most of the nicotinic acid and phosphorus (mainly found in the outer layers) and protein of relatively high biological value. The outer layers also contain most of the non-starch polysaccharide (NSP), and a pigment which is responsible for the colour of higher-extraction flours. The removal of this pigment results in the production of a white flour.

It will be seen, then, that the lower the extraction rate, the whiter the flour will be, but the less it will contain of certain important nutrients, notably thiamin, nicotinic acid, iron and NSP. The extraction rates for flours are given in Table 9.1.

The term 'wheatmeal' is sometimes used for brown flour.

Table 9.1 Extraction rates for flours

Type of flour	Extraction rate
White flour	60–70%
Brown flour	85–95%
Wholemeal flour	100%

Fortification of flour

Since the Second World War, the nutritive value of flour has been to a certain extent safeguarded by legislation. The Bread and Flour Regulations 1963, at present in force, provide that all flour sold for human consumption in the UK shall contain not less than certain specified minimum amounts of thiamin, nicotinic acid and iron. Thus the lower-extraction flours are fortified with these nutrients. The Regulations also provide for the addition of calcium to all flours other than those derived from the whole of the products of the milling of the wheat (i.e. wholemeal flour).

When comparison is made between flours of varying extraction rates, it must be remembered that the higher-extraction flours contain more phytic acid than white flour, and that phytic acid combines with minerals such as iron and calcium to form insoluble salts which are not readily available to the body. On the other hand, high-extraction flours contain most of the NSP, and are better sources of vitamins than white flour, even when the latter is fortified to the required level.

Much of the iron, B vitamins and calcium in flour and its products are the result of fortification.

Bread is a valuable source of the various important nutrients present in flour and contributes 12% of the energy content of the average UK diet. In the preparation of biscuits, scones, cakes and puddings, the nutritive value is modified by the inclusion of ingredients such as eggs, fat, milk, sugar and fruit.

Effect of cooking on cereals

Cereals are usually milled to a flour, which is then either baked into a type of bread or cooked into a porridge, depending on the type of cereal and availability of fuel.

Raw starch is insoluble in cold water, but when it is heated in water, as when cornflour is used for thickening sauces and milk puddings, the starch granules swell and absorb water, and gelatinisation occurs.

When water is added to wheat flour, for the making of bread, the proteins glutenin and gliadin present in the flour combine to form gluten. This makes the

---

Box 9.1 Nutrients obtained from cereals

- Carbohydrate in the form of starch
- NSP
- Minerals, especially iron and phosphorus
- Vitamins of the B complex, especially thiamin and nicotinic acid
- Vitamin E
- Protein—this is present in a relatively small amount when compared with high-protein foods such as meat. However, because of the quantity eaten, bread and other cereal products make a significant contribution to protein intake.

These nutrients are not uniformly distributed throughout the grain, and the nutritive value of the cereal depends upon the degree of refinement which has taken place during milling.

dough elastic and enables it to increase in size. The expansion of the gluten is brought about by incorporating a raising agent. One commonly employed is yeast, the growth of which in the dough results in the production of carbon dioxide gas.

Chemical raising agents are also used. These consist of bicarbonate of soda in conjunction with an acid, such as cream of tartar or sour milk. Chemical agents also give rise to the production of carbon dioxide in the dough. Air, incorporated during the preparation of the mixture, also acts as a raising agent, as does steam which is produced in the mixture during baking. The air, carbon dioxide or steam, or a combination of these, bring about expansion of the gluten, which is fixed by heat in this expanded position. Partial gelatinisation of the starch also occurs.

Dry heat converts starch to dextrins, which are intermediate products in the breakdown of the complex starch molecule to glucose and are slightly sweet; some caramel is also formed. These changes take place when bread is toasted and in the crust of bread during baking, the brown appearance being due to the caramel.

During the baking of bread, some loss of thiamin occurs and a further loss results from the use of chemical raising agents. The toasting of bread causes considerable loss of thiamin.

DAIRY PRODUCTS

Milk

Milk for human consumption is obtained from a variety of animals, for example the cow, goat, reindeer, ewe and mare. Custom varies in different parts of the world, depending upon which animal is most readily available. All types of milk resemble one another in composition, but the constituents are present in varying proportions, depending upon the species from which the milk has been obtained. Thus cow's milk contains a higher proportion of protein than mare's milk. Cow's milk will be considered here as it is the most frequently used (Box 9.2). All types of milk contain lactose as the carbohydrate source.

Although of high nutritive value, milk is not the perfect food, as is sometimes supposed. Certain nutrients are poorly represented, notably iron, ascorbic acid and vitamin D—this is of particular importance during the weaning period (see Chapter 15).

Milk can be served in many different ways, requires the minimum of preparation, and is inexpensive when compared with other foods of comparable nutritive

---

> **Box 9.2** Nutrients obtained from cow's milk
>
> Milk is one of the most nutritious of foods. The most important constituents are:
>
> - *proteins*, principally casein and lactalbumin; milk proteins supply the essential amino acids in especially good proportions for tissue building
> - *carbohydrate*, in the form of lactose
> - *fat* in a finely emulsified form
> - *calcium* and *phosphorus*, in readily absorbable forms
> - *vitamin A*, in largest amount when the cow is eating green fodder high in β-carotene
> - *vitamins of the B complex*, especially riboflavin.

value. These considerations, along with the high biological value of its proteins, make it of particular value when a high-protein diet is required. 250 ml of semi-skimmed milk contains approximately:

- 8 g protein
- 3 g fat
- 12 g carbohydrate
- 300 mg calcium.

Skimmed milk is similar to whole milk in its content of carbohydrate, protein, minerals and water-soluble vitamins, but is of course lacking in fat and fat-soluble vitamins as these are removed with the cream. Because of its lower fat content, skimmed milk has a lower energy content than whole milk.

Some skimmed milk products are fortified with vitamins A and D.

Semi-skimmed milk

Only half of the fat has been removed in its preparation, so semi-skimmed milk has a fat and energy content which is lower than whole milk, but higher than skimmed milk.

Changing from ordinary pasteurised milk to semi-skimmed or skimmed milk is a good way of reducing the daily fat intake. Skimmed milk should not be used for children under 5 (see Chapter 15).

Dried milk

Dried milk is prepared by passing the milk in a film between heated rollers, or by spraying it through a fine nozzle into a heated drying chamber.

Dried milk, when reconstituted, is similar to fresh milk in nutritive value. There is some loss of thiamin and ascorbic acid. These losses, however, are not nutritionally significant.

Dried skimmed milk. When reconstituted, this has a similar nutritional content to fresh skimmed milk. Exceptions to this are those dried skimmed milks with added vegetable fat. The fat added is not always polyunsaturated. These milks have the advantage of being easy to reconstitute but are neither low in fat nor low in saturated fat.

Condensed and evaporated milks

In the preparation of condensed milk, the milk is pasteurised, sugar is added and a proportion of the water is removed by evaporation. Unsweetened condensed milk is also obtainable and is usually referred to as evaporated milk. The sweetened product owes its preservation to condensation and to the high sugar content, which inhibits bacterial growth. The preservation of the unsweetened condensed milk depends upon its having been sterilised after the sealing of the can.

Condensed milk, like the dried product, shows some loss of thiamin and ascorbic acid. These losses, however, do not significantly affect the nutritional value of the total diet, as these vitamins are readily available from other dietary sources.

Cream

In the preparation of cream, the fat is removed from milk either by a mechanical separator or by skimming by hand after the cream or fat-containing portion has risen to the surface. The residue is known as skimmed milk or separated milk. Cream has a high saturated fat content and is of value principally as a source of energy.

Milk products

Butter and buttermilk

In the preparation of butter, cream is subjected to continuous agitation known as churning. During this process the particles of fat come together to form butter.

Traditionally, butter was prepared from milk which had first been scoured, the liquid remaining after removal of the fat being known as buttermilk. At the present time, butter is prepared from fresh cream. Buttermilk available commercially has been made by adding to skimmed milk a culture of organisms which ferment lactose, resulting in lactic acid formation and imparting a characteristic sour flavour.

Butter has a high content of vitamin A, varying with the diet of the cow. The vitamin D content is moderate or low, being greater in summer than in winter.

Buttermilk is similar to skimmed milk in nutritive value.

Yoghurt

Yoghurt is made by adding to milk a specially prepared culture of bacteria which ferment the lactose, giving rise to the production of lactic acid. Clotting takes place when a certain degree of acidity is reached. Flavour and nutritional content are sometimes modified by the addition of such items as sugar, flavouring and fruit.

In general, the nutritional content of yoghurt is similar to that of the milk from which it was made, milk being the basic constituent, but the information given on the container should be consulted in each case for details of additional ingredients, as there may be a high sugar content. Fromage frais is similar in nutritional value to yoghurts but has a different physical texture, being more like cream.

Probiotic Yoghurts

These are yoghurts which contain large numbers of live non-toxic and non-pathogenic microorganisms which survive in the gastrointestinal tract. By altering the composition of the intestinal microflora it is suggested that these foods have a range of health benefits, which include the alleviation of lactose intolerance symptoms, prevention and treatment of rotavirus diarrhoea and enhancement of the immune system (Salminen et al 1998).

Cheese

In the preparation of cheese, milk is treated with rennet, an enzyme which brings about clotting of the milk. The clot is then broken up and separated into the liquid part (the whey) and the solid part (the curd). Cheese is formed when the curd, which has been salted, is compressed and left for a period of time to ripen.

During the ripening process, chemical changes take place which modify the flavour of the cheese. In the preparation of most cheese, the milk undergoes a preliminary ripening before the addition of the rennet. This is usually effected by adding a bacterial starter, consisting of a culture of organisms which ferment lactose to produce lactic acid. A distinctive flavour can be imparted to a cheese by encouraging the penetration of specific moulds, as is done in the case of Stilton, Danish Blue and Gorgonzola.

Most cheeses are excellent sources of protein, fat, calcium, phosphorus and vitamin A. Some riboflavin is also present. When cheese is prepared from skimmed milk, the fat and vitamin A contents are much reduced. When including cheese in any diet, it is important to remember the high saturated fat and high calorie content.

Cottage cheese is prepared from skimmed milk. Some fat may be added to improve the texture. Fat content, however, is low, but will depend on how much fat has been added.

Ice-cream

Ice-cream is a frozen dessert consisting largely of milk or dried milk powder with the addition of sugar, flavourings and often vegetable oil. When the fat of ice-cream consists solely of butter fat, the product is referred to as 'dairy ice-cream'.

MARGARINE, COOKING FATS AND OILS

Margarine and cooking fats are prepared by the hydrogenation of vegetable oils, such as palm and maize oils (see Chapter 3). Fish oils and other animal fats such as lard are occasionally used. Not all margarines are low in cholesterol and high in polyunsaturated fats. Those margarines manufactured from a polyunsaturated vegetable oil are labelled 'high in polyunsaturates'.

The flavour of margarine is mainly determined by the addition of milk which has been cultured with selected organisms.

By law, margarine intended for the retail trade is fortified with vitamins A and D, and is similar to butter in vitamin A content. It is a better source than butter of vitamin D and for this reason the housebound should be encouraged to use margarine instead of butter.

Margarines which have been enriched with plant sterols are now manufactured. Including these margarines in the diet can contribute to the lowering of blood cholesterol levels (Hendriks et al 1999).

Margarine, cooking fats, cooking oils, and butter are similar in fat content and energy value. The ratio of polyunsaturated:saturated fat content of vegetable oils varies with the vegetable type. Low-fat spreads contain less fat than margarine or butter and have a lower energy content, and so can be useful as part of a reducing diet.

Fats slow the rate of gastric emptying—this can contribute to the feelings of nausea and fullness experienced in some disorders of the gastrointestinal tract. Fried foods always retain some of the cooking fat and so have a high energy content and should be discouraged wherever possible.

EGGS

Eggs have a high nutritive value. They are of particular importance as a source of iron, and protein of high biological value. They contain considerable amounts of fat, calcium, phosphorus, vitamins A and D, thiamin and riboflavin. Most of these nutrients are present either wholly or principally in the yolk, the white contributing mainly protein and riboflavin. The protein of egg white is egg albumin, and the principal protein of the yolk is vitellin. Of all the dietary proteins, those found in eggs have the highest biological value. Egg yolk is a rich source of cholesterol, each yolk containing approximately 250 mg.

Egg white coagulates at a temperature below boiling point and becomes toughened as the temperature increases. Raw eggs should not be eaten because they are frequently microbiologically contaminated—the yolks should always be thoroughly cooked, so that they are hard, before they are eaten by the elderly, children, pregnant women and those who are unwell.

MEAT AND FISH

Meat

The term meat usually implies beef, pork, mutton, veal, lamb, poultry, game or rabbit. Most meat is skeletal muscle, but the term may be extended to include offal.

Muscle meats consist of muscle fibres, connective tissue which holds the fibres together, and fat. The degree of tenderness of the meat depends upon the density of the connective tissue and the toughness of the muscle fibre. This, in turn, is related to the age of the animal and the degree of activity associated with the particular cut of meat.

The most important constituents of meat are protein, iron and B-group vitamins, especially nicotinic acid. Varying amounts of fat are also present. Pork is a good source of thiamin.

The characteristic flavour and aroma of meat are due to the presence of organic substances known as extractives. These are of negligible nutritive value, but are important as they stimulate the appetite and encourage the flow of digestive juices.

Deposits of fat within the muscle, giving a marbled appearance, are associated with the more tender cuts. Maturing or hanging of the carcase results in the formation of acids which assist the tenderising process.

Lengthy cooking is necessary to tenderise connective tissue, while the muscle fibres are hardened if high temperatures are used. Cooking of meat should aim at tenderising the connective tissue while avoiding, as far as possible, overcooking the muscle fibres.

Offal

Liver and brains have a high cholesterol content.

Liver, kidney and heart have a comparatively high content of riboflavin, thiamin, nicotinic acid and iron. Liver, especially, is a good source of iron. It also has a high content of vitamin A. Because of fears of the teratogenic effect of high doses of vitamin A, pregnant women should be advised not to eat liver.

Many different methods for cooking meat are used (Box 9.3). The method which is chosen depends on the cut of meat, facilities available and personal preference of the cook.

Fish

The flesh of fish is comparable with meat in composition. Like meat, it is a valuable source of protein and vitamins of the B group, especially nicotinic acid. Iron is also present, but to a lesser extent than in meat.

In the case of dark-fleshed fish such as herrings, mackerel, sardines and salmon, fat is present between the muscle fibres. These are known as the fatty or oily fish, and supply not only fat, but valuable amounts of the fat-soluble vitamins A and D. The flesh of white fish such as cod, haddock, whiting, plaice and sole has a very low fat content and contains a greater proportion of water than that of the dark-fleshed fish. It is therefore relatively lower in energy value. Some fish-liver oils contain very high concentrations of vitamins A and D, e.g. cod and halibut liver oils.

The cooking of fish in fat, as in frying and grilling, adds greatly to its energy value.

Substituting fish for meat in the diet is a good way of reducing saturated fat intake and increasing the intake of omega-3 fatty acids.

VEGETABLES

All vegetables have a structural framework of cellulose which is not digested.

Unless artificially dried, vegetables have a high water content of:

- around 90% in green vegetables
- 80–90% in root vegetables
- 70–80% in potatoes, peas and beans.

Green vegetables and tomatoes

Green vegetables contain varying amounts of vitamin C. Cabbage, cauliflower, broccoli, Brussels sprouts and tomatoes are important sources of this vitamin.

Tomatoes and vegetables with dark-green leaves, such as cabbage and spinach, are good sources of β-carotene, the precursor of vitamin A.

Green vegetables also contribute to the intake of folic acid, iron and calcium.

The members of this group are of negligible energy value, which is why they are allowed freely in weight-reducing diets.

The mineral content of vegetables depends on the mineral content of the soil in which they were grown.

Potatoes

Potatoes, when eaten in considerable amounts, make a useful contribution to the energy value of the diet. One small potato is of approximately the same energy value as one thin slice of bread—about 335 kJ (80 kcal).

The ascorbic acid content of potatoes is not great and decreases during storage. Potatoes can be an important source of this vitamin, because of the quantity and regularity with which they are eaten. They also contain small but significant amounts of protein, iron and B-complex vitamins.

Box 9.3 Methods of cooking meat

Boiling and stewing

Heat is conducted from the water into the meat. Water-soluble nutrients and flavour are lost into the water.

Pressure cooking

Heat is conducted into meat from the steam. Higher temperatures are reached, so cooking times can be shortened. Nutrients are lost into the cooking liquid.

Roasting and grilling

Convection from hot air and radiant heat cook the meat. As the meat shrinks, the juices are expelled and dry on the surface of the meat, so fewer nutrients are lost.

Microwave cooking

This method of cooking generates heat inside the food. The food is bombarded with electromagnetic radiation, which causes the water molecules inside the food to oscillate. This oscillation generates heat energy which cooks the food. Because the food is not subject to direct heat, it is not browned.

Root vegetables

Root vegetables such as carrot, parsnip and beetroot contain some ascorbic acid, but are not as good a source of this vitamin as the green vegetables. Turnips and swedes are the only really valuable sources of ascorbic acid in this group.

Carrots and sweet potato are of value as a source of β-carotene.

Root vegetables have a slightly higher energy value than green vegetables, owing to the presence of a higher proportion of starch and sugar. Their contribution to the energy intake is nevertheless not very significant. Beetroot and parsnips contain more carbohydrate than carrots, turnips or swedes.

Yam is an important source of carbohydrate in the traditional African and Afro-caribbean diets.

Pulse vegetables

Peas, beans and lentils contain more carbohydrate and protein than most other vegetables. Their protein, however, is of low biological value. They also contain considerable amounts of iron and B-complex vitamins, especially thiamin, so are very important in the vegetarian diet. The disadvantage of their low biological value can be overcome by mixing them with other types of pulses, cereal or nuts. Fresh green peas and beans are a source of ascorbic acid.

FRUITS

Fruits contain varying amounts of ascorbic acid, so not all are good sources of this vitamin.

Citrus fruits, such as oranges and grapefruit, have a high ascorbic acid content. Blackcurrants, strawberries, kiwifruit, raspberries and gooseberries are also good sources. The ascorbic acid content of blackcurrants is well retained in commercially prepared blackcurrant syrup.

Peaches, apricots and prunes are rich in β-carotene.

Some fruits have a high iron content, notably canned and dried peaches, dried apricots and figs, prunes, raisins, currants and sultanas. The extent to which this iron is available for absorption is, however, uncertain.

Fruits contain some carbohydrate, principally in the form of fructose. As with vegetables, they have a structural framework of cellulose. The water content of the edible portion is usually high, e.g. approximately 94% in the case of melon, 84% in the case of apple and 86% in the case of orange.

PRESERVING NUTRIENT VALUE OF VEGETABLES AND FRUITS

The cooking of vegetables softens their cellulose framework and makes them more easily masticated and more accessible to digestive enzymes. If the cooking water is discarded, the water-soluble vitamins and minerals which have been leached into it will also be lost. Fruit and vegetables are the only source of ascorbic acid in the diet. This nutrient is easily destroyed and care should be taken to preserve as much of it as possible. It is not unusual for 75% of this vitamin to be lost.

Destruction of ascorbic acid

1. Ascorbic acid is oxidised by the oxygen in the atmosphere to an inactive form. This process is speeded up by light, heat and the metals zinc, iron and copper.

2. Ascorbic acid is very soluble in water.

3. Plant cells contain the enzyme ascorbic acid oxidase, which increases the rate of ascorbic acid oxidation. This enzyme is normally separated from the vitamin. However, if the plant cells are damaged by chopping, bruising or wilting, then the enzyme will come into contact with the ascorbic acid and it will be destroyed.

4. Ascorbic acid is unstable in alkaline conditions. Sodium bicarbonate is sometimes added to cooking vegetables to improve the colour. This makes the cooking water alkaline and so destroys the ascorbic acid.

Loss of ascorbic acid from vegetables can be minimised by following the steps listed in Box 9.4.

Some loss of vitamins occurs when vegetables are canned, dried or frozen. In general, losses resulting from drying are greater than from canning or freezing.

> **Box 9.4** Steps necessary to minimise ascorbic acid losses
>
> 1. Use vegetables while they are fresh.
> 2. Prepare them immediately before cooking.
> 3. Use a sharp knife and, if possible, avoid peeling, grating and shredding.
> 4. Cook in boiling water; this destroys the enzyme ascorbic acid oxidase quickly.
> 5. Use only a small amount of water.
> 6. Cook for the shortest possible time.
> 7. Have a lid on the saucepan to keep oxygen out.
> 8. If possible, use the cooking water for gravies, sauces and soups.
> 9. Serve vegetables immediately after cooking.

At the same time, vegetables preserved by modern methods retain much of their vitamin content, and can be superior to so-called fresh vegetables which have been kept in the kitchen until they are wilted, or which have been damaged by careless cooking and serving.

Fruits, like vegetables, are rendered more digestible by cooking, because of softening of the cellulose. Losses of ascorbic acid in cooking water are less important, as fruits, other than the citrus fruits, are not as important a source of this vitamin as vegetables and, in any case, the cooking liquor is usually eaten along with the fruit.

Raw vegetables and fruits served in the form of salads introduce a variety of textures and flavours and add interest to meals. The food value of a salad is, of course, that of the ingredients used in its preparation. However, if the vegetables have been shredded, grated or stored, there will be a considerable loss of ascorbic acid.

NUTS

Nuts, with the exception of the chestnut, have a high content of fat and protein and are moderately low in carbohydrate. They therefore have a high energy value. Other constituents include iron and B-group vitamins. Chestnuts are comparatively low in fat and protein and high in carbohydrate.

Nuts are not eaten to any great extent in the UK, but can be of great importance in vegetarian and vegan diets.

BEVERAGES

Tea and coffee are of no energy value without the addition of milk, cream or sugar. They contain caffeine and theobromine, which are mild stimulants and are not harmful in moderation. Taken in excess they sometimes cause sleeplessness and irritability.

Tea is a rich source of bioflavenoids, particularly catechins and quercetin which have antioxidant activity so may have a role in preventing cardiovascular disease.

Cocoa contains significant amounts of iron, protein, fat and carbohydrate, but in the amounts in which cocoa is normally consumed it is of little value as a source of these nutrients.

Meat extracts are stimulating to the appetite and encourage the flow of digestive secretions. They contain a considerable amount of certain of the vitamins of the B group. Their protein content is insignificant. They are used for flavouring soups and gravies and also, diluted with water, as a beverage. Bovril™ is an example of a preparation which has a basis of meat extract.

Yeast extracts are similar in flavour to extracts of beef and have similar uses. They are good sources of the vitamins of the B group. An example of yeast extract is Marmite™.

Meat and yeast extracts have a high salt content.

Alcoholic beverages

On metabolism, alcohol yields 29 kJ (7 kcal) per gram.

The alcohol content of beverages is variable, being approximately 5% in the case of beer, cider and stout, around 10% in the case of light wines and about 15% in the case of sherry and port. Whisky, prepared by distilling a liquor resembling beer, and brandy, a distillate of wine, contain 30–40% alcohol.

Sweet wines, beer and stout have a considerable carbohydrate content. Cider, ale, beer and stout have a high energy value, e.g. 500 ml stout provides approximately 840 kJ (200 kcal).

The regular, heavy and prolonged consumption of alcohol over a period of years can cause damage to certain organs, particularly the liver and brain.

SOME ASPECTS OF FOOD PRODUCTION

The continual evolution of new and improved methods of agriculture and food processing is essential to the feeding of a world population which is increasing rapidly. Some examples of developments which were thought to have benefited humankind are the use of pesticides, the introduction of inorganic fertilisers, the intensive rearing of livestock, and the use of antibiotics in animal husbandry. However, there is now increasing concern about the safety of food in the UK.

Developments such as these require careful study in order to ensure the maximum benefit to humankind and to reduce potential health hazards to the minimum. For example, pesticides help to secure maximum crop yields. Some of them, however, remain in the crop after harvesting and processing and are eventually found in food. Small amounts of pesticide residues can be detected in human fat and the result of long-term ingestion of this material is not yet known. Some pesticides have come under suspicion and have been withdrawn from use.

Antibiotics are used in the treatment of infectious diseases in livestock. If recommended procedures are not followed on the farm, this may give rise to residues in foodstuffs. For example, milk containing a trace of penicillin has been known to cause reactions in sensitised persons, although such cases are rare.

Certain antibiotics have been found to accelerate growth, for example in broiler fowls and in pigs, and for this reason have been used as components of feeding mixtures. Statutory control is exercised over which antibiotics are permitted and how much may be fed. So far, there is little evidence to suggest that this practice gives rise to harmful residues in foods derived from these animals. Nevertheless, concern about pesticide and drug residues in food has led to a rapid expansion in the range and availability of organic food in supermarkets.

Many of the foods we eat contain additives, for example preservatives, colouring or flavouring agents, and emulsifiers. Careful control is exercised, and enforced by legislation where necessary. Without these measures toxic materials, including possible carcinogens, could be introduced into the diet.

Developments such as these must be considered in the light of expected benefits and any risks taken must be calculated ones. It is also relevant to note that certain foods which we eat regularly, and which we take entirely for granted, contain harmful material, for example the goitrogens present in members of the cabbage family (p. 33), and the toxic substance solanin which is found in potatoes.

GENETICALLY MODIFIED FOODS

The use of biotechnology, to change the genetic characteristics of food plants and the microorganisms used in food manufacture, is being developed. For example the genetic make-up of plants has been altered to make them more resistant to disease or pesticide treatment, to improve the flavour of the fruit or to lengthen the storage time. In the UK, foods which contain genetically modified soya or maize are required to be labelled.

FOOD ADDITIVES

The 1984 Food Labelling Regulations, which have been implemented since July 1986, describe as a food additive, 'any substance, not commonly regarded or used as food, which is added to or used in or on any food at any stage to affect its qualities, texture, consistency, appearance, taste, odour, alkalinity or acidity, or to serve any other technological function in relation to food'.

It is now compulsory for all prepared foods to have all additives, except flavourings, listed on the packaging. Additives are used to enhance the taste and appearance of products and to increase the length of

time that they can be stored. It has been estimated by the World Health Organization that 20% of the world's food supply is destroyed by the growth of bacteria, moulds and yeasts during storage. Any additive must be shown to be technologically necessary and safe before it is included in the UK Government list of permitted additives.

A new additive is only included in the Government's permitted list after a lengthy process of research and consultation; the process is in three stages (see Box 9.5).

If the new additive belongs to one of the categories which requires approval by the European Community, it must then undergo a further lengthy approval process before the prefix 'E' can be used before its designated serial number.

The list of additives on a food package must show the category of the additive used (see Table 9.2) and its chemical name or serial number (frequently an E number). Most additives are harmless and many are beneficial, e.g. ascorbic acid (vitamin C), which is used as an antioxidant and has serial number E300. The link between disease and food additives is discussed in Chapter 28.

Box 9.5 Stages of research and consultation required before inclusion of a new additive in the Government's list of permitted additives

1. The food manufacturer who wants to use the additive must convince the independent Food Advisory Committee that the new additive will be of benefit to the consumer, and that no other substance or process which has already been approved provides a suitable alternative.

2. If the Food Advisory Committee agrees that there is a need for a particular new additive, it is then up to the Committee on Toxicity of Chemicals in Food, Consumer Products and the Environment (COT), which consists of expert toxicologists, to assess the safety of the new additive.

3. The COT recommends to Government ministers whether or not the new additive should be used and the types of products and concentrations in which it should be used. They may, for example, recommend that it is not used in baby foods.

FOOD LABELLING

In the UK, all prepacked food in packages greater than 10 cm^2, and most non-prepacked food, must by law be labelled to tell the consumer:

- the name of the food
- the condition of the food, e.g. fresh or dried
- if the food has been treated in any way

Table 9.2 A summary of the major uses of food additives

Category	Function	Comments
Flavours	Create new flavours of products Restore flavour lost in processing Ensure all food in a batch tastes the same	Flavours do not have serial numbers
Sweeteners	Sweeten foods	The two sweeteners with serial numbers are sorbitol (E420) and manitol (E421). Others are saccharine and aspartame which are extremely sweet (naturally occurring sugars such as sucrose or fructose are not classified as additives)
Colours	Improve appearance of food Restore colour lost during processing Ensure batch uniformity	There is an increasing use of naturally occurring food dyes, e.g. betanin extracted from beetroot, instead of artificial colours Colours usually have serial numbers in the 200s
Preservatives	Prevent the growth of bacteria, mould and yeast Prevent formation of 'off' flavours of fermentation	Preservatives, e.g. salt and vinegar, have been used for centuries Most have serial numbers in the 100–122 group
Antioxidants	Prevent rancid taste and smell Preserve content of some vitamins	
Emulsifiers	Allow oil and water and stabilisers to mix Prevent separation of these mixtures, e.g. in mayonnaise	Modified starches are frequently used as emulsifiers
Solvents	Dissolve colour or flavour additives so that they can be incorporated in food	The only solvent currently permitted is glycerol, E422
Mineral oils	Prevent food from drying out Improve appearance of food	Frequently added to dried fruit to prevent further drying out
Miscellaneous	Acids, bases, anti-caking agents, buffers, bulking agents, humectants, packaging gases, liquid freezants	Assorted numbers

- the ingredients listed in descending order by weight (this list will include any additive, unless it was used in the preparation of a single ingredient, for example a bleaching agent added to flour which is used for biscuit making; pesticide residues do not have to be listed)
- the quality of the food

Most food must also be date-marked. It is usual for this to be prefixed with the phrase 'Best before' and the date is based on the minimum period of time that the manufacturer would expect the food to remain wholesome and pleasant to consume. The date-mark is only applicable if the food is stored in the conditions recommended by the manufacturer and printed on the packaging.

It would be inappropriate to list all the approved additives and their functions in this text. More details about the serial numbers, chemical names and common uses of the permitted additives are available from Food Standards Agency (See Further Reading Section).

REFERENCES

Hendriks H F J, Westrate J A, Van Vliet T, Meijer G W 1999 Spreads enriched with three different levels of vegetable oil sterols and the degree of cholesterol lowering in normocholesterolaemic and mildly hypercholesterolaemic subjects. European Journal of Clinical Nutrition 53: 319–327

Salminen S, Bouley M C, Boutron-Rualt M C et al 1998 Functional food science and gastrointestinal physiology and function. British Journal of Nutrition 80 (Suppl 1): 147–181

Stanton B R 1971 Meals for the elderly. King Edward's Hospital Fund for London, London

FURTHER READING

British Nutrition Foundation 1999 Nutrition and Food Processing. British Nutrition Foundation, London.

Lobstein T 1988 Fast food facts. Camden Press, London

National Consumer Council (NCC) 1992 Your food: whose choice? (Chapters 9 and 10) HMSO, London

MAFF 1999 Food sense booklets (available from the Food Standards Agency):
- About food additives (PB0552)
- Food and pesticides (PB0863)
- Understanding radioactivity in food (PB1212)
- genetic modification and food (PB2052)
- Organic food (PB2085)
- Understanding food labels (PB0553)
- Use your label: making sense of nutrition information (PB2362)

USEFUL WEBSITE

Food Standards Agency: www.food.gov.uk

Public health and community nutrition

10

An introduction to public health nutrition

LEARNING OBJECTIVES

After studying this chapter you should be able to:

- discuss the contribution good nutrition makes to public health
- describe the techniques used to collect dietary information
- contribute to public health iniatives designed to reduce inequalities in health caused by poor nutrition.

Public health workers have been interested in nutritional status and dietary intake, and how these contribute to the maintenance of good health and prevention of disease in the populations they serve, for centuries.

Everyone who is involved in public health and health care has a contribution to make towards improving public health. Specific examples of the ways the skills and knowledge of nutritionists and dietitians are used include:

- the promotion and maintenance of good health by good nutrition
- the prevention of diet-related disease
- involvement in nutritional epidemiological research
- contributing to the development of diet policy, particularly food-based dietary guidelines at both local and national levels
- evaluating the effectiveness of dietary interventions.

DIETARY INVESTIGATION METHODS

The technique used to investigate dietary intake depends on the population and the specific nutritional issue which is being researched. The techniques

Box 10.1   Dietary investigation methods

Diet recall involves interviewing all subjects. During the interview subjects are asked to recall everything that has been eaten or drunk in a defined period of time, often the last 24 hours. This method provides information about habitual dietary intake in populations. It is used where a limited range of foods is available and there is little daily variation in the types of food eaten. The disadvantage of this method is that it relies on the recall ability of the person being interviewed and it is therefore possible that those foods that are not routinely eaten every day might not be recalled.

Diet history also involves an interview. The detailed interview contains both open-ended and closed questions lasting 2–3 hours. From the results of this interview the investigator constructs a typical 7-day eating pattern for the individual. This method highlights individual daily variations in meal patterns and nutrient intake. This method is very time-consuming but is used in large studies looking at all the nutrients that are eaten.

Weighed diet history is the most accurate method of collecting dietary information. It is, however, very demanding as subjects are asked to record in a food diary a description including the weight of everything that is eaten and drunk over the study period, which is usually 1 week. This is the method used for the National Diet and Nutrition Surveys (Gregory et al 1990, Gregory 2000). While providing very good quality data about actual nutrient intake, this method is very time-consuming for both participants and investigator.

Food frequency questionnaire is used by researchers who are interested in the intake of specific nutrients or foods. It identifies dietary habits that impact on the intake of a specific nutrient or nutrients. A situation where this method might be used is to investigate dietary intake of iron. The investigator would quantify the frequency with which iron-rich foods were eaten and also any foods that inhibit iron absorption.

commonly used for dietary assessment and nutritional research are shown in Box 10.1

PUBLIC HEALTH NUTRITION IN THE UK

The specific aspect of nutrition and diet that is topical and being researched at a particular time depends on existing medical and scientific knowledge, the nutritional and health status of the population, political pressures and the concerns of the population. In the UK the importance of the concerns of the population has been responded to by the Food Standards Act 1999 with the establishment of the Food Standards Agency, which includes in its remit a commitment to provide independent nutritional information. This is further discussed in Chapter 11.

During the last 150 years major nutritional advances have been made which include the understanding of the role of diet in the aetiology of disease, in the maintenance of good health and also in the prevention of and recovery from disease (this is further discussed in Chapter 12). These advances have often been followed by public health interventions. This was demonstrated, for example, by:

- the introduction of school meals in 1906 in response to Boer War recruitment problems which had identified malnutrition as a problem among recruits
- the success of the food-rationing programme of 1940–1945, the intention of which was to ensure that the entire population was well nourished by an equitable distribution of essential foods to all. The

allocation was based on a scientific assessment of nutrient requirements of specific population groups. This was the first time that women and children were specifically targeted as vulnerable groups and their particular nutritional needs identified.

Health workers hoping to change dietary habits need to understand the context within which people live their lives and the factors which influence the choices that they make about their diet (Margetts & Nelson 1997). For, not only has the understanding of the role of nutrition in the maintenance of health changed, so have many other factors which influence diet. These include the roles and occupations of members within family units, levels of disposable income, types of housing, cooking facilities, availability of foods, new advances in food manufacturing and improved ease of travel, so it can hardly be a surprise that the diet that is habitually eaten by many people in the UK shows little resemblance to that eaten 100 years ago.

In 1901 the diet of a working class family was monotonous and deficient in protein, most vitamins and minerals, as it was based on bread, bacon, cheese and tea (Johnston 1977). The meals eaten on a weekday were typically:

- Breakfast: bread, butter and tea
- Dinner: bread, bacon and tea
- Tea: bread, butter and tea.

In contrast to this, the most recent Diet and Nutrition survey of UK adults (Gregory et al 1990), which looked at 51 food groups and types, showed that a wide range of foods were now included in the average UK diet. Although bread remains an important food, being eaten by 87% of the group within the 7-day study period, a range of foods were also eaten, for example:

- 26% ate pasta
- 33% ate yoghurt
- 48% ate baked beans
- 26% ate burgers and kebabs.

These major changes in dietary intakes have been accompanied by changes in the nutritional status of the population. This can be illustrated by a comparison of two nutritional reports on school children published approximately 95 years apart.

Johnston (1977) cites the report of the Committee on Physical Deterioration 1904, which reported that a third of all children were under-nourished and that 12-year-old boys attending public schools were 5 inches taller than those attending council schools.

In contrast to this, the World Health Organization has suggested that 25% of children are now overweight (WHO 1998a). The recent National Diet and Nutrition Survey of Children (Gregory 2000) has shown that there was no widespread evidence of malnutrition and the heights and weights are higher than in previous surveys. There were still causes for concern about the diet, as 8% of boys and 11% of girls had a plasma cholesterol at or above 5.20 mmol/l and children in lower socioeconomic groups had low intakes of calcium and vitamin C.

These two reports highlight the need for different public health solutions to different problems. In the past, public health nutrition policy has been very successful in eliminating deficiency diseases and ensuring equitable distribution of food when resources were limited. In the UK it has now moved on to improving access and availability of healthy foods to reduce inequalities in health, in particular the increased prevalence of cardiovascular disease, cancer and obesity in low-income groups (DoH 1999).

The McGovern Report

The first major report to signify the important shift for nutritionists from the prevention of deficiency diseases to prevention of degenerative diseases was the McGovern report (Senate Select Committee 1977). This report showed that the diets of most Americans contained too much fat, sugar and salt and that this was linked to increased death rates from cardiovascular disease. This report stimulated other countries to look at their national diet and publish similar reports.

The NACNE Report

In the UK the National Advisory Committee on Nutrition Education (NACNE) was established in 1979. This working group included representatives from the Ministry of Agriculture, the Department of Health and Social Security, the Health Education Council and the food industry. Their report was eventually published in 1983 (HEC 1983).

The report was unpopular particularly with the food industry and was published amidst considerable acrimony. This was because it suggested that the entire population was eating badly and that this had health implications. It set clear dietary goals about the amount of fat and sugar that should be eaten.

Committee on Medical Aspects of Food Policy (COMA) Reports

This controversy was repeated, but to a lesser extent, when the COMA reports on Nutritional Aspects of Cardiovascular Disease (DoH 1994) and Nutritional Aspects of the Development of Cancer (DoH 1998) were published, when again the dietary recommendations that they proposed triggered debate. Nevertheless, it was the publication of the NACNE report that stimulated a new era of nutrition education and research.

The key dietary recommendations of these reports are summarised in Chapters 12 and 14.

The National Food Survey

This is a report produced annually which provides national data on food expenditure, consumption and nutrient intakes. It was first produced in 1950 and the results are derived from a random sample of 6000 private households in the UK. The results are classified according to various geographical and household characteristics, so provide valuable information about patterns of consumption and expenditure in different types of households.

DIET AND HEALTH INEQUALITIES

'Diet affects the health of socially disadvantaged people from the cradle to the grave. The social and economic reasons are complex, but the potential for health gain through improved diet is enormous. A poor diet, physical inactivity, and smoking are a lethal triad for the lower social class, leading to an intergenerational spiral of ill-health and handicap. Modern nutritional and sociological research is now providing a basis for targeted action to reverse this cycle.'

(James et al 1997)

Box 10.2   The consequences of a poor diet that leads to the development of inequalities in health

Poor maternal diet prior to birth

Low folic acid intake
- Neural tube defects

Low n-3 fatty acid intake
- Impaired brain development

Low energy intake
- Low birth-weight
- Hypertension, diabetes and coronary heart disease in adulthood

Low intake of iron rich foods
- Low iron stores at birth can lead to iron deficiency anaemias

Infancy

Not breast-fed
- Increased incidence of infection and allergy
- Not exposed to substances in breast-milk which stimulate the immune system and enhance the development of the brain and gastrointestinal tract.
- Iron deficiency anaemia

Poor choice of weaning foods and early weaning
- Iron deficiency anaemia
- Dental caries
- Obesity
- Poor dietary habits established leading to disease in later life
- Preference for salty and sugary foods established

Pre-school child

High intake of sugary foods
- Dental caries
- Obesity
- Preference for energy dense sweet foods in adulthood

High intake of savoury snacks
- Obesity
- Preference for energy dense, salty, high fat snacks in adulthood

Low intake of fruit and vegetables
- Vitamin and mineral deficiencies

- Reduced resistance to infection
- Constipation
- Poor dietary habits established leading to ill-health in later life

Low intake of iron rich foods
- Iron deficiency anaemia

School child/adolescent

High intake of confectionery/soft drinks
- Dental caries
- Obesity

High intake of fatty and fried foods
- Raised blood lipids

Low intake of iron-rich foods
- Iron deficiency anaemia

Low intake of calcium rich foods
- Osteoporosis

Low intake of fruit and vegetables
- Poor intake of vitamins and minerals
- Poor dietary habits established leading to obesity, diabetes, hypertension and cancer in later life

Adults

High salt intake
- Hypertension and cerebrovascular disease

High fat intake
- Cardiovascular disease
- Obesity

Low intake of fruit and vegetables
- Cardiovascular disease and some cancers

High intake of alcohol
- Some cancers
- Liver disease

Older adults

As adults get older, however, the incidence of deficiencies of energy, vitamins and minerals increases:
- reduced resistance to infection
- increased repair and recovery times → increased hospital stays
- deficiency diseases.

The Acheson report (Acheson 1997) documented these inequalities and current UK public health policy is focused on addressing them. Box 10.2 summarises the consequences of a poor diet that lead to the development of inequalities in health.

The NHS plan (DoH 2000) has identified improving diet and nutrition as one of six key areas for reducing inequalities and improving health. The strategy identified for improving diet and nutrition acknowledges that local availability and affordability of food frequently influences the food choices people make. The Plan identifies areas for action before 2004, which include:

- a new national fruit scheme, where every child in nursery and aged 4–6 years in infant schools will receive a free piece of fruit each school day
- a 5-a-day programme to increase fruit and vegetable consumption
- work with industry and retailers to provide better provision of fruit and vegetables to communities
- initiatives with the food industry to improve the overall diet including salt, fat and sugar
- tackling obesity and physical inactivity
- a hospital nutrition policy to improve the outcome for patients

- a reform of welfare foods, with increasing support for breast-feeding and parenting.

Adequacy, availability and accessibility of the food supply

In order for individuals and populations to have a healthy diet, the food supply must be available, adequate and accessible to all.

Adequacy of food supply. This relates to the nutritional content of the diet. For example, is the amount of food that is available adequate to meet the needs of the entire population or is there insufficient to meet everyone's nutritional needs, even if it is distributed equitably?

Availability of food supply. This relates to where the food actually is and whether or not it is available to the local population, assuming that they have the resources to purchase it.

In the UK, although the food supply is adequate, there are some areas where, because of lack of public transport or limited choice in small local shops, foods that are needed for a healthy diet, such as fresh fruit and vegetables, are unavailable. Another situation where food is unavailable would be if it were stored in a central depot but there was no means of transporting it to the surrounding settlements. This occurs during wartime and is then a cause of malnutrition.

Accessibility of food supply. This is the cause of malnutrition for much of the world's population. An adequate supply of food is available but only if the people have enough money to buy it, or they are not required to sell the food they have produced to another individual or an organisation.

Local food projects

Health improvement programmes have incorporated local food projects as part of the multidisciplinary strategy to meet the specific needs in addressing health inequalities of a particular community. Local food projects are initiatives developed by the local community, usually with the support of local health or community workers, to enable members of the community improve their diet. There is a wide range of different types of local food project. The particular type of project that is developed will depend on the specific strengths and needs of the community that it is developed to support. Examples of the types of local food projects that have developed are:

- establishment of local food cooperatives to increase the choice of fresh produce available and to reduce price

- bulk-buying groups to reduce the purchase price of food
- community gardens and allotments for growing fresh vegetables
- cooking and tasting sessions to enable people to experiment with different foods and cooking methods
- cookery courses for all age groups
- community cafes for the provision of meals, and to provide a community meeting place and opportunities for skills training.

McGlone et al (1999) reviewed 25 local food projects and concluded that, although the types of projects differed in that they were developed to meet different community needs and were organised in different ways, no particular type was best. Not only do the projects improve diet by improving access to food, increasing the variety of foods eaten and improving cooking skills, they also offer social support to the individuals involved and provide common ground for local people and health professionals to meet upon.

Local food projects are not the sole answer to reducing the existing inequalities of health, but they are a valuable component of a wider strategy and as such are often included in Health Improvement Programmes. Their success should not be judged solely on long-term changes in nutritional status and health, but also on changes in shopping and eating behaviour and increased cooking skills within the community. Successful food projects raise the levels of skill and training in the community, help to overcome social isolation and increase an individual's self-worth, as well as enabling individuals to eat a healthier diet.

Obesity

Overweight and obesity develop when there is an imbalance between the energy intake and energy expenditure of an individual for a period of time, leading to an energy intake that exceeds energy expenditure. A range of genetic, metabolic, socioeconomic and behavioural factors all contribute to the development of the energy imbalance and are not the same for every individual.

The prevalence of obesity has more than doubled in the last 30 years. The Health Survey for England (Prescott-Clarke & Primatesta 1999) showed that 53% of women and 62% of men had a BMI (body mass index) of greater than 25 kg/m^2, so were overweight, and that 1 in 5 women and 1 in 6 men were obese (BMI greater than 30 kg/m^2). Current data shows that this trend continues (Moore 2000).

In the UK there is evidence to show that decline in physical activity is crucial in the development of obesity. The average energy intake has declined since the 1970s (MAFF 1991), while the incidence of obesity has risen. It has been shown using proxy measures of inactivity, such as hours spent watching television and car ownership (Prentice & Jebb 1995), that there is a strong relationship between obesity and inactivity.

However, the role of diet in the development of overweight and obesity should not be ignored. A diet in which a high proportion of its energy is provided by fat is more energy-dense, therefore smaller in volume and considered by many to be more palatable than a low-fat diet of the same energy content. Diets with a high fat content encourage over-consumption of energy (Poppitt 1995) and it has been suggested that the high fat content in some way undermines the appetite regulatory mechanisms. Manipulation of an individual's habitual diet to increase the fat, and therefore the energy content, has been shown to result in a passive over-consumption of energy because the individual does not reduce the quantity of food eaten to compensate for this (Blundell & Macdiarmid 1997). Therefore, it seems likely that for susceptible individuals a high-fat diet will result in an energy imbalance and weight-gain, particularly if it is accompanied by physical inactivity.

Healthy eating guidelines

It would seem that establishing the link between diet and disease and producing dietary guidelines is relatively easy compared with changing long-established eating habits of the population so that their diet is healthier. Evaluation has shown that healthy eating interventions can achieve dietary change in a variety of settings and populations (Roe et al 1997), but the diet and obesity targets set by the 'Health of the Nation' document (DoH 1992) remain difficult to achieve. One of the reasons identified for this is confusion among the general public as to what a healthy diet actually is. This was because there was so little agreement between the information provided by health care professionals and the media. The consequence of this is that people feel that the 'experts' are always changing their minds.

To help eliminate confusion and to support dietary change, standardised dietary guidelines were produced by the Health Education Authority (1994) (see Chapter 14). These guidelines were disseminated widely and the Nutrition Task Force document 'Eat Well 2' (DoH 1995) encouraged all those involved in nutrition education to use them (See Chapter 14).

It is now the situation that these guidelines are used along with the 'Balance of Good Health' (HEA 1994), a pictorial representation of the types and amounts of foods that make up a healthy diet. This information can be seen in schools, supermarkets, workplace canteens, hospitals, clinics and surgeries, as it is also the basis of nutrition education literature produced by the food industry.

PUBLIC HEALTH NUTRITION IN DEVELOPING COUNTRIES

In 10 000 BC, the population of the world has been estimated as 6 million and life-expectancy at birth as 20 years. As we enter the second millennium, the world's population exceeds 6 billion and the 'World Health Report' (WHO 1998b) records a global life-expectancy of 66 years. This global life-expectancy at birth has increased dramatically in the last 45 years. The global average was only 48 years in 1955 and it is projected that it will reach 73 years in 2025.

While these figures seem very optimistic, there are still enormous variations in life-expectancy both internationally and within national populations. In approximately 83% of the population the life-expectancy at birth is over 60 years. This covers over 120 countries.

The changes in the world population are a consequence of changes in the mortality and fertility rates, and population growth in developing countries is much greater than in the developed ones. Reasons for these rapid changes are improvements in sanitation, nutrition and health care and the changes in economies caused by industrialisation.

In order for a population to be well nourished, they must have a secure food supply which ensures that all people have a nutritionally adequate diet. A range of different methods are used to assess food security, including measuring household food stocks and the cost of an average (defined) basket of food.

Malnutrition is the physical deterioration that occurs due to an inadequate or inappropriate intake of nutrients. Four types of malnutrition have been identified (Mayer 1976). These are over-nutrition, dietary deficiency, secondary malnutrition and under-nutrition.

Over-nutrition causes the 'diseases of affluence' first identified by Trowell (1960) and it occurs when a diet high in fat and sugar and low in non-starch polysaccharides is consumed. There is much epidemiological evidence to show how the incidence of heart disease and stroke and some cancers has increased when populations have moved from a rural area to an urban one and the composition of their diet has changed showing an increase in the fat and sugar content. This type of malnutrition is becoming increasingly important as countries become industrialised.

Dietary deficiency occurs when the diet does not contain an adequate amount of a specific micronutrient (vitamin or mineral). Dietary deficiencies are relatively easy to prevent or correct using fortification and supplements. Examples of nutrients which may be deficient are vitamin A, iron and iodine.

Secondary malnutrition develops as a consequence of disease, For example, in diarrhoeal disease and measles, when the infant is unable to consume adequate nutrients to meet its increased requirements. It is often the case that a child who is marginally malnourished will enter a downward spiral into severe malnutrition as a consequence of disease.

Under-nutrition occurs when there is not enough food, and is found predominantly in low-income countries of the developing world. It results in low birth-weight, high infant mortality, low height for age, low weight for height, low weight for age, increased maternal mortality and decreased work capacity.

The WHO report 'Health in Europe 1997' (WHO 1998b) revealed that Europe's overall health was deteriorating for the first time for 50 years. The top health problems, cardiovascular disease, obesity, diabetes, osteoporosis and cancer, share common risk factors which are unhealthy nutrition, lack of physical activity, smoking and heavy drinking.

Commenting on this report Sjöstrom et al (1999) state that for the majority of European adults who neither smoke nor drink excessively, the most significant controllable risk factors affecting their long-term health are what they eat and how physically active they are. This is an assertion which is supported by many others and is influencing health policy in 'developed countries' (DoH 1999). As people migrate from rural to urban areas and move from their traditional diet and employment to a different way of life, every effort needs to be made to ensure that this issue is not ignored.

In the 'developed world' the general public's perception of malnutrition is of the terrible suffering and loss of life caused by famine, whereas in reality the number of people who suffer starvation as a consequence of famine is much smaller than the number who suffer an increased morbidity and decreased life-expectancy because of a lifetime of under-nutrition leading to reduced immunity and failure to achieve their full potential both physically and intellectually. This results in a lifetime of poverty and the inability to achieve their potential economically. Obviously it would be too simplistic to assume that being adequately nourished would mean that poverty and ill-health could be eradicated, but nevertheless it is a significant piece of the jigsaw.

Famine is the most extreme form of food insecurity (Yip 1997) and often the result of transitory or acute deterioration of access to food. Increased malnutrition and mortality are the consequences of mass starvation during famine.

One of the challenges of the new millennium has to be: can famines, which involve not only hunger and death from malnutrition as well as the breakdown of normal social relationships and disintegration of families, be prevented and, if not prevented, then anticipated and the suffering caused significantly reduced.

Prevention of malnutrition

There are well-documented cases in which major food shortages have been managed to ensure that famine did not develop, for example, Collins (1993) reported that famine was averted in 1992 in Southern Africa. At this time a severe drought affecting virtually all the countries in Southern Africa resulted in crop-failure rates of up to 80%. Famine was averted by cooperation between countries within the region, and external assistance coming as shipments of grain and help to distribute the grain.

Famines which result from natural disasters are easier to anticipate and so reduce the severity of, than those caused by political instability and war. While famine monitoring systems that include weather surveillance, monitoring of the price of food, income levels, agricultural production and food indices are relatively easy to develop and respond to, famines caused by political unrest and war are far more difficult to predict and respond to. This is particularly because interventions based on the development of community programmes, such as food for work, cash for work and food price stabilisation, are difficult to implement and in these situations, the reliance has to be on food aid.

The prevention of malnutrition is complex. It has already been shown that malnutrition results from a complex interplay of factors, which include household access to food, access to basic health care, safe water and sanitation and literacy, particularly for women. These factors have been summarised into categories in Figure 10.1 to show their inter-relationships.

The policy dilemma for governments is how to ensure that nutrition is adequate for all in the next century—should resources be spent on treating causes or treating symptoms or a combination of both?

Nutrition intervention programmes intended to treat symptoms include:

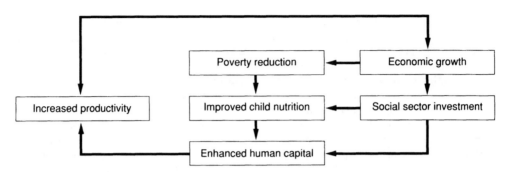

Figure 10.1 The inter-relationship between factors that contribute to the development of malnutrition.

- food aid either as general food distribution programmes or selective feeding programmes
- restricting the sale and movement of locally produced food
- limiting the price of food and, if necessary, subsidising the cost

Programmes that treat the causes address the following issues:

- improving sanitation
- increasing employment
- improving literacy/education, particularly for women
- improving transport and infrastructure
- better methods of food production
- population limitation
- land reform.

REFERENCES

Acheson D (1997) Independent inquiry into inequalities in health. HMSO, London

Blundell J E, Macdiarmid J I 1997 Passive over-consumption. Fat intake and short term energy balance. Annals of the New York Academy of Sciences 827: 392–407

Collins C 1993 Famine defeated: Southern Africa, UN wins battle against drought. Africa Recovery August 9: 1–13

Department of Health (DoH) 1992 The health of the nation. HMSO, London

Department of Health (DoH) 1994 Nutritional aspects of cardiovascular disease. Report of the Cardiovascular Review Group Committee on Medical Aspects of Food Policy (Report on Health and Social Subjects 46). HMSO, London

Department of Health (DoH) 1995 Nutrition Task Force Eat Well 2. HMSO, London

Department of Health (DoH) 1998 Nutritional aspects of the development of cancer. Report of the Working Group on Diet and Cancer of the Committee on the Medical Aspects of Food and Nutrition Policy (Report on Health and Social Subjects 48). HMSO, London

Department of Health (DoH) 1999 Saving lives: our healthier nation. HMSO, London

Department of Health (DoH) 2000 The NHS plan: A plan for investment, a plan for reform. HMSO, London

Gregory J 2000 The diet and nutritional survey of 4 to 18 year olds. HMSO, London

Gregory J, Foster K, Tyler H, Wiseman M 1990 The dietary and nutritional survey of British adults. HMSO, London

Health Education Authority (HEA) 1994 The balance of good health. Health Education Authority, London

Health Education Council (HEC) 1983 National Advisory Committee on Nutrition Education (NACNE) Proposals for nutritional guidelines for health education in Britain. Health Education Council, London

James W P T, Nelson M, Ralph A, Leather S 1997 Socioeconomic determinants of health: The contribution of nutrition to inequalities in health. British Medical Journal 314: 1545–1553

Johnston J P 1977 A hundred years eating. Gill and Macmillan, Dublin

Margetts B M, Nelson M 1997 Design concepts in nutritional epidemiology, 2nd Edn. Oxford University Press, Oxford

Mayer J 1976 The dimensions of human hunger. In: Food and agriculture. Freeman, San Francisco

McGlone P, Dobson B, Dowler E, Nelson M 1999 Food projects and how they work. Joseph Rowntree Foundation, York

Ministry of Agriculture, Fisheries and Food (MAFF) 1991 Household food consumption and expenditure 1940–1990. HMSO, London

Moore MS 2000 Interactions between physical activity and diet in the regulation of body weight. Proceedings of the Nutrition Society 59 (2): 193–198

Prentice A M, Jebb S A 1995 Obesity in Britain: gluttony or sloth? British Medical Journal 311:437–439

Poppit S D 1995 Energy density of diets and obesity. International Journal of Obesity 19 (Suppl 5): S20–S26

Prescott-Clarke P, Primatesta P 1999 Health Survey for England 1997 Volume 1: Findings. HMSO, London

Roe L, Hunt P, Bradshaw H, Rayner M 1997 Health promotion interventions to promote healthy eating within the general population—a review. Health Education Authority, London

Senate Select Committee on Nutrition and Human Needs 1977 Dietary goals for the United States. US Senate, Washington DC

Sjöstrom M, Yngre A, Poorvliet E, Warm D, Ekelund U 1999 Diet and physical activity—interactions for health: public health nutrition in the European perspective. Public Health Nutrition 2(3a): 453–459

Trowell H 1960 Non-infective disease in Africa. Edward Arnold, London

United Nation's Children's Fund (UNICEF) 1998 The state of the world's children. UNICEF, New York

World Health Organisation (WHO) 1998a Consultation on obesity. Global prevalence and secular trends in obesity. In: WHO (Ed) Obesity: preventing and managing the global epidemic. WHO, Geneva: 17–40

World Health Organisation (WHO) 1998b The World Health Report 1998. WHO, Geneva

Yip R 1997 Famine. In: Noji E K (Ed) The public health consequences of disasters. Oxford University Press, New York

FURTHER READING

Baggott R 2000 Public health policy and politics (Chapter 8). Macmillan Press, London

Foster P 1992 The world food problem—tackling the causes of undernutrition in the third world. Adamantine Press, London

United Nations 1993 Human Development Report 1993. United Nations, New York

11

Food-borne diseases and their prevention

LEARNING OBJECTIVES

After studying this chapter you should be able to:

- explain the mechanisms that cause food-borne diseases and how these diseases can be prevented
- discuss the importance of the Food Standards Agency in ensuring safe food for consumers.

FOOD POISONING

The term 'food poisoning' is applied to acute inflammation of the gastrointestinal tract following the consumption of food which contains harmful material. The condition can be caused by ingestion of:

- food contaminated with bacteria and their toxins
- poisonous plants or fish
- chemicals
- viruses
- mycotoxins.

Sometimes the food is infected at the source, as in the case of meat from a diseased animal. Alternatively, infection may take place during handling of the food if certain precautions (to be discussed later) are not observed. It has been estimated that 75% of cases of food poisoning in the UK are associated with meat and meat products.

Bacteria in food

Most species of bacteria are not harmful to humankind and many perform useful functions. Examples of the latter are the lactobacilli, which ferment lactose with the production of lactic acid and thus bring about the souring of milk. Other examples are the bacteria which synthesise vitamins in the intestine, and the bacteria of the soil, which break down waste material and convert it to plant foodstuffs.

Some bacteria, however, are pathogenic. These pathogenic species demand our attention, as some may be taken into the body along with food and may give rise to food poisoning (see Box 11.1). It is important to know how food becomes infected with these bacteria and what precautions should be taken to guard against such infection. Food poisoning is a preventable illness which causes pain and distress to individuals, time away from work and cost to health services. It is particularly harmful for those people who are already unwell.

Campylobacter infection

The number of recorded outbreaks of gastroenteritis caused by *Campylobacter jejuni* now exceeds those caused by *Salmonella* (Garrow et al 2000). Symptoms occur 2–11 days after ingesting infected foodstuff. Sources of infection are listed in Box 11.2.

Salmonella species

There are approximately 2200 serotypes of *Salmonella* known as a cause of food poisoning. These bacteria occur in the intestinal tract of birds and animals. The sources of human infection are listed in Box 11.3.

Salmonella bacteria are destroyed by thorough cooking. They like moisture and warmth and, provided the medium is suitable, will multiply rapidly in food which is being kept warm for some time before being eaten. This food will cause food poisoning but will not taste, smell or look different from other foods.

Staphylococcus aureus

Certain strains of *staphylococci* are also known to cause food poisoning, the most common being *Staphylococcus*

Box 11.2   Sources of *Campylobacter jejuni* infections

- Unpasteurised milk
- Poultry
- Manufactured foods that have been contaminated during processing
- Dogs, cats and birds act as the source of infection

Box 11.3   Sources of *Salmonella* infection

- Cooked meat which has been handled by a person suffering from the condition, or who is a carrier, is a common source of infection. Healthy carriers are individuals who recovered from *Salmonella* food poisoning but have bacteria remaining in the intestinal tract for some time after recovery has taken place. These carriers may, through faulty personal hygiene, be the means of spreading the disease
- Meat or milk from infected animals, and milk and milk foods infected by a food handler
- Eggs and poultry can also be sources of *Salmonella* infection. The way in which poultry are processed means that the infection from one diseased animal can be spread to many
- Flies may be the means of spreading the disease
- Rats and mice are particularly susceptible to *Salmonella* infections and may transmit the disease to humankind by contamination of food with excreta

---

aureus. The symptoms are brought about as a result of the ingestion of a toxic substance formed by the bacteria during their period of growth in the food.

Staphylococcal food poisoning is associated with foods which have been infected during preparation and have then been set aside for some hours before being eaten cold (see Box 11.4). During this period, the bacteria grow in the food and the toxin is produced. Such foods include meats such as ham, tongue, meat pies and brawn, and to a lesser extent, milk and milk dishes and artificial cream. Staphylococcal food poisoning may therefore be contracted at a cold buffet.

Staphylococci are destroyed by cooking, but this is not always true of the enterotoxin.

E. coli

This organism is found in the intestines of humans and most of the serotypes are not pathogenic. The serotype *E. coli 0157* is pathogenic and an outbreak of food poisoning which occurred in Scotland in 1996 and resulted in 21 deaths and over 500 people having symptoms of food poisoning was traced back to cooked meat

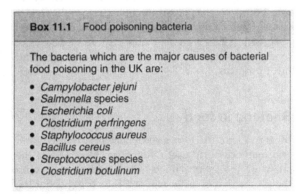

Box 11.1   Food poisoning bacteria

The bacteria which are the major causes of bacterial food poisoning in the UK are:

- *Campylobacter jejuni*
- *Salmonella* species
- *Escherichia coli*
- *Clostridium perfringens*
- *Staphylococcus aureus*
- *Bacillus cereus*
- *Streptococcus* species
- *Clostridium botulinum*

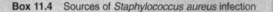

Box 11.4   Sources of *Staphylococcus aureus* infection

- Septic conditions such as boils and abscesses in people concerned with the handling of food—such lesions harbour staphylococci which are transmitted to the food from the hands of the infected person
- Respiratory infections in food handlers, the organisms being transmitted to the food from the hands, or directly in droplets discharged from the respiratory tract while speaking or coughing
- Staphylococci present in the respiratory tract and on the skin of healthy persons

---

purchased from one butcher's shop (Penington Group 1997).

Clostridium perfringens

This organism can also give rise to food poisoning. Food can become infected from either of the sources given in Box 11.5, the bacteria then forming spores which are not always destroyed by cooking. For example, when a large quantity of meat is cooked at one time and allowed to cool slowly, the heat penetration may be insufficient to kill the spores, which later germinate and multiply. The poisoning is due to a toxin which the bacteria produce while they multiply in the host's intestine after they have been eaten.

Bacillus cereus

Bacillus cereus occurs in a wide variety of foods, especially cereals, and causes a form of food poisoning which is associated particularly with rice which has been cooked, re-heated and served in restaurants, as the organism forms spores which can survive cooking.

The rice is parboiled some hours before it is required and kept at room temperature, during which time the spores germinate and produce a toxin in the food. The final heating of the rice prior to serving is insufficient to destroy this toxin, which is subsequently ingested, resulting in food poisoning. It can be prevented by reducing the interval between parboiling and frying to

less than 2 hours. Rice should be parboiled in small batches, cooled quickly, and kept in a refrigerator.

Listeria monocytogenes

Listeria monocytogenes is a bacterium which can multiply rapidly at the low temperatures of domestic and commercial refrigerators and chilled storage cabinets. It is found naturally in soil, vegetation and the faeces of animals and humans. Eating food infected with these bacteria leads to the disease listeriosis. The symptoms are those of a mild flu-like illness. The infection can be much more serious and in some situations leads to septicaemia and meningitis.

Patients with reduced immunity, such as those receiving immunosuppressive drugs and those with cancer of the lymphatic system, are particularly at risk of listeriosis and should be advised to avoid foods which are likely sources of the bacteria (see Box 11.6).

The bacteria are destroyed by heat, so if chilled foods are re-heated correctly the bacteria will be killed.

Listeriosis in pregnancy. There is a risk that if a pregnant woman suffers listeriosis, the developing baby will also become infected. This can lead to miscarriage, stillbirth or severe illness in the newborn. It is for this reason that pregnant women should be advised to avoid food which may be contaminated with *Listeria monocytogenes*.

Table 11.1 summarises the characteristics of bacterial food poisoning.

Some other diseases resulting from bacterial infection of food

Information on the food sources of infection with the following diseases is summarised in Table 11.2.

Tuberculosis and brucellosis (undulant fever). These may be transmitted by unpasteurised milk, the original source of the infection being the udder of the cow.

Bovine tuberculosis has been almost totally eradicated from the UK. Brucellosis monitoring programmes are implemented and outbreaks are infrequent.

Typhoid fever and paratyphoid fever. These are often associated with poor sewage disposal, which results in a contaminated water supply. Oysters and other shell-

---

Box 11.5   Sources of *Clostridium perfringens* infection

- These organisms are present in soil
- They are also normal inhabitants of the intestines of both animals and humans

---

Box 11.6   Sources of *Listeria monocytogenes* infection

- Soft cheeses
- Chilled pâtés
- Chilled ready-to-serve meals

Table 11.1   Characteristics of bacterial food poisoning (Garrow et al 2000)

Organism	Common sources of infection	Site of toxin production	Incubation period (hours)	Mode of transmission	Reservoir of organism
Staphylococcus aureus	Ham, poultry and egg salads, cream-filled bakery produce, ice cream, cheese	Food	2–6	Food	Skin and mucous membranes of food handlers
Bacillus cereus	Cooked rice, cooked meats, vegetables, starchy puddings	Food (rapid onset) Intestine (slow)	1 16	Food	Soils, airborne spores
Clostridium botulinum	Fish, meat, home-preserved vegetables	Food, heat-labile	12–96	Food	Soil, mammals, birds, fish
Clostridium perfringens	Cooked meats and poultry, gravy, beans	Food	18–20	Food	Soils, animals, humans
Salmonella spp.	Poultry, meat, eggs, dairy produce, chocolate	Intestine	3–36	Food, some transmission from water and person-to-person	Poultry, most animals, humans
Campylobacter jejuni	Raw milk, poultry	Intestine	3–5 days	Water, food, person-to-person	Chickens, dogs, cats, cattle, pigs, wild birds
Escherichia coli	Salads, raw vegetables	Intestine	12–36	Water, food, person-to-person	Humans, water contaminated by sewage
Listeria monocytogenes	Soft cheeses, milk, paté, coleslaw	Intestine	1–90 days	Water, food, person-to-person	Very widely distributed in the environment

Note: undercooked meat, raw milk, cheese row — Escherichia coli appears before; the row "Undercooked meat, raw milk, cheese | Intestine | 12–36 | Water, food, person-to-person | Cattle, poultry, sheep"

Table 11.2 Sources of some food-borne diseases

Disease	Food sources of infection
Tuberculosis	Unpasteurised milk
Brucellosis	Unpasteurised milk
Typhoid fever	Contaminated shellfish
Paratyphoid fever	Contaminated shellfish
Botulism	Tinned food

fish may be a source of 'typhoid bacteria' if they have been obtained from water which is contaminated with sewage.

In the UK, legislation relating to the gathering and sale of shellfish helps to prevent the spread of infection in this way.

Botulism. This is a serious and often fatal disease which occurs only rarely in the UK. It results from the ingestion of a toxin produced by the bacterium *Clostridium botulinum*. This organism is present in soil. Therefore vegetables, fruit, meat and fish are susceptible to contamination by *Clostridium*. These bacteria multiply in food in the absence of oxygen, and the toxin produced is a product of their growth. In adverse conditions they develop spores, in which form they are able to survive until conditions once more become favourable for growth. The toxin is destroyed by heat but the spores are heat-resistant, requiring very high temperatures to destroy them.

No harm would result from the ingestion of infected food while fresh because spores and toxin have not been produced, but in the case of tinned or bottled food, if sterilising procedures have not been correctly carried out, spores may survive. Finding conditions in the can favourable for growth, they subsequently multiply in the food, making it poisonous. The spores are more heat-resistant in non-acid foods such as carrots, peas, beans and most vegetables than in the acid conditions associated with some fruits. Manufacturers of canned meats and other susceptible foods exercise great care, and foods heat-processed commercially may be considered safe.

PARASITIC INFESTATION OF FOOD

Food containing animal parasites can be a means of transmitting the parasites to humans. Tapeworm infestation can result from eating beef or pork which contains the organisms in the form of cysts. The cysts are destroyed by thorough cooking of the meat.

The eggs of roundworms and threadworms may be present in food which has been contaminated with human faeces. These are also destroyed during cooking. This type of infestation is particularly liable to

occur in countries where crops are fertilised with human excreta.

POISONOUS CHEMICALS IN FOODS

Poisoning may result from the presence in food of chemicals, traces of which are not necessarily harmful, but which could become harmful if present in sufficient quantity, for example:

* traces of pesticides used in agriculture can remain in the crop after harvesting
* antibiotics given to animals could possibly be present in animal products in significant amounts
* many foods contain chemical additives which are necessary for technical or other reasons
* certain plastic packaging material, in direct contact with the food, can leave a residue
* The concentration of heavy metals can build up in shellfish growing in polluted water.

In the UK the presence of chemicals in food is constantly monitored, and such matters as the presence of a particular material in a specific food (whether or not it is potentially harmful), the amount likely to be ingested, and the setting of safe limits, are the responsibility of bodies such as the Food Standards Agency. The Government has powers under the Food and Drugs Act of 1955 to make and enforce regulations when necessary to ensure safe food for the consumer.

In the home, chemicals such as weed-killers and cleaning materials may be added to food in error. Care should therefore be taken in the labelling and storage of such material.

POISONS PRESENT IN SOME FOODS

Red kidney beans contain the poison haemagglutinin, which is destroyed by boiling for 10 minutes, but not if beans are cooked slowly.

Cereals and nuts which have been infected with the moulds *Aspergillus flavus* and *Aspergillus parasiticus* contain the poison aflatoxin.

BSE AND CJD

Bovine spongiform encephalopathy (BSE) was first identified in cattle in 1986. The investigation into the cause of the infection concluded that it was caused by giving to cattle food that included, as the protein source, meat and bone meal from sheep that were infected with the spongiform encephalopathy scrapie. In 1990 the National CJD surveillance unit was established to identify changes in the pattern of human Creutzfeldt–Jakob disease (CJD) that might be attributable to BSE-infected cattle. In 1996 atypical cases of CJD were identified and it was proposed that they resulted from the eating of beef infected with BSE (Will et al 1996). By 1999 it was apparent that the prion strain which had caused BSE in cattle was causing the human prion disease new variant CJD.

Prions are infective agents which are proteins that are resistant to sterilising treatments. In the UK programmes of killing infected animals and changes in butchery practice have been introduced to prevent infected material from entering the food chain.

It is not known how many people will develop new variant CJD, estimates vary from a few hundred to hundreds of thousands. This uncertainty exists because the amount of infected material that needs to be eaten to cause infection, and the incubation period of the infection, are still unknown.

SAFE FOOD HANDLING

Once food has been infected with bacteria, the rate at which the bacteria multiply and the effectiveness with which they are destroyed are both dependent upon temperature (Table 11.3). This is why food stored in a refrigerator should be kept at 1–4°C and re-heating of food should be thorough. Food which is being kept warm should be kept at a temperature above 63°C.

Table 11.3 Increase of bacteria with change in temperature

Temperature (°C)	Effect
0	Food may freeze Bacteria not destroyed but do not multiply
1–4	Bacteria multiply very slowly
5–30	Rate of multiplication of bacteria increases with increases in temperature
30–45	Rate of multiplication of bacteria is optimal at some temperature in this range 37°C is the optimum for many bacteria
63–100	Food poisoning bacteria start to die: death rate increases with increase in temperature Toxins are not destroyed by this heat

National legislation sets compulsory standards for the production, distribution and sale of foodstuffs, and provides local authorities with the power to make by-laws to meet the special needs of each area. For example:

- Control is exercised over the circumstances in which milk may be produced or distributed, and there are standards with regard to bacteriological contamination to which all milk sold for human consumption must conform.
- Animals intended for slaughter must be free from disease and carcasses are subject to inspection.
- There are specifications covering the handling, wrapping and sale of foods, and premises used for the sale of food or the production of food intended for sale must conform to certain specifications.
- Control is exercised over the addition of chemicals to foods, for example as preservatives or as colouring matter.

It will be seen, then, that legislation relating to the production and distribution of foodstuffs affords a very considerable degree of protection to the consumer. Although recent legislation has made food-hygiene enforcement more effective, it should be appreciated that legislation is of necessity limited in its scope, and that its ultimate effectiveness depends upon the cooperation of each individual concerned in food handling.

Guidance for the food-handler

Food may be heavily contaminated with pathogenic organisms, and yet show no visible signs of spoilage, being unaffected in appearance, odour or taste.

Poisonous chemicals may easily be mistaken for foods and used as such if tins and bottles are not labelled, or if both chemicals and foods are kept in the same store cupboard. The presence of such poisonous material in food may be unsuspected until the food has been sampled and then, probably, the damage will have been done.

It will be seen, therefore, that food which appears in every way wholesome may yet contain pathogenic organisms or other harmful material. Safety depends upon the adoption of safe methods of handling food. The rules in Box 11.7 should be observed.

FOOD STANDARDS AGENCY

The Food Standards Agency is a new organisation created by Act of Parliament with a remit to:

Box 11.7   Safe food-handling

1. Wash the hands before preparing food and cover lesions such as cuts and burns with waterproof dressings.
2. Wash the hands after blowing the nose or going to the toilet; do not allow persons with septic skin conditions, respiratory infections or diarrhoea to handle food.
3. Do not touch food with the fingers unnecessarily.
4. See that food is protected from rats, mice, flies and domestic pets.
5. Do not leave crumbs and food particles lying around the kitchen; keep refuse bins covered.
6. Cooked and raw foods should be covered and kept separately. Wherever possible, food should be stored in a refrigerator. Refrigerators should be kept at 1–4°C and defrosted regularly. The lower the temperature, the lower the bacterial content.
7. The refrigerator must be cleaned regularly and its contents checked. Cooked food must be kept apart from raw food.
8. Avoid partial cooking of joints of meat intended for use on the following day, as this results in a temperature in the centre favourable to bacterial growth. A similar effect occurs in frozen chickens if these have not been completely thawed before cooking.
9. Food not used by Its 'use by' date should be discarded. Do not attempt to assess the condition of suspected food by tasting it. This practice is both dangerous and ineffective.
10. Store chemicals such as insecticides, cleaning materials and medicines away from food, and out of the reach of children. See that containers are clearly labelled.

---

protect public health from risks which may arise in connection with the consumption of food, and otherwise to protect the interests of consumers in relation to food.

It was established as a response to growing concerns about the safety of food in the UK, and the need for independent advice about food safety issues.

The Agency is led by a Board who have been appointed to act in the public interest and it is accountable to parliament through health ministers. The statutory functions of the Food Standards Agency are listed in Box 11.8.

In order to ensure that the Agency provides independent advice it publishes the advice that it gives to government. Further information about the Agency and its UK food surveillance programme can be found on its website (http://www.foodstandards.gov.uk).

Box 11.8   Functions of Food Standards Agency

1. To provide advice and information to the public and government on food safety from farm to fork, and nutrition and diet.
2. To protect consumers through effective enforcement and monitoring.
3. To support consumer advice through promoting accurate and meaningful labelling.

REFERENCES

Garrow J S, James W P T, Ralph A 2000 Human nutrition and dietetics, 10th edn. Churchill Livingstone, Edinburgh
Penington Group 1997 Report on the circumstances leading to the 1996 outbreak of infection with E. coli 0157 in Central Scotland, the implications for food safety and the lessons to be learned. HMSO, Edinburgh
Will R G, Ironside J N, Zeidler MZ 1996 A new variant of Creutzfeldt-Jakob disease in the UK. Lancet 347: 921–930

FURTHER READING

Collinge J 1999 Variant Creutzfeldt-Jakob disease. Lancet 354 (9175): 317–323
Patterson W J, Painter M J 1999 Bovine Spongiform encephalopathy and new variant Creutzfeldt-Jakob disease: an overview. Communicable Disease and Public Health 2(1): 5–13.
Wall P G 1999 Food poisoning. In: Truswell A S (ed) ABC of nutrition, 3rd Edn. London, British Medical Journal: pp. 89–95

12

Diet-related diseases

LEARNING OBJECTIVES

After studying this chapter you should have a clearer understanding of the:

- different relationships between diet and disease
- role of diet in the development and prevention of cardiovascular disease
- role of diet in the development and prevention of cancers
- foetal origins of disease hypothesis.

The association of diets deficient in essential nutrients with specific dietary deficiency diseases, and the use of diet as the treatment for certain diseases, are both accepted and well established. However, the role of diet in causing, or contributing to the causation of disease, is less well understood. This relationship is important in the aetiology of many of the non-infectious diseases which are the major causes of death and ill-health in the western world.

Diets and disease are related in four ways:

1. the use of diet as a treatment for disease
2. diseases which are caused by diet
3. diseases whose incidence is associated with diet
4. those diseases whose incidence appears to be related to foetal growth and birth-weight.

DIET AS A TREATMENT FOR DISEASE

Diet therapy is used to treat a wide range of diseases. The type of diet used depends on the nutritional status of the individual and the condition that is being treated. The types of diet therapy used can be divided into three broad categories:

1. Diet is used to reduce or prevent symptoms, for example a high-fibre diet for the treatment of constipation.

103

2. Diet is used to compensate metabolic abnormality, for example a low-phenylalanine diet for phenylketonuria.
3. Diet is used to promote recovery and repair, for example nutritional support to meet the increased nutrient needs of a patient following surgery.

There are many other ways in which diet is used to treat disease; they are explained in detail in Section 3 of this book.

DISEASES CAUSED BY DIET

Diet can cause disease when it contains too little or too much of a specific nutrient, if it contains dietary toxins, or when the food eaten is contaminated. One of the first diseases proven scientifically to be caused by diet was scurvy, which was common among sailors in the 18th century. James Lind (1753) was able to show that the addition of citrus fruits to the diet both cured and prevented scurvy. He also showed that other dietary and medicinal treatments were ineffective.

Excessive intakes of nutrients which cannot be metabolised and excreted, such as the fat-soluble vitamins and some minerals and trace elements, also cause disease. These disorders, along with the deficiency diseases, are described in the chapters on specific nutrients.

The presence of poisonous substances in the diet can also cause disease. These can be naturally occurring substances in the food or they can be formed in the food by processing, or added to food unintentionally. Some foods contain chemicals which can be toxic when consumed in large amounts. In the processing of food, substances may be formed which are harmful, for example hydrocarbons formed during the smoking of foods and by high-temperature frying. Chemical additives are frequently accused of causing disease, though they rarely do. In the UK, the EEC, North America and most westernised countries, food processing is controlled by legislation and food additives undergo an intensive programme of tests for toxic effects before they are used.

During storage and preparation, food can become contaminated with toxic substances such as bacteria, pesticides and heavy metals. Bacterial food poisoning is an acute disease which is easily identified. Other contaminants are less easily identified because the symptoms are less well known and take longer to develop (see Chapter 11).

DIET-ASSOCIATED DISEASES

The disease pattern of the western world has changed considerably in the last 150 years. Better hygiene, improved living standards and treatment with antibiotics have reduced the incidence of infectious diseases. It is now necessary to identify the causes of the large group of degenerative diseases, such as diseases of the cardiovascular system, and various malignant diseases. The incidence of these diseases is increasing and has been linked to diet. It is unlikely that these diseases are due to any one nutritional factor but rather to a combination of factors, some of which are nutritional. Most of the evidence to associate diet with disease is epidemiological.

The links between diet, socioeconomic status, disease and public health responses to this are discussed in Chapter 10, 'Public Health and Community Nutrition'.

Epidemiology

Early epidemiologists studied outbreaks of diseases such as cholera and typhoid. By studying these epidemics, they were able to understand the disease better by identifying both the source of infection and the way in which it was spread.

Epidemiologists study the distribution of all diseases, not only infectious ones, within a population and try to identify factors which influence them. These factors include geographical location, climate, age, income, occupation, ethnic group and diet. It is always difficult to identify one particular factor because many may be involved.

For example, the incidence of bowel disease among African bushmen is lower than among western businessmen. This could be because the diet of businessmen is different, or because they drive to work, or even that they own a personal computer, or any of a host of other factors. Epidemiological evidence can suggest causes which are also factors associated statistically with a disease and may identify relationships between disease and environment, but it rarely provides conclusive proof. Experimental evidence is needed to confirm a hypothesis. This is very difficult to obtain because the degenerative and malignant diseases take a long time to develop in humans and evidence from animal experiments is not always available or directly applicable to humans.

Evidence from epidemiological studies does not necessarily mean that an individual exposed to a specific environmental factor will develop a disease. It indicates that the incidence of a disease among the population exposed to that factor is higher than the incidence in a population not exposed, and identifies risk factors. Increased incidence of both cardiovascular disease and some malignant diseases has been associated with diet and are discussed below.

DIET AND CARDIOVASCULAR DISEASE

Cardiovascular disease (CVD) is a term which includes coronary heart disease (CHD), stroke and peripheral atherosclerosis. The major form of CVD is CHD.

The term CHD includes sudden death, acute myocardial infarction and angina pectoris. It is a major cause of death in western countries and the incidence is increasing in some developing countries and some eastern European countries.

Although the death rates from CHD and stroke in England have fallen they continue to be among the worst in Europe. In 1997 41% of adult deaths before the age of 75 years were due to circulatory disease (DoH 1998a). The *Our Healthier Nation* target for coronary heart disease and stroke is to reduce the death rate from CHD, stroke and related diseases by at least two fifths by 2010 (DoH 1999).

Incidence of CHD in the UK

Life-expectancy in the UK is among the highest in the world, but so is the incidence of CHD.

However, not every adult in the UK will suffer a heart attack. Factors have been identified which appear to increase the risk of cardiovascular disease.

These factors have been divided into four categories in *The Health of the Nation Key Area Handbook* (DoH 1993) (see Box 12.1).

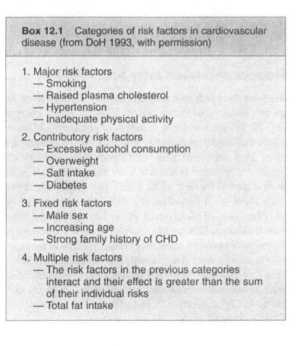

Box 12.1 Categories of risk factors in cardiovascular disease (from DoH 1993, with permission)

1. Major risk factors
   — Smoking
   — Raised plasma cholesterol
   — Hypertension
   — Inadequate physical activity

2. Contributory risk factors
   — Excessive alcohol consumption
   — Overweight
   — Salt intake
   — Diabetes

3. Fixed risk factors
   — Male sex
   — Increasing age
   — Strong family history of CHD

4. Multiple risk factors
   — The risk factors in the previous categories interact and their effect is greater than the sum of their individual risks
   — Total fat intake

Of these risk factors, only six can be considered to have a dietary component and it is only these six that will be discussed in this book. For further information on the other factors, see the handbook (DoH 1993).

Raised plasma cholesterol

Evidence for the link between raised plasma cholesterol and increased incidence of CHD comes from many studies including those of Rose & Shipley (1986) and Pocock et al (1989), which showed that the higher the plasma cholesterol level the greater the risk of CHD.

As improved methods of measuring plasma cholesterol have been developed, it has become possible to differentiate between different sorts of cholesterol.

There is a considerable variation in the mean plasma cholesterol for different populations and within these populations there will also be variations. Two populations with a low plasma cholesterol are Kalahari Bushmen and Masai tribespeople. They have a mean value of 3.0 mmol/l compared with an average value for UK adults of 5.8 mmol/l (Gregory et al 1990) and higher values in some other places, e.g. 7.2 mmol/l in East Finland.

It is only in countries where the average cholesterol figure exceeds 5.2 mmol/l that CHD is common. Martin et al (1986) state that people with a cholesterol level of higher than 6.5 mmol/l are at high risk of CHD, and the European Atherosclerosis Society recommends intervention to lower the level for individuals with a plasma cholesterol of higher than 6.5 mmol/l (EAS 1987).

A level of 5.2–6.5 mmol/l constitutes a moderate risk of coronary disease. The UK government's white paper *The Health of the Nation* (DoH 1992) concluded that the plasma cholesterol sets a baseline of CHD risk within the population.

Total plasma cholesterol can be divided into two fractions:

- LDL cholesterol
- HDL cholesterol.

The major portion of the plasma cholesterol is carried on low-density lipoproteins and so is known as LDL cholesterol. It is this portion that is associated with increased CHD risk. A reduction of LDL cholesterol is associated with a reduced risk of CHD.

It has been proposed that the HDL (high-density lipoprotein) has a protective role against CHD and the ratio of HDL to total cholesterol or to LDL is sometimes used as a marker of CHD risk.

It has been suggested by Bingham (1991) that if *Health of the Nation* targets were achieved the average serum cholesterol would be reduced to 5.4 mmol/l and that this would result in a corresponding reduction in the mortality from cardiovascular disease over time.

Many nutritional factors affect cholesterol levels, some more than others. They are listed in Box 12.2.

Total fat

In the UK diet, fat provides approximately 40% of the food energy. It comprises saturated, polyunsaturated and monounsaturated fat (see Chapter 3 for chemical structures). There is epidemiological evidence to link the death rate from CHD in different countries with the national fat intake (Keys 1980). This can be partly explained by the link between saturated fatty acid (SFA) intake and plasma cholesterol and the link between total fat intake and obesity, both CHD risk factors. Romieu et al (1988) and Dreon et al (1988) observed a positive correlation between the proportion of dietary energy provided by fat and incidence of obesity. Foods which have a high fat content are more energy dense, so overconsumption of these foods can rapidly lead to the development of obesity. There is also some evidence to suggest that a high fat intake increases the tendency of the blood to clot (Miller et al 1989).

In the light of the evidence, the Committee on Medical Aspects of Food Policy (COMA) report (DoH 1994) recommends that the current proportion of dietary energy provided by total fat, currently about 40%, should be reduced to 35%.

Saturated fatty acids (SFA)

The National Food Survey (MAFF 1994) shows that in the UK saturated fats contribute 16% of the food energy and that the principal sources of this are dairy and meat products and fat spreads.

Box 12.2 Nutritional factors that affect cholesterol levels

- Saturated fat intake (SFA)
- Monounsaturated fat intake (MFA)
- Polyunsaturated fat intake (PUFA)
- n-6 polyunsaturated fatty acids (n-6 PUFA)
- *Trans* fatty acids
- Balance of fatty acids
- Carbohydrate intake
- NSP intake
- Sodium
- Potassium
- Antioxidant nutrients
- Alcohol

An early study which showed the link between the percentage of dietary energy provided by fat and CHD mortality was the 'Seven Countries' study (Keys 1980), which showed that two-thirds of the variation in plasma cholesterol concentration could be predicted by dietary intakes of SFA and cholesterol. It is known that when people migrate from a country where the dietary fat and SFA intake is low to one where it is higher, and the migrants adopt the new diet, their plasma cholesterol level also changes to be in line with that of the rest of the population.

As has already been mentioned, meat products are a significant contributor to the saturated fatty acid content of the diet. A comparison between the blood cholesterol levels of strict vegetarians and meat eaters (Sanders & Roshanai 1984) has shown that the vegetarian group had the lowest cholesterol levels and that this could be explained almost entirely by the differences in SFA intake. The evidence for the links between SFA intake and plasma cholesterol has led to the COMA recommendation that dietary intake of SFA should be reduced to no more than about 10% of dietary energy (DoH 1994).

As the amount of SFA in the diet increases, so do the levels of LDL cholesterol and total cholesterol (Grundy 1991). However, all SFA do not have the same effect on plasma cholesterol levels, there being no evidence to show that SFA with a chain-length of less than 12 or greater than 16 (see Chapter 3) raise plasma cholesterol. The SFA which have been shown to raise plasma cholesterol are: lauric (12 carbon atoms in chain), myristic (14), and palmitic (16) acids (Mensink 1993).

Monounsaturated fatty acids (MFA)

MFA are the predominant class of fatty acids present in most foods, providing about 15% of food energy (MAFF 1994). The most commonly occurring MFA is oleic acid, which is found at particularly high levels in olive and rapeseed oils. LDL and total cholesterol levels are reduced when MFA are substituted for SFA in the diet (Hegsted et al 1965), but enriching diets with oleate-rich fats does not result in a reduction in the plasma total cholesterol. It has been proposed that substitution of SFA by MFA is better than substitution by polyunsaturated fatty acids (PUFA). This is because PUFA also lower HDL cholesterol, which is not desirable (see below). Among Mediterranean populations, who consistently consume a diet richer in MFA and lower in SFA than the UK population, the incidence of CHD is lower.

Polyunsaturated fatty acids (PUFA)

The PUFA can be divided into two classes which have different biological effects. These are the n-3 PUFA and n-6 PUFA.

n-6 PUFA

This group is found in seed oils and polyunsaturated margarines and includes the essential fatty acids. When substituted for SFA, they lower both LDL cholesterol and HDL cholesterol.

Many n-6 PUFA seed oils are also a rich source of vitamin E, an antioxidant which may have a protective role by preventing the peroxidation of lipids in the artery wall. There has been a trend for n-6 PUFA to replace SFA in the national diet, the average UK intake of n-6 PUFA now being 6%. Because there is as yet no evidence as to the safety of a lifetime's diet containing more than 9–10% of dietary energy as PUFA, it is recommended that the average intake of n-6 PUFA does not increase beyond 6%.

n-3 PUFA

Currently, less than 1% of food energy is provided by n-3 PUFA. There is much interest in the role of long-chain n-3 PUFA. These have a chain of 20 or 22 carbon atoms and their most common dietary source is oily fish. Salmon, trout, sardine, pilchard, herring, tuna and mackerel are oily fish. Currently only about one-third of adults eat oily fish in any week, so the current average intake of long-chain n-3 PUFA is about 0.1 g/day.

The long-chain n-3 PUFA have an antithrombotic and antiinflammatory effect but have only a minimal effect on LDL and HDL cholesterol levels.

There is evidence to show an inverse relationship between fish consumption and CHD mortality (Kromhout et al 1985). Increasing the consumption of oily fish by men who had already had a heart attack resulted in a reduction in mortality from CHD (Burr et al 1989) and it seems reasonable to suppose that increasing the consumption of oily fish not only reduces the risk of death from recurrent heart attacks but also reduces the risk of a first heart attack.

It is recommended by COMA that the population average consumption of n-3 PUFA be doubled to 0.2 g/day and that this is done by increasing oily fish consumption.

Trans fatty acids (TFA)

Most naturally occurring fatty acids are in the *cis* form. Fatty acids which are hydrogenated exist in the *trans* form. Currently, the average intake of *trans* fatty acids is 2% of food energy (about 5 g/day). This comes from confectionery, biscuits, margarines and some dairy and meat products.

Mensink et al (1992) have shown that *trans* fatty acids raise LDL cholesterol and lower HDL cholesterol. Other workers have also shown *trans* fatty acids from hydrogenated vegetable oils to be the most harmful, and a study by Ascherio et al (1994) on the intake of *trans* fatty acids showed that people with the highest intake had twice the risk of myocardial infarction as did those with the lowest intakes.

Dietary cholesterol

Public awareness and confusion is great about the role that dietary cholesterol plays in the development of heart disease. The average UK intake has fallen and is now 245 mg/day.

Increasing the cholesterol level in the diet increases the LDL cholesterol, but there is a wide variation in response between individuals. The response appears only to occur within the range of dietary intakes 95–450 mg/1000 kcal. When the cholesterol intake exceeds this level, the excess cholesterol either suppresses endogenous cholesterol production or is not absorbed.

Dietary cholesterol is generally found in foods with a high SFA content, so reduction of SFA will automatically reduce cholesterol intake. Egg yolks are an exception to this, having a high cholesterol content without a correspondingly high fat content. It is recommended that the average dietary intake of cholesterol should not rise above the current level of 245 mg/day (DoH 1994).

OTHER DIETARY FACTORS AFFECTING CHD

Dietary antioxidants

Oxygen-derived free radicals (for further explanation see Garrow et al 2000) are released during most normal physiological processes and are important in the cause of cancers, and cardiovascular and cerebrovascular diseases. They act by attacking DNA, proteins and the unsaturated fatty acids in lipoproteins and cell membranes.

Foods which are rich sources of polyunsaturated fatty acids, such as seeds and some grains, are also rich sources of vitamin E. This antioxidant vitamin is present to prevent the polyunsaturated fatty acids from being oxidised.

Other antioxidants found in the diet are selenium, vitamin C and carotenoids (precursors of vitamin A, see Chapter 6), which are found in fruit and vegetables. Low plasma levels of vitamins C and E and low dietary intakes of fruit and vegetables are associated with a higher incidence of CHD (Gey et al 1991). There is evidence to suggest that a diet rich in the antioxidant vitamins C and E is protective against heart disease (Steinberg 1993).

NSP

Some forms of non-starch polysaccharides (NSP), particularly the soluble ones found in pulses, reduce the plasma total cholesterol levels (Mehta 2001). Ripsin et al (1992) showed that including oat bran or oatmeal in the diet had a modest effect on the plasma cholesterol level, with the greatest reduction being seen in those subjects with plasma cholesterol levels higher than 5.9 mmol/l. Three mechanisms have been suggested for the way in which plasma cholesterol is reduced by NSP (Ashwell 1993):

1. Cholesterol and bile acids in the small intestine may bind to NSP, so preventing them from being reabsorbed.
2. Soluble NSP are fermented by colonic bacteria producing, among other things, proprionate which may inhibit cholesterol formation by the liver.
3. NSP slows the rate of glucose absorption in the small intestine, which results in lower concentrations of blood insulin which may decrease cholesterol synthesis in the short term.

Water

There is a lower level of CHD in areas where the water is hard, but the size of this effect is small. Nevertheless, it is recommended that it is prudent for people living in hard-water areas not to artificially soften their drinking water.

Coffee and tea

The evidence linking coffee and caffeine consumption with CHD is inconsistent. Brown et al (1993) have shown that in the UK coffee consumption does not affect CHD risk. Tea drinkers consume a similar amount of caffeine to coffee drinkers but there is little evidence to show any effect of tea consumption on either CHD or plasma cholesterol. Tea is a rich source of flavenoids which are antioxidant nutrients, so may be beneficial.

Garlic and onions

Alliin is the principal bioactive constituent of garlic and onions. Garlic contains more alliin than onions but onions also contain antioxidant flavenoids, which may have potential to influence atherogenesis. There is no conclusive evidence for an effect of fresh garlic or onions (or commercial preparations) on cardiovascular risk factors or clinical events (Kleijnen et al 1989, Mansell & Reckless 1991).

HYPERTENSION AND STROKE

Stroke is a major cause of disability among elderly people in the UK and, in 1991, approximately 12% of all UK deaths resulted from stroke. The most important risk factor for stroke is raised blood pressure (DoH 1992). Dietary factors which contribute to raised blood pressure are:

- sodium intake
- excessive alcohol intake
- excessive energy intake leading to obesity.

Sodium intake

Sodium is an essential nutrient and contained in a wide range of foods. The majority of sodium in the diet comes from salt added to food. In the UK, the average daily salt intake is 9 g/day and the predominant source is salt added in the manufacturing and processing of foods, estimated at between 60–85% of total salt intake (Gregory et al 1990).

Internationally there is a wide range in salt intake. Hypertension is virtually unknown in Kalahari Bushmen who have an average intake of 2 g/day, whereas in northern Japan, where the average intake is 25 g/day, the incidence of hypertension and stroke is very high.

There is much evidence to show that restricting the amount of salt in the diet reduces the blood pressure of people who have mild to moderate hypertension (MacGregor et al 1989, Weinberger et al 1988), but the evidence that restricting the salt intake of people whose blood pressure is within the normal range lowers blood pressure has been inconsistent. However, the COMA report *Nutritional Aspects of Cardiovascular Disease* (DoH 1994) concluded that, 'sodium intake appears to be an important determinant of blood pressure in the population as a whole at least partly by influencing the rise in blood pressure with age'. The degree of an individual's sensitivity to salt appears to be greater with increasing age and higher initial blood pressure.

Potassium intake

Increased dietary potassium intakes may reduce blood pressure (Cappuccio & MacGregor 1991). Fruit and vegetables are rich sources of potassium and this may be a further reason for the benefit of increasing fruit and vegetable consumption.

Alcohol and blood pressure

Blood pressure rises with acute alcohol consumption but blood pressure is also related to habitual alcohol consumption, heavy drinkers having a higher blood pressure than light drinkers (ICRG 1988).

Obesity and blood pressure

Obesity inevitably develops when the energy intake is greater than energy expenditure. As foods which have a high fat content are more energy-dense, an overconsumption of these foods can lead to the development of obesity.

Stamler et al (1978) have shown that hypertension is 50% more prevalent in older obese subjects and twice as prevalent in young obese subjects, as in those subjects with normal weight. Weight loss is an effective treatment for hypertension and all overweight hypertensive patients should be encouraged to lose weight (Hovell 1982). If hypertensive obese patients lose weight, they can be expected to show blood pressure reductions of 10 mmHg systolic/5 mmHg diastolic for 5 kg weight loss (Truswell 1992).

DIET AND THE DEVELOPMENT OF CANCER

Diet is an important lifestyle factor in the development of cancer. It has been estimated that diet is the most important lifestyle factor in the development of up to 80% of cancers of the large bowel, breast and prostate (Willett 1995). Diet also contributes, but to a lesser and varying extent, to the risk of developing other cancers including those of the lung, stomach, pancreas and oesophagus (Cummings & Bingham 1998).

In 1997 cancers accounted for 21% of deaths before the age of 75 years in England (DoH 1998a) and diet accounted for about one quarter of the cancer deaths (DoH 1998b). It is suggested that the lifestyle changes of stopping smoking and adopting a diet that is rich in cereals, fruit and vegetables could reduce cancer death rates in those under 75 by 10% by 2010 in England (DoH 1998b).

The evidence to link diet with specific cancers is briefly reviewed in the next sections. For more detail the reports, *Nutritional Aspects of the Development of Cancers* (DoH 1998b) and *Food, Nutrition and the Prevention of Cancer: a Global Perspective* (WCRF 1997) should be consulted.

Gastric cancer

The nitrite content of the diet correlates with the incidence of gastric cancer. Nitrites and nitrates are used to preserve food, particularly meat. They are converted in the stomach to nitrosamines, which are known to be carcinogenic under some circumstances. The countries with the highest incidence of gastric cancer are Chile and Colombia, where the water has a high nitrate content, and Japan, where the diet is rich in salted and smoked dried foods. Its incidence in England and Wales has declined in recent years (Howson et al 1986), though the reason why is not clear. It may be due to the change to refrigeration as a means of food preservation. A diet rich in fruit and vegetables is associated with a low incidence of this disease. Laboratory experiments have shown that ascorbic acid inhibits nitrosamine formation and this may be part of the explanation. Diets which contain a lot of preserved foods have a low vitamin C content and it may be that the increased incidence of gastric cancer is due to the lack of protection provided by vitamin C, rather than the nitrates and nitrites in the food. Many studies have shown the relationship between fruit and vegetable intake and incidence of stomach and oesophageal cancers (Burr 1994).

Helicobacter pylori infection of the stomach is a cause of chronic gastritis which is a precursor of gastric cancer. This infection results in increased production of free radicals. Vegetables are good sources of the antioxidants beta-carotene and vitamin E and so may be important in preventing damage by these free radicals.

Breast and endometrial cancers

Epidemiological evidence shows that these diseases are more common among women eating a western-type diet than in women eating an unrefined, low-fat diet (Armstrong & Doll 1973). These diseases are oestrogen-dependent, and are also associated with obesity, which causes an increase in oestrogen production (Herschopf & Bradlow 1987). Dietary fat does not act directly as a carcinogen but acts indirectly by altering hormonal balance and by contributing to the development of obesity.

High intakes of meat and alcohol are associated with increased risk of breast cancer (Smith-Warner et al 1998) and low intakes of vegetables, non-starch polysaccharide and phytoestrogens have also been implicated (Bingham et al 1998).

Prostate cancer

There is evidence of a modest increase in risk of prostate cancer, associated with a high consumption of red meat and a modest decrease in risk associated with a high intake of vegetables and salads (DoH 1998b).

Colorectal cancer

Population studies have related the prevalence of diverticular disease, appendicitis, large bowel cancer, haemorrhoids and constipation to dietary fibre intake (Trowell et al 1985). Diets which have a high NSP content generally have a low fat and animal protein content. Willett et al (1990) reported a reduced risk of colonic cancer among vegetarians and an increased risk with high saturated and monounsaturated fat intakes. Bingham et al (1979) reported that the death rates from colon cancer in different regions of the UK were negatively correlated with the local consumption of vegetables excluding potatoes. The COMA report, *Nutritional Aspects of the Development of Cancer* (DoH 1998b), reports that there is moderately consistent evidence that diets with less red and processed meat and more vegetables and NSP are associated with reduced risk of colorectal cancer.

NSP reduces the risk of colorectal cancer in two ways. These are:

1. By increasing stool bulk and reducing transit time NSP prevents constipation. Constipation is a risk factor for colorectal cancer (DoH 1998b).
2. Its fermentation by the colon microflora produces short-chain fatty acids, in particular butyrate, which has a protective effect against colorectal cancer.

It has been proposed that the link between dietary intake of red and processed meats and colorectal cancer are due to:

1. The heterocyclic amines formed when meat is browned during cooking.
2. The increased level of ammonia in the bowel that is associated with high meat intake.
3. The formation of N-nitrosocompounds, which are possible carcinogens, in the bowel from the meat residues in the bowel contents.

Other dietary factors which have been implicated in colorectal cancer are obesity and intakes of iron, calcium, flavenoids, phytoestrogens and carotenoids.

Other cancers

Mouth, pharynx, pancreatic and liver cancers are associated with a high alcohol intake.

The six key components of dietary advice to reduce cancer risk are summarised below:

- Eat plenty of fruit and vegetables (at least five portions a day)
- Eat plenty of cereal foods, mainly in the unprocessed form (as a source of NSP)
- Maintain ideal body-weight (BMI 20–25) (avoid fatty foods)
- Eat red meat and processed meat in moderation (no more than 140 g/day)
- Alcohol in moderation (a maximum of two units a day for women and three units a day for men)
- Avoid highly salted and mouldy foods.

DIET AND CONSTIPATION

Constipation is characterised by infrequent bowel habits (less than three times a week), a stool weight of below 50 g/day and a transit time of 5 days or more. It is more common in women than men and is more common in those aged over 65 years. It is the cause of considerable morbidity in the UK.

In the UK, the median stool weight is about 100 g/day with 18% of the population passing less than 50 g/day.

There is individual variation in the response of bowel habit to NSP intake. Experimental studies show that as NSP intake increases so does stool weight, and that on an NSP-free diet stool weight falls to 30–60 g/day and constipation develops (see Chapter 8).

Dietary NSP are not digested in the human stomach and small intestine. Once they enter the large intestine, most forms of NSP are fermented by the anaerobic flora to produce short-chain fatty acids, carbon dioxide, hydrogen and methane.

The type of NSP found in cereals has a greater effect on stool weight than that present in fruit and vegetables (Cummings et al 1978), because of its greater water-holding capacity.

THE FOETAL ORIGIN OF DISEASE

The foetal origin of disease hypothesis was proposed following an investigation into the cardiovascular mortality of a cohort of men for whom accurate records of birth-weight and weight during the first year of life had been kept. This study showed that ischaemic heart disease was commoner in those men who had been both small at birth and at 1 year (Barker & Osmond 1986). Further work published in 1991 linked reduced interuterine growth to high blood pressure, impaired glucose tolerance and non-insulin dependent diabetes (Hales et al 1991).

It is hypothesised that the foetus undergoes permanent metabolic and endocrine changes as a response to under-nutrition. These changes would be beneficial if nutrition continued to be inadequate after birth.

However, if nutrition after birth is plentiful then these metabolic and endocrine changes make the individual more likely to become obese and have impaired glucose tolerance. While this theory is plausible, the need for further research into the complex interactions between prenatal and postnatal environmental and social factors has been identified (Lucas et al 1999) and will continue.

REFERENCES

Armstrong B, Doll R 1973 Environmental factors and cancer incidence in different countries with special reference to dietary practices. International Journal of Cancer 15: 617–631

Ascherio A, Hennekens C H, Buring J E, Master C, Stampfer M J, Willett W C 1994 Trans fatty acids intake and risk of myocardial infarction. Circulation 89: 94–101

Ashwell M (ed) 1993 Diet and heart disease: a round table of factors. British Nutrition Foundation, London

Barker D J P, Osmond C 1986 Infant mortality, childhood nutrition and ischaemic heart disease in England and Wales. Lancet (i) 1077–1081

Bingham S 1991 Dietary aspects of a health strategy for England. British Medical Journal 303: 353–355

Bingham S, Williams D R R, Cole T J, James W P T 1979 Dietary fibre and regional large-bowel cancer mortality in Britain. British Journal of Cancer 40: 456–463

Bingham S A, Atkinson C, Liggins J, Bluck L, Coward A 1998 Phytoestrogens: where are we now? British Journal of Nutrition 79: 393–406

Brown C A, Bolton-Smith C, Woodward M, Tunstall-Pedoe H 1993 Coffee and tea consumption and the prevalence of coronary heart disease in men and women: results from the Scottish Heart Health Study. Journal of Epidemiology and Community Health 47: 171–175

Burr M L 1994 Antioxidants and cancer. Journal of Human Nutrition and Dietetics 7: 409–416

Burr M L, Fehily A M, Gilbert J F et al 1989 Effects of changes in fat, fish and fibre intakes on death and myocardial reinfarction: Diet and Reinfarction Trial (DART). Lancet (ii): 757–761

Cappuccio F P, MacGregor G A 1991 Does potassium supplementation lower blood pressure? A meta-analysis of published trials. Journal of Hypertension 9: 465–473

Cummings J H, Southgate D A T, Branch W J et al 1978 The colonic response to dietary fibre from carrot, cabbage, apple, bran and guar gum. Lancet (i): 5–8

Cummings J, Bingham S A 1998 Diet and the prevention of cancer. British Medical Journal 317: 1636–1640

Department of Health (DoH) 1992 The health of the nation: a strategy for health in England. HMSO, London

Department of Health (DoH) 1993 The health of the nation key area handbook: coronary heart disease and stroke. Department of Health, Heywood, Lancashire

Department of Health (DoH) 1994 Nutritional aspects of cardiovascular disease. Report of the cardiovascular review group of the committee on medical aspects of food policy (COMA) (Report on Health and Social Subjects 46). HMSO, London

Department of Health (DoH) 1998a Public health common data set. Office for National Statistics, HMSO, London

Department of Health (DoH) 1998b Nutritional aspects of the development of cancer. Report of the working group on diet and cancer of the committee on medical aspects of food and nutrition policy (COMA) (Report on Health and Social Subjects 48). HMSO, London

Department of Health (DoH) 1999 Saving lives: our healthier nation. HMSO, London

Dreon D M, Frey-Hewitt B, Ellsworth N, Williams P T, Terry R B, Wood P D 1988 Dietary fat: carbohydrate ratio and obesity in middle-aged men. American Journal of Clinical Nutrition 47: 995–1000

European Atherosclerosis Society Study Group (EAS) 1987 Strategies for the prevention of coronary heart disease: a policy statement of the European Atherosclerosis Society. European Heart Journal 8: 77–88

Garrow J S, James W P T, Ralph A 2000 Human nutrition and dietetics, 10th edn. Churchill Livingstone, Edinburgh

Gey K F, Puska P, Jordan P, Moser U K 1991 Inverse correlation between plasma vitamin E and mortality from ischemic heart disease in cross-cultural epidemiology. American Journal of Clinical Nutrition 53 (1 Suppl): 326S–334S

Gregory J, Foster K, Tyler H, Wiseman M 1990 The dietary and nutritional survey of British adults aged 16 to 64 living in Great Britain. Office of Population Censuses and Surveys, Social Survey Division. HMSO, London

Grundy S M 1991 Multifactorial etiology of hypercholesterolemia: implications for prevention of coronary heart disease. Arteriosclerosis and Thrombosis 11: 1619–1633

Hales C N, Barker D J, Clark P M et al 1991 Fetal and infant growth and impaired glucose tolerance at age 64. British Medical Journal 303(6809): 1019–1022

Hegsted D M, McGandy R B, Myers M L, Stare F J 1965 Quantitative effects of dietary fat on serum cholesterol in man. American Journal of Clinical Nutrition 17: 281–295

Herschopf R J, Bradlow H L 1987 Obesity, diet, endogenous estrogens and the risk of hormone-sensitive cancer. American Journal of Clinical Nutrition 45 (Suppl 1): 354–360

Hovell M F 1982 The experimental evidence for weight loss treatment of essential hypertension: a critical review. American Journal of Public Health 72: 359–368

Howson C P, Hiyama T, Wynder E L 1986 The decline in gastric cancer: epidemiology of an unplanned triumph. Epidemiology Review 8: 1–27

Intersalt Cooperative Research Group (ICRG) 1988 Intersalt: an international study of electrolyte excretion and blood pressure. Results for 24-hour urinary sodium and potassium excretion. British Medical Journal 297: 319–328

Keys A 1980 Seven countries: multivariate analysis of death and coronary heart disease. Harvard University Press, Cambridge MA

Kleijnen J, Knipschild P, ter Riet G 1989 Garlic, onions and cardiovascular risk factors: a review of the evidence from human experiments with emphasis on commercially available preparations. British Journal of Clinical Pharmacology 28: 535–544

Kromhout D, Bosschieter E B, De Lezenne Coulander C 1985 The inverse relation between fish consumption and 20-year mortality from coronary heart disease. New England Journal of Medicine 312: 1205–1209

Lind J 1753 A treatise of the scurvy (Reprinted 1953) Edinburgh University Press, Edinburgh

Lucas A, Fewtrell M S, Cole T J 1999 Fetal origins of adult disease—the hypothesis revisited. British Medical Journal 319: 245–249

MacGregor G A, Markandu N D, Sagnella G A, Singer D R, Cappuccio F P 1989 Double-blind study of three sodium intakes and long-term effects of sodium restriction in essential hypertension. Lancet 2: 1244–1247

Mansell P, Reckless J P 1991 Garlic: effects on serum lipids, blood pressure, coagulation, platelet aggregation and vasodilation. British Medical Journal 303: 379–380

Martin M J, Hulley S B, Browner W S, Kuller L H, Wentworth D 1986 Serum cholesterol, blood pressure and mortality: implications from a cohort of 361 662 men. Lancet 2: 933–936

Mehta D 2001 BNF42 British National Formulary. British Medical Association and the Royal Pharmaceutical Society, London (www.bnf.org)

Mensink R P 1993 Effects of the individual saturated fatty acids on serum lipids and lipoprotein levels. American Journal of Clinical Nutrition 57(S): 711S–714S

Mensink R P, Zock P L, Katan M B, Hornstra G 1992 Effects of dietary *cis* and *trans* fatty acids on serum lipoprotein(a) levels in humans. Journal of Lipid Research 33: 1493–1501

Miller G J, Cruickshank J K, Ellis L J et al 1989 Fat consumption and factor VII coagulant activity in middle-aged men: an association between a dietary and thrombogenic coronary risk factor. Atherosclerosis 78: 19–24

Ministry of Agriculture, Fisheries and Food (MAFF) 1994 Household food consumption and expenditure 1993. Annual Report of the National Food Survey Committee. HMSO, London

Pocock S J, Shaper A G, Phillips A N 1989 Concentrations of high density lipoprotein cholesterol, triglycerides and total cholesterol in ischaemic heart disease. British Medical Journal 298: 998–1002

Ripsin C M, Keenan J M, Jacobs D R et al 1992 Oat products and lipid lowering—a meta-analysis. Journal of the American Medical Association 267: 3317–3325

Romieu I, Willett W C, Stampfer M J et al 1988 Energy intake and other determinants of relative weight. American Journal of Clinical Nutrition 47: 406–412

Rose G, Shipley M 1986 Plasma cholesterol concentration and death from coronary heart disease: 10-year results of the Whitehall study. British Medical Journal 293: 306–307

Sanders T A B, Roshanai F 1984 Assessment of fatty acid intakes in vegans and omnivores. Human Nutrition: Applied Nutrition 38A: 345–354

Smith-Warner S A, Spiegelman D, Yaun S S et al 1998 Alcohol and breast cancer in women. Journal of the American Medical Association 279: 535–540

Stamler R, Stamler J, Reidlinger W F, Algera G, Robers R H 1978 Weight and blood pressure. Journal of the American Medical Association 240: 1607–1610

Steinberg D 1993 Antioxidant vitamins and coronary heart disease. New England Journal of Medicine 328: 1487–1489

Trowell H, Burkitt D, Heaton K (eds) 1985 Dietary fibre, fibre-depleted foods and disease. Academic Press, London

Truswell A S 1992 ABC of nutrition, 2nd Edn. British Medical Journal, London

Weinberger M H, Cohen S J, Miller J Z, Luft F C, Grim C E, Fineberg N S 1988 Dietary sodium restriction as adjunctive treatment of hypertension. Journal of the American Medical Association 259: 2561–2565

Willett W C, Stampfer M J, Colditz G A, Rosner B A, Speizer F E 1990 Relation of meat, fat and fiber intake to the risk of colon cancer in a prospective study among women. New England Journal of Medicine 323: 1664–1672

Willett W C, 1995 Diet, nutrition and avoidable cancer. Environmental health perspectives 103 (Suppl 8): 165–170

World Cancer Research Fund (WCRF) 1997 Food, nutrition and the prevention of cancer: a global perspective. World Cancer Research Fund, American Institute of Cancer Research, Washington DC

FURTHER READING

Ashwell M (ed) 1993 Diet and heart disease: a round table of factors. British Nutrition Foundation, London

Department of Health 1993 The health of the nation key area handbook: coronary heart disease and stroke. Department of Health, Heywood, Lancashire

Garrow J S, James W P T, Ralph A 2000 Human nutrition and dietetics, Chapter 13, 10th edn. Churchill Livingstone, Edinburgh

Health Education Authority 1999 Nutritional aspects of the development of cancer. Health Education Authority, London

Sanders T (for the Health Education Authority) 1994 Dietary fats: nutrition briefing paper. Health Education Authority, London

Scottish Intercollegiate Guidelines 1999 Lipids and the primary prevention of coronary heart disease. A National Clinical Guideline. SIGN, Edinburgh

USEFUL ADDRESSES

Cancer Research Campaign
10 Cambridge Terrace
London NW1 4JL
Tel: 020 7224 1333
Website: www.crc.org.uk

British Heart Foundation
14 Fitzhardinge Street
London W1H 6DH
Tel: 020 7935 0185
Website: www.bhf.org.uk

13

Factors which influence food choice

LEARNING OBJECTIVE

After studying this chapter you should have a clearer understanding of the range of factors which influence the food choice of individuals and groups.

Food is perceived to be fundamental to life in all societies. There is no universal diet consumed by everyone or even by everyone in the same geographical location.

The food supply for some people is so limited that there is no opportunity to exercise any choice at all. However, cultural taboos will still exist and some foods will never be eaten. For other people there is an enormous range of foods from which to choose.

It is important that health workers know what their patients and clients eat and the factors which have led them to choose their diet. It is only by understanding what an individual eats and why that particular diet is chosen, that a health worker can offer acceptable, realistic advice about changing the diet to a healthier one.

For those people who have a wide range of foods from which to choose the choice is influenced by a range of factors (see Fig. 13.1).

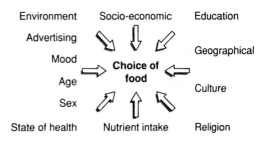

Figure 13.1 Factors influencing food choice.

For most individuals all of these factors are inter-related but are of differing significance for each person. For example, the cost of an item may mean that it is excluded from the diet of someone on a low income, or it may be included in the diet of someone with a higher income because it is perceived as a food that successful people with high incomes consume. In a similar way, people on higher incomes may not want to be seen eating foods that they consider are eaten by people with a lower income.

INDIVIDUAL CHARACTERISTICS

Age

This is of key importance because infants have no choice over what they eat, but as they become older they exert more and more control over the food that they consume. This normal process of development, as toddlers start expressing their individual food preferences, starts the establishment of the food preferences of a lifetime. Although it may not seem like it to the carers, it is they who still exert overwhelming control over their children's consumption. Once children start school, peer-group pressure starts to influence food choice. Old age also influences food choice; as the frailty of an individual increases so do the limitations that the frailty imposes on the ability to purchase, prepare and consume food.

Gender

Males have higher energy requirements than females and, in those societies where they are seen as the 'breadwinners', they are likely to be given the largest portion of a meal and the choicest parts of the food (Devault 1991).

State of health

An individual's health affects choice in a number of ways:

- A food that causes discomfort will be avoided.
- Anorexia and nausea usually mean that people choose small portions of familiar foods.
- Physical difficulty in obtaining, preparing and eating food all restrict choice.
- Foods that are believed to be health-giving or beneficial for a specific condition will be chosen. The 'hot' and 'cold' beliefs present in many cultures are very complicated and are reviewed in Thomas (1994).
- Foods that are associated with comfort will be chosen.

Mood

Mood affects an individual's choice of food. For example, someone may choose confectionery because he or she feels that he or she should be indulged.

SOCIOECONOMIC FACTORS

Advertising

Huge amounts of money are spent on food advertising, the main aims of which are to persuade people to:

- buy a new product
- buy more of a particular product
- change brand of a particular product
- maintain loyalty to a specific product.

No group of the population is excluded from the influences of advertising and it has profound effects on food choices.

A lot of advertising on television is intended to change children's eating habits and it has been suggested that children are unable to differentiate between television programmes and advertisements. One study found that three-quarters of 4-year-olds and 20% of 10-year-olds were unable to differentiate between advertisements and programmes (Zuckerman & Gianinno 1987). It is particularly confusing for children when familiar cartoon characters, television personalities and sports celebrities are used to promote a product. More than half of the advertisements on children's television are for food and, of these, more than 80% are for high-fat or high-sugar products (Food Magazine 1990).

Environment

The environment in which a food is to be prepared affects food choice, as does the environment in which it is to be consumed. If the cooking and storage facilities are limited, then the choice of foods is restricted by whether or not it is actually feasible to prepare and cook a particular item. The same applies to where the food is to be eaten. For example, it is more difficult to eat a plate of spaghetti bolognaise balanced on your knee than to eat a cheese sandwich. Environment is also influenced by socioeconomic factors.

Income

Surveys show that those with a low income have a poorer diet than those with a higher income. Examples include:

1. The *Dietary and Nutritional Survey of British Adults* (Gregory et al 1990) showed that the dietary intakes of fibre, sugar and protein tended to be higher among men and women in socioeconomic groups I and II than those in groups IV and V, but that there was no consistent trend from group to group. It did, however, show that those surveyed in groups I and II had higher intakes of vitamins and minerals than those in groups IV and V, the most obvious of these being the difference in vitamin C intake. This is not surprising as:

2. The National Food Survey for 1991 (MAFF 1992) showed that the richest fifth of the population consume 70% more fresh fruit, 20% more green vegetables and 400% more fruit juice than the poorest third.

3. The impact of low income on diet was highlighted by a survey conducted for the National Children's Home (NCH 1991) of 354 families using NCH family centres. This survey found a direct relationship between the lowest income and poorest diet among those surveyed, and that 20% of parents and 10% of children had gone without food because of lack of money.

Any dietary advice given to people on low incomes should be carefully considered and meet the following criteria:

- Is it realistic given the other pressures and constraints acting on the family?
- Would it be acceptable to the whole family?
- Would it be acceptable for a period of time?
- Are there any hidden extra costs, e.g. fuel?
- Are the foods easily available?

Those on low incomes may have a diet that is high in fat and sugar and contain many manufactured foods, but they generally get better nutritional value for their money than those on higher incomes, e.g. bread is a far more economical source of energy than fresh fruit.

The Health Education Authority report (HEA 1989) showed that, when given nutritional advice, people on low incomes changed their cooking methods. However, further reductions in fat intake and increase in NSP intake were not made due to the cost of basic ingredients. Advice useful when working with individuals on a low income is included in Chapter 14 (p. 122).

Group activities which promote food cooperatives and bulk buying can be helpful in facilitating people with lower incomes to improve their diets.

Transport

Superstores stock a wide variety of goods that are generally at lower prices, but are only accessible to those with their own transport or good public transport. Local corner shops usually stock a limited range of goods at higher prices. This may mean that foods like fruit, vegetables and wholemeal bread are expensive.

Storage/cooking facilities

If storage and cooking facilities are poor, then it is inevitable that people will have to rely on manufactured and prepacked foods which require little more than unwrapping and re-heating, or buy their food at restaurants or take-away food shops. This is of particular significance to those living in bed and breakfast accommodation.

Social status

In every culture there are foods that are perceived as high-status foods and those that are considered low-status. For example, in the UK cabbage is seen as a low-status food while broccoli is seen as a high-status food.

Peer-group pressure

Individuals want to belong to a group and so conform to the dietary pattern of those around them. This is particularly so among children.

Education

Individuals acquire knowledge from a host of sources and people. Not only do they obtain nutritional knowledge from people who influence them, such as family and teachers, but they also acquire attitudes as to whether or not this information is important and should be acted upon.

GEOGRAPHICAL AND CULTURAL FACTORS

Geographical location

This influences the availability of foods. The staple food of a population depends on the climate, and the way in which food is cooked depends on the availability of fuel. For example, if there is very little fuel for cooking, food is cut into small pieces and cooked rapidly. Nutritional deficiencies can develop when people move from one area to another where the food is unfamiliar and familiar foods are unavailable or very expensive. This can occur among immigrants to the UK who are unfamiliar with the vegetables that are traditionally available here; although their traditional vegetables are imported, they are not eaten in the customary amounts because they are expensive.

Culture

Culture is defined as, 'the customs and civilisation of a particular people or group' (from the *Oxford Paperback Dictionary*). The dietary habits of any group of people conform to a culturally standardised set of behaviours. These are acquired from the family and surrounding community and show considerable variation. An example of this is that it is usual in British culture to have bread/toast or cereal for breakfast, while it is usual in China to have soup and noodles for breakfast. Children grow up in a particular culture and accept and adapt to the cultural tradition that surrounds them.

Culture will also govern food intake. In some cultures, the ideal body shape is very thin, whereas in others, obesity is striven for as it signifies wealth and success.

Religion

Food has differing significance in different religions, and some adherents need to abide by different dietary laws (see Chapter 18). The significance of religious dietary rules depends on the individual. Not all adherents to the same religion will follow the religious dietary laws as strictly as each other.

REFERENCES

Devault M L 1991 Feeding the family: the social organization of caring as gendered work. Chicago University Press, Chicago
Food Magazine 1990 Are children fed a diet of junk food ads? Food Magazine April–June: 13–18
Gregory J, Foster K, Tyler H, Wiseman M 1990 The dietary and nutritional survey of British adults. Office of Population, Censuses and Surveys. HMSO, London
Health Education Authority (HEA) 1989 Diet, nutrition and 'healthy eating' in low income groups. HEA, London

Ministry of Agriculture, Fisheries and Food (MAFF) 1992 Household food consumption and expenditure 1991. Annual Report of the National Food Survey Committee. HMSO, London
National Children's Home (NCH) 1991 Poverty and nutrition survey. NCH, London
Thomas B (ed) 1994 Manual of dietetic practice, 2nd Edn. Blackwell Scientific Publications, Oxford
Zuckerman P, Gianinno L 1987 Measuring children's response to television advertising. In: Esserman J (ed) Television advertising and children.

FURTHER READING

Baggot R 2000 Food, diet and health in public health policy and politics. Macmillan Press, Hampshire
Charles N, Kerr M 1988 Women, food and families. Manchester University Press, Manchester
Conway J (ed) 1988 Prescription for poor health. London Food Commission, Maternity Alliance, SHAC, Shelter, London
Food Commission 1990 Sweet persuasion. Food Magazine: 4
Henson S, Gregory S, Hamilton M, Walker A 1998 Food choice and diet change within the family setting. In: Murcott A (ed) (1998) The nation's diet—the social science of food choice. Longman, London
Holmes S 1993 Force of habits. Nursing Times 89(35): 48–50
Mennell S, Murcott A, van Otterloo A H 1992 The sociology of food: eating, diet and culture. Sage Publications, London

Murcott A (ed) 1998 The nation's diet — the social science of food choice. Longman, London
National Consumer Council (NCC) 1992 Your food: whose choice? HMSO, London
National Dairy Council 1992 Healthy eating on a budget. National Dairy Council, London
Price S, Sephton J 1991 Just desserts? Influencing food choice: food behaviour and strategies for change. Horton Publishing, Bradford
Rogers P J, Blundell J E 1990 Psychological bases of food choice. In: Ashwell M (ed) Why we eat what we eat. British Nutrition Foundation Nutrition Bulletin 15 (Suppl): 21–40
Shephard R (1999) Social determinants of food choice. Proceedings of the Nutrition Society 58: 807–812

14

Dietary recommendations for adults

LEARNING OBJECTIVES

After studying this chapter you should be able to:

- discuss the development of current recommendations for a healthy diet for adults
- explain the *Balance of Good Health* guide to healthy eating
- provide adults with practical advice on how to achieve a healthy diet and understand how this advice should be altered for pregnant women.

The nutritional value of food is not the major influence governing the food choices of most people. Their choice is influenced by cost and availability of food, by their culture and by personal preferences. Any attempt to change dietary habits is difficult because long-standing preferences and opinions must be overcome. For dietary advice to be effective, it must be both practical and acceptable. The best way to achieve this is to base advice on simple modifications of existing habits. It is both impractical and unreasonable to expect anyone, except in the most extreme situations, to adopt a completely new diet.

It is now well established that diet has an important part in maintaining health and in the prevention of disease. It also has an important role in the treatment of disease. Preceding chapters of this book have treated nutrients as separate entities. In this chapter, general nutritional advice is given which applies to most adults. More specific nutritional advice for groups with special nutritional needs, such as the elderly and minority ethnic groups, is given in later chapters.

RECOMMENDATIONS FOR A HEALTHY DIET

Reference nutrient intakes (RNIs)

RNIs for specific nutrients, as published by the Department of Health (1991) are reproduced in

Appendix 2 and referred to in the sections on specific nutrients (see Chapters 1–8). They are not intended to be used rigidly as a guide to an individual's diet, because individual dietary requirements vary greatly. They are used as a reference point in population nutritional surveys, in planning food supplies, in large-scale catering operations in institutions and as a tool in assessing the adequacy of an individual's intake.

Many countries have prepared individual national nutritional guidelines. In doing this, the enormous amount of research into diet and disease, much of which was conflicting, has been reviewed to produce reports which provide a consensus of informed opinion.

The NACNE report

The policy background and reasons for publishing this influential report are explored in Chapter 10.

In 1979, the National Advisory Committee on Nutrition Education (NACNE) was instituted by the British Nutrition Foundation and the Health Education Council. A discussion paper entitled *Proposals for Nutritional Guidelines for Health Education in Britain* was prepared by an ad hoc working party under the chairmanship of Professor W.P.T. James and published by the Health Education Council (NACNE 1983). This paper, frequently referred to as the NACNE report, presents a consensus of views on what is a healthful diet and quantitative values as to how this should be achieved. It was a precursor to Committee on Medical Aspects of Food Policy (COMA) Report 28 on diet and cardiovascular disease (DHSS 1984).

The dietary changes advocated were for the entire population, not specific individuals. This feature should be considered when interpreting the NACNE paper, which was intended for use by those concerned with health education rather than the general public. Because permanent dietary change is difficult to achieve, the paper's proposals were presented as long-term and short-term goals. It was hoped that the short-term goals would be accomplished by the end of the 1980s. This report has now been superseded by Report 46 (DoH 1994), which includes improvements and has a slightly different format.

A criticism of the COMA Report 28 (DHSS 1984) was that it was difficult for the lay person to interpret because its recommendations were quantitative targets for dietary intake of specific nutrients, and needed to be interpreted into food terms before it could be used as a working document.

To overcome this problem, the COMA Report 46 (DoH 1994) presented its recommendations in two forms: quantitative targets for the intake of particular nutrients; and patterns of food intake. Their recommendations are summarised below.

COMA diet and recommendations for healthy eating

Nutrient recommendations

These targets are intended to be used by public health workers in the development and monitoring of diet and nutrition policy. The targets set are believed by the authors of the report to be both moderate and achiev-

Table 14.1 Summary of recommendations of COMA Report 46 on diet and cardiovascular disease (from DoH 1994, with permission)

Nutrient recommendations	Food recommendations
Total fat intake should be reduced to about 35% of dietary energy	Use reduced-fat spreads and low-fat dairy products
Saturated fatty acid intake should be reduced to no more than about 10% of dietary energy	Replace saturated fats and oils with those low in saturates, rich in polyunsaturates
The n-6 PUFA intake should stay the same	
The long-chain n-3 PUFA intake should double to about 1.5 g/week	Eat two portions of fish a week, one of which should be oily
Cholesterol intake should not rise	
No more than 2% of dietary energy should be provided by *trans* fatty acids	
The proportion of dietary energy provided by complex carbohydrates should be increased by 50%	Consumption of fruit, vegetables, bread and potatoes should be increased by 50%
Potassium intake should be increased to about 90 mmol/day	This will result from increased fruit and vegetable consumption
Reduce sodium intake from 150 to 100 mmol/day	
Manufacturers and caterers should explore ways of reducing sodium content of foods	

able and should not be 'over-interpreted' as targets for the nutrient composition of a biologically optimal diet.

Food recommendations

Advice about healthy eating for individuals is of far greater value if it is given as patterns of food intake, rather than as nutrient targets. The food recommendations include changes in the amounts of particular foods and food groups eaten. This results in a change to a different, but practical and enjoyable, eating pattern which conforms to the nutrient recommendations.

The nutrient and food recommendations are summarised in Table 14.1.

The report also includes an example of the changes in consumption of foods normally eaten during 1 week that would be needed to achieve the nutrient targets. This is reproduced as Appendix 5. The figures represent national averages of intake from the National Food Survey (MAFF 1993), so do not include food and drink consumed away from home. They are intended as an example of what a diet could look like, not as a prescription for a better diet—and should not be interpreted as such—but are a useful, understandable illustration of what could be eaten.

The Balance of Good Health

This publication has been produced by the Health Education Authority to give consistent and practical messages about healthy eating (HEA 1994). It is hoped that, if it is consistently used within schools, workplaces, health centres and retail outlets, the previous confusion will be overcome.

Box 14.1 Guidelines for a healthy diet (HEA 1994)

- Enjoy your food.
- Eat a variety of different foods.
- Eat the right amount to be a healthy weight.
- Eat plenty of foods rich in starch and fibre.
- Don't eat too much fat.
- Don't eat sugary foods too often.
- Look after the vitamins and minerals in your food.
- If you drink alcohol, keep within sensible limits.

The Balance of Good Health aims to help people understand and enjoy healthy eating. It shows that people don't have to give up the foods they most enjoy for the sake of their health, but variety and a change towards more vegetables, fruit, bread, breakfast cereals, potatoes, rice and pasta is what matters. Snacks as well as meals count towards the healthy balance (HEA 1994).

The guide consists of three sections:

1. Eight guidelines for a healthy diet (Box 14.1).
2. Classification of foods commonly eaten in food groups (Table 14.2).
3. A plate divided into five sections, the size of each section showing the relative amounts of food that should be eaten (see Fig. 14.1). For example:
   — fatty and sugary foods should not be eaten too often and should be eaten in small amounts
   — bread, other cereals and starchy foods— something from this group should be eaten at every meal.

Dietary advice is much easier to follow if it is given as practical advice rather than vague statements which

Table 14.2 The five food groups

Food group	What's included	How much to choose	What types to choose
Bread, other cereals and potatoes	Breakfast cereals, pasta, rice, chapattis	Eat lots	Eat wholemeal or high-fibre versions if possible
Fruit and vegetables	Fresh, frozen, tinned and dried	Eat lots	A wide variety
Milk and dairy foods	Milk, cheese, yoghurt and fromage frais (but not butter and eggs)	Eat or drink moderate amounts Choose lower-fat versions if possible	Semi-skimmed or skimmed milk, low-fat yoghurts or fromage frais, lower-fat cheeses
Meat, fish and alternatives	Meat, poultry, fish, eggs, pulses and nuts	Eat moderate amounts Choose lower-fat versions if possible	Meat with fat cut off, poultry without skin, fish without batter Cook these foods without fat
Fatty and sugary foods	Margarine, low-fat spread, butter, oils, cream, chocolate, crisps, biscuits, pasties, cake, puddings, ice-cream, sweets, sugar	Eat sparingly–infrequently	Small amounts: margarine/low-fat spread/butter, cooking oils Occasional: other items on list

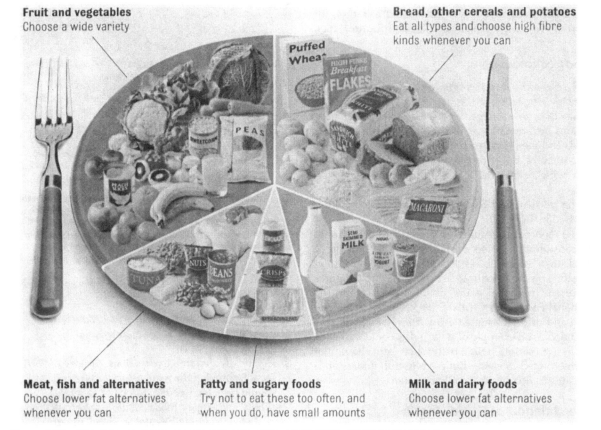

Figure 14.1 *The Balance of Good Health* (reproduced from HEA 1994 with kind permission).

need interpreting. For example, the suggestion, 'eat an apple at lunch time instead of a chocolate biscuit', is easier to follow than either of the statements, 'eat less chocolate', or 'eat more fruit'. The publication *Eight Guidelines for a Healthy Diet—a Guide for Nutrition Educators* (HEA 1997) is a helpful and practical resource for health care workers. The next section includes ways in which healthy eating information can be interpreted.

Practical hints for eating the healthier way

Eat more starchy foods

- Serve larger portions of bread, potato, pasta, rice or chapatti.
- Include pasta, potatoes, rice and cereals such as pearl barley in soups, stews and casseroles.
- Cut bread more thickly or buy thickly sliced bread.

- Serve bread in addition to potatoes/pasta at a main meal.

Eat more fruit

- Have fruit as a between-meal snack.
- Include tinned, fresh or dried fruit with breakfast, e.g. sliced banana with breakfast cereal, or dried fruit included in muesli.
- Base desserts on fresh fruit or fruit tinned in fruit juice. These can be served with jelly, custard or milk pudding that has been made from low-fat milk.

Eat more vegetables

- Include salad vegetables in sandwiches.
- Add vegetables to casseroles and stews.
- Add extra cooked vegetables to soups, e.g. add sweetcorn to mushroom or chicken soup.

- Serve more than one vegetable at a meal. Include a side salad as well as cooked vegetables with a main meal.

Eat less fat

- Identify those foods which contain 'hidden' fat. Cakes, biscuits, pies and pastries all have a high fat content and should be eaten as a special occasion food rather than routinely.
- Avoid chips and fried potatoes. Try to eat roast potatoes only once a week.
- Spread fat on bread or chapattis more thinly, or eat them without it sometimes.
- Cut the fat off meat before cooking.
- Remove the skin from chicken before cooking.
- Use skimmed milk wherever possible, e.g. in sauces or custard.
- Use skimmed or semi-skimmed milk for drinks and breakfast cereals.
- Use lower-fat cheeses, e.g. reduced-fat Cheddar or Edam, and lower-fat spreads in preference to full-fat ones.
- Change to lower-fat between-meal snacks. Have fresh fruit, dried fruit, dry-roasted or raw nuts, plain currant buns, bread or cracker-type biscuits, instead of crisps and biscuits.
- Grill, braise or microwave foods instead of frying them.
- Reduce the amount of fat used in recipes. This particularly applies to minority ethnic recipes where fat is used in the preparation of spices.

Eat fewer sugary foods

- Do not add sugar to drinks.
- Drink sugar-free squashes and fizzy drinks instead of the sugar-containing alternatives.
- Reduce the amount of sugar added during cooking and used in baking.
- Use fruit tinned in fruit juice, rather than syrup.
- Eat fewer sweets.
- Try to have fruit instead of a pudding.

Eat less salt

- Reduce the amount added to food during cooking.
- Taste foods before adding extra salt at the table.
- Experiment with flavourings other than salt, such as lemon juice, herbs and spices.
- Buy vegetables tinned in water rather than tinned in brine. Buy lower-salted alternatives of tinned products such as baked beans and spaghetti.

Meal ideas

Box 14.2 gives an example of the meals for a family that is trying to eat healthily. It is intended as an example of the variety of foods that are included in a healthy diet and how enjoyable healthy eating can be. It does not include high-fat, high-sugar snack foods. It is not assumed that they will be excluded from the diet totally, but rather that they are not routinely eaten every day.

Box 14.2 Examples of healthy meals

Snack meals	Main meals
Tuna-filled rolls Pear, low-fat yoghurt	Chicken casserole, Potatoes, sprouts, carrots Tinned fruit and custard
Cottage cheese and pineapple sandwiches Banana, fruit loaf	Chilli con carne and rice Side salad Low-fat fruit yoghurt
Egg salad and roll Orange Currant bun	Spaghetti bolognaise Side salad Fresh fruit salad
Chicken and sweetcorn filled pitta Apple	Chick pea/vegetable curry Chapattis/rice Tomato/onion salad Fresh fruit
French bread filled with ham and salad Banana and grapes	Jacket potato with fish filling Celery and carrot sticks Fresh fruit in jelly
Baked beans, pizza and jacket potato	Grilled trout Mashed potatoes, broccoli and carrots Sliced oranges and lemon sorbet
Lentil and vegetable soup Crusty rolls	Roast meat Boiled and roast potatoes, green beans and peas Summer pudding

Desserts

The desserts chosen depend on individual preference, time available for food shopping and fruit availability. Some people will find fresh fruit an easy, acceptable dessert, while others will feel that a meal is incomplete without 'pudding'. Desserts should be fruit-based and use low-fat dairy products, e.g. tinned fruit and custard, milk puddings and fruit mousses. Pies, crumbles and sponge puddings should not be encouraged because of their high fat content.

HEALTHY EATING ON A BUDGET

As has been shown in the previous chapter on food choices, the amount of money individuals have to spend on food is a key factor affecting how good their diet is. It is usual in the UK for those on lower incomes to have less fresh fruit and vegetables in their diet and more fatty and sugary foods. Box 14.3 outlines some of the ways in which the restrictions imposed by a limited budget can be overcome.

Many local initiatives are being developed in England as part of Health Improvement Programmes to reduce the inequalities of access to and availability of healthy food (See Chapter 10).

HEALTHY EATING DURING PREGNANCY

There is a correlation between maternal nutrient intake during pregnancy and birth-weight (Naeye 1979). With low birth-weight goes an increased risk of neurological and other handicaps (OPCS 1988). Maternal malnutrition is a modifiable risk factor in the prevention of low-birth-weight babies (Kramer 1987). Other risk factors include maternal age, smoking and the interval between pregnancies.

Studies of the effect of undernutrition have shown that it depends on the period during the pregnancy when the undernutrition occurred (Stein et al 1975). If the mother was malnourished prior to conception and during the early stages of her pregnancy, there is a higher risk of congenital abnormality, whereas if the undernutrition occurs at a later stage of the pregnancy, foetal growth is affected.

Pre-conception advice

Ideally, nutritional advice should be given prior to conception so that the mother's nutrient status is satisfactory and any nutritional deficiencies that are identified can be corrected. In their position paper on pre-conceptional nutrition, the British Dietetic Association (1994) recommend that the following groups of women are targeted for nutritional advice:

- those with poor obstetric history, e.g. previous low-birth-weight baby and/or history of miscarriage
- very underweight or overweight women
- those with eating disorders
- those with birth intervals of less than 18 months
- mothers of more than four children
- adolescents

Box 14.3   Guidelines for healthy eating on a budget

1. *Try to plan at least a day ahead and always make a shopping list.* This avoids the impulse-buying of foods you don't really need and ensures you buy the food you do need.
2. *Only buy food in quantities that you will use.* Large packets are not always economical if you are unable to store the food and have to waste some of it. Greengrocers and butchers are generally happy to provide the amount you want.
3. *Try to compare the prices and weights of similar products when shopping.* Supermarket own-brands are often the cheapest.
4. *Buy fruit and vegetables regularly.* They are usually cheaper at market stalls than in supermarkets. Fruit and vegetables that are in season are usually the best value. Store them carefully when you get home to get the best nutritional value from them and reduce wastage.
5. *Only buy small portions of new foods.* Buy larger ones when you know you like the food.
6. *Include generous helpings of starchy foods at all meals.* Breakfast cereals, bread, potatoes, rice, pasta and chapattis are all cheap, filling and healthy.
7. *Buy the leanest meat you can afford.* By adding pulses and vegetables to casseroles and stews a

small amount of meat can be made to serve more people.
8. *Tinned fish like pilchards, mackerel and tuna are cheaper than fresh fish.* They can be served in a sauce with pasta, a sandwich filling, in a fish pie or used to fill a jacket potato.
9. *Frozen poultry is often cheaper than fresh poultry and meat.* Remember it **must** be thawed properly and cooked thoroughly before serving.
10. *Careful cooking can use less fuel.*
    - Only heat the amount of water you need in the kettle.
    - Using an electric toaster instead of a grill to make toast uses less fuel.
    - If you are using the oven, make the most of the heat by cooking several dishes at once in the oven, e.g. a casserole, jacket potatoes and a milk pudding.
    - When cooking in a saucepan, bring the food to the boil, put the lid on and turn the heat down so that the contents simmer.
11. *Share the cooking and shopping.* It may be more economical to cook and shop with a friend. You will use less fuel and the more economical large packets of food can then be shared.

- low-income women
- those living in bed and breakfast accommodation with poor cooking facilities
- vegans and vegetarians with an inadequate diet
- smokers
- those with pre-existing conditions such as diabetes, food allergies, malabsorption states and phenylketonuria.

The nutritional advice given to pregnant women should be based on normal healthy eating which will ensure an adequate intake of all nutrients. Topics which should be included are:

- general nutrition
- appropriate weight gain
- folate and iron supplements
- avoidance of foods rich in vitamin A
- food hygiene
- alcohol consumption.

For most people, their pre-pregnant diet is sufficient during pregnancy, when the body becomes more efficient at utilising the nutrients in the diet. Although the requirements for protein, vitamins and minerals are increased, the increased energy required is less than might be expected, because of a reduction in activity and physiological adaptation. Thus it is *quality* of the diet that is important, not increased quantity.

Weight gain

Weight gain occurs during pregnancy due to the increase in size of the reproductive tissues, the foetus and the maternal fat stores. During her pregnancy, a woman will gain about 12.5 kg in weight; 3.5 kg of this will be in the first 20 weeks and then the rate is about 0.5 kg per week. If a pregnant woman's diet is varied and provides adequate energy for sufficient weight gain, the increased requirements of most nutrients will be met. Additional milk is recommended to provide the extra calcium required during the third trimester and during lactation—300 ml a day is the recommended amount.

Weight loss prior to pregnancy

Being overweight or underweight, and attempts to lose weight, can all cause infertility (Bates et al 1982, Wynn & Wynn 1990). Ideally, a woman should not be trying to lose weight in the 2–3 months prior to conception or during her pregnancy, and her pre-pregnant weight should be within the normal body mass index (BMI) range of 20–25 (see p. 198).

Folate supplementation

Genetic and environmental factors interact to cause neural tube defects. There is evidence to show that folic acid supplementation of the diets of women who have already had a baby with a neural tube defect reduces the incidence of neural tube defects, and supplementation may reduce the incidence in first-time mothers (Wald et al 1991).

Current recommendations are that women who are planning to become pregnant should take a dietary supplement of 400 µg folic acid from attempting to conceive until the twelfth week of pregnancy (DoH 1992). Women with a previous pregnancy affected by a neural tube defect should take a daily supplement of 5 mg folic acid (DoH 2000). The way in which the folic acid acts to prevent neural tube defects is not yet understood. Folate (folic acid)-rich foods normally included in the diet are vegetables and fortified breakfast cereals. Women should be advised to include these in their diet and not over-cook vegetables, as this destroys the folic acid in them.

Iron supplements

Routine supplements of iron are no longer given to all pregnant women in the UK. Many women find that they cause nausea, constipation or diarrhoea. The RNI for iron does not increase during pregnancy (DoH 1991) and the menstrual iron loss ceases. However, if the maternal iron stores were low before the pregnancy started, because of a low dietary intake, then iron supplementation will be necessary.

Vitamin A

High intakes of vitamin A are associated with an increased incidence of birth defects (see Chapter 6). Pregnant women are therefore advised not to eat liver and liver products (such as liver sausage) because of their high vitamin A content.

Food hygiene

See Chapter 11.

Toxoplasmosis. The parasite causing this infection can occur in raw meat, unpasteurised goat's milk and milk products, unwashed fruit and vegetables and cat faeces. Pregnant women should take care when handling these to avoid contact with this parasite.

Listeriosis. The foods which may contain the bacteria *Listeria monocytogenes* include unpasteurised milk and cheeses, pâté, pre-cooked meals and cook–chill meals. Unpasteurised milk and cheese should not be eaten. If pre-cooked and cook–chill meals are bought, they must be heated thoroughly—heated to 70°C and kept there for 2 minutes—and should not be re-heated.

Alcohol consumption

An association between congenital malformations and high maternal alcohol intake has been identified (Beattie 1988). This foetal alcohol syndrome (FAS) was seen in the children of mothers who drank more than 80 g pure alcohol per day. The symptoms include growth retardation and developmental problems. A safe level of alcohol consumption during pregnancy has not been identified but a study of 952 pregnancies found that alcohol consumption of less than 100 g (10 standard drinks) per week produced no ill effects (Sulaiman et al 1988). Women who are planning to become pregnant or who are pregnant are advised only to drink one or two units of alcohol once or twice a week (HEA 1997).

Problems during pregnancy which may influence nutritional status

Nausea and vomiting

For many women this is accepted as an unpleasant, but normal, part of their pregnancy, occurring in about half of all pregnant women (Fairweather 1968). Its incidence decreases after the end of the first trimester. Many cures have been suggested, different ones working for different women.

Small, frequent meals and avoiding being hungry may help, as may avoiding the smells of food and food preparation. Some women find avoiding drinking with meals beneficial. As antiemetics are not prescribed, women need to develop a strategy for ensuring that they eat small, nourishing snacks such as sandwiches, fruit, yoghurts and plain biscuits rather than depending on high-fat, high-sugar snacks such as crisps and confectionery, for eating between and instead of meals.

Hyperemesis gravidarum

This is very severe nausea and vomiting that develop during pregnancy, the cause of which is still not understood. It can be so serious that hospital admission is necessary to prevent dehydration and to correct for vitamin and mineral deficiencies which have occurred. Once clear fluids have been tolerated for 24 hours, sip-feeds can be introduced, followed by a return to normal eating habits.

Constipation

Constipation develops in many pregnant women. It is caused by decreased physical activity, depressed gut motility, decreased absorption of fluid from the colon and dietary changes. It can be overcome by increasing the amount of non-starch polysaccharide (NSP) in the diet, by including a high-fibre breakfast cereal, wholemeal bread, fruit and vegetables, and by increasing fluid consumption.

Heartburn

This is caused by increased abdominal pressure and slower gastric emptying. It can be overcome by small frequent meals, the use of antacids and avoiding foods such as spicy foods, citrus fruits and fatty foods.

HEALTHY EATING FOR VEGETARIANS

There is a general trend for people who include meat in their diet to eat less meat, and the number of people choosing to eat a vegetarian diet is increasing.

Like meat eaters, vegetarians do not conform to one particular stereotype. Surveys of vegetarians in the UK show that they come from a wide variety of backgrounds. Some, brought up as vegetarians, retain this lifestyle in adulthood, whereas others, having been brought up in meat-eating families, choose not to eat meat. Women are more likely to be vegetarian than men and there are higher rates of vegetarianism among younger adults, teenagers and children than in older adults.

Types of vegetarian diet

- *Partial vegetarian*—diet includes fish, excludes red meat, may eat poultry.
- *Lactoovovegetarian*—diet includes plant foods, dairy products and eggs.
- *Lactovegetarian*—diet includes plant foods and dairy produce.
- *Total vegetarian* (vegan)—diet includes plant foods only.

In this book the term vegetarian will be used to describe lactoovovegetarians and lactovegetarians but not vegans. The majority of people in the UK who are not meat eaters are vegetarians, rather than vegans. Other vegetarian diets which are sometimes eaten and are usually nutritionally inadequate, particularly for children, are macrobiotic and fruitarian diets (Roberts et al 1979).

Macrobiotic (ZEN) diets. There are 10 levels of macrobiotic diet, from -3 to +7; they become increasingly restrictive as they approach level 7 and also stress the importance of natural, organically grown, unprocessed foods. The lowest-level diets include some meat and fish, while the highest-level diet consists entirely of wholegrains and liquids used sparingly. In practice, most macrobiotic diets are vegan and there is a risk of developing calcium, iron and vitamin B_{12} deficiencies. The higher the level of the diet, the greater the risk of malnutrition. Modified macrobiotic diets are sometimes used as part of the holistic treatment of some diseases (Pike 1988).

Fruitarian diet. This diet excludes cereals and pulses as well as animal products. The diet consists of fruits, nuts and seeds which are usually eaten uncooked. This diet can lead to protein–energy malnutrition, as well as vitamin and mineral deficiencies.

Reasons for choosing a vegetarian diet

A vegetarian diet is chosen by individuals for a variety of reasons which can be grouped into three categories:

- religious and moral views
- economic and environmental circumstances
- health benefits.

Religious and moral views

Many people who have an abhorrence of killing and causing suffering choose not to eat meat as a way of reducing suffering to animals.

- *Hinduism*—pork and beef are not eaten, because pork is considered unclean and the cow is a sacred animal. In practice, many Hindus are strict lactovegetarians.
- *Seventh Day Adventists*—lactoovovegetarian diet.
- *Jainism*—lactovegetarians who fast frequently.
- *Buddhism*—usually lactoovovegetarians.
- *Bahai*—vegan diet including obligatory fasting for those aged 15–70 years.
- *Hare Krishnas*—lactovegetarians who avoid processed foods.

Economic and environmental circumstances

Meat is an expensive food to buy and can require a lot of fuel to cook (depending on the type of meat bought). This means that some people cannot afford to buy meat or feel that they can spend their money more wisely by choosing not to buy meat.

Meat is an expensive and inefficient source of protein to produce. For example, it takes 30 kg of cattle food to produce 1 kg of beef. Some people choose not to eat meat because they feel its production involves an unwise use of environmental resources, causing unnecessary environmental damage.

Health benefits

Lower rates of coronary heart disease, stroke and certain cancers have been found in vegetarians than in meat eaters (Burr & Butland 1988). A vegetarian diet has a lower saturated fat content and higher content of complex carbohydrates, NSP and the natural antioxidants contained in fruit and vegetables, and it has been proposed that the reduced rates of disease are a consequence of this. However, it has been suggested (Dwyer 1991) that the health benefits are not due to the diet but to the lifestyle generally adopted by vegetarians. Those vegetarians studied tend to be more health conscious, smoke less, exercise more and have a higher socioeconomic status than their meat-eating counterparts.

Work by Thorogood et al (1994), in which he followed a group of British meat eaters and a group of British vegetarians for 12 years, showed that after adjusting for the effects of smoking, variations in BMI and socioeconomic status, all causes of premature mortality were 20% lower in the vegetarian than in the meat-eating group. This was higher than the reduction found by Key et al 1996.

Nutritional content of vegetarian diets

Most vegetarian diets are nutritionally adequate as long as a range of foods are eaten (Draper et al 1993). The risk of malnutrition is far greater among vegans than among vegetarians. It is generally the case that those people who care about healthy eating and the nutritional content of their diet, and who have the resources to provide it, have a better diet than those who do not, irrespective of whether or not they eat meat. Some vegetarians rely heavily on full-fat dairy products, particularly cheese, and eat a lot of high-fat snack foods; this group, therefore, has a poor-quality high-fat diet. The cheese eaten by lactoovovegetarians and lactovegetarians must be vegetarian cheese made with animal-free rennet, ordinary cheese made with rennet from calves being unsuitable.

Individuals who are at particular risk of having an inadequate diet are vegans and vegetarians with an increased nutrient requirement, e.g. pregnant and lactating women, children and adolescents who need to

Table 14.3 Nutrients which may be deficient in vegetarian and vegan diets

Nutrient	Dietary sources suitable for vegetarians	Dietary sources suitable for vegetarians and vegans	Comments
Vitamin D	(Sunlight) Egg yolk Oily fish	(Sunlight) Fortified vegan margarine Fortified vegan soya milk, e.g. Pramil, Unisoy Gold Fortified breakfast cereals	Sunlight is the most important source of this vitamin Fortified foods and a dietary supplement will be necessary for those who are housebound
Vitamin B_{12}	Milk Dairy products	Fortified soya milk Fortified soya products, e.g. soya mince, burger mix Fortified yeast extracts, e.g. Tastex, Barmene, Natex	B_{12} is only found in animal products The Vegan Society recommends that all vegans include B_{12}-fortified foods in their diet
Riboflavin	Milk Dairy products	Fortified breakfast cereals Wheatgerm Nuts and seeds Pulses Fortified products	Riboflavin deficiency is rare in vegetarians
Calcium	Milk Dairy products	Hard water Green vegetables Nuts, cereals, sesame seeds White bread (fortified with calcium) Fortified soya milk	An adequate vitamin D intake is important to ensure calcium balance
Iron	Eggs	Pulses Nuts and seeds Fortified breakfast cereals Green vegetables Dried fruit	Although haem iron (that found in meat) is much better absorbed than non-haem iron (that found in plants), including vitamin-C-rich foods in the meal greatly increases the iron absorption, and vegetarian diets are generally rich in vitamin C Draper et al (1993) have shown in a study of the iron intake of vegetarians and vegans that the mean intake was greater than the UK dietary reference value for iron
Zinc	Eggs Shellfish	Pulses Nuts and seeds Fortified breakfast cereals Wholemeal bread	
Iodine	Milk Dairy products	Vegetables Cereals Seaweed Seaweed products	The iodine content of vegetables and cereals depends on the iodine of the soil in which they were grown

fulfil their nutrient requirements for optimum growth, and those vegetarians who are the sole vegetarian member of a meat-eating family and so may have difficulty obtaining the right sorts of foods. Also, people who have recently chosen to become vegetarian, but are unaware of the nutritional implications of this decision, may be at risk. Table 14.3 lists the nutrients which may be deficient and food sources of these nutrients that are suitable for vegetarians and vegans.

The food-group approach based on *The Balance of Good Health* can be used to ensure the nutritional adequacy of a vegetarian or vegan diet.

The intake of starchy foods should be the same, as should the intake of fresh fruit and vegetables. If dairy products are excluded from the diet, fortified soya products should be used instead and pulses, nuts and seeds used to replace the meat in the diet. The key to an adequate vegetarian/vegan diet is not just the exclusion of animal products, but their substitution by an alternative food such as pulses, nuts or seeds, and the consumption of a wide variety of different foods. Box 14.4 provides examples of a day's vegetarian meals.

Pulses

Care must be taken when cooking dried pulses. Salt should not be added while they are cooking as this stops the pulses from softening. Kidney beans should always be boiled for 15 minutes to destroy the haemagglutinins and toxins present in the beans. If cooking facilities are limited, the preparation of beans may be difficult. Many beans can now be bought tinned in water, overcoming this problem.

Vegetarian diets and mineral absorption

A vegetarian diet contains high levels of NSP, phytates, oxalates and tannins, which can combine with minerals and reduce their bioavailability and hence their absorption. This appears not to affect mineral utilisation in vegetarians (Kelsay et al 1988) and it may be that the gastrointestinal tract adapts to increase absorption. This may be the reason why new vegetarians are at greater risk of developing iron deficiencies

Box 14.4 Examples of vegetarian meals for a day
Breakfast Fortified breakfast cereal (most breakfast cereals are fortified with minerals and vitamins) Milk or soya milk Fruit juice Bread or toast with spread **Lunch** Sandwiches: — vegetarian cheese or nut butter and yeast extract — salad — fruit **Evening meal** Mixed bean casserole, vegetables and potatoes Yoghurt and fruit or soya-based yoghurt and fruit

than long-term vegetarians (Helman & Darnton-Hill 1987).

Vegetarian infants and children

See Chapter 15.

REFERENCES

Bates G W, Bates S R, Whitworth N S 1982 Reproductive failure in women who practice weight control. Fertility and Sterility 37(3): 373–378

Beattie J O 1988 Alcohol and the child. Proceedings of the Nutrition Society 47(2): 121–127

British Dietetic Association (BDA) 1994 Preconceptional nutrition: Position Paper. BDA, Birmingham

Burr M, Butland B 1988 Heart disease in British vegetarians. American Journal of Clinical Nutrition 48: 830–832

Department of Health (DoH) 1991 Dietary reference values for food energy and nutrients for the United Kingdom. Report of the Panel on Dietary Reference Values of the Committee on Medical Aspects of Food Policy (COMA) (Report on Health and Social Subjects 41). HMSO, London

Department of Health (DoH) 1992 Folic acid and the prevention of neural tube defects. Report from an Expert Advisory Panel. HMSO, London

Department of Health (DoH) 1994 Nutritional aspects of cardiovascular disease. Report of the Cardiovascular Review Group of the Committee on Medical Aspects of Food Policy (COMA) (Report on Health and Social Subjects 46). HMSO, London

Department of Health (DoH) 2000 Folic acid and the prevention of disease: report of the committee on medical aspects of food and nutrition policy (Report on Health and Social Subjects 50). The Stationery Office, London

Department of Health and Social Security (DHSS) 1984 Diet and cardiovascular disease. Committee on Medical Aspects of Food Policy (COMA) (Report on Health and Social Subjects 28). HMSO, London

Draper A, Lewis J, Malhotra N et al 1993 The energy and nutrient intakes of different types of vegetarian: a case for supplements? British Journal of Nutrition 69: 3–19

Dwyer J T 1991 Nutritional consequences of vegetarianism. Annual Review of Nutrition 11: 61–91

Fairweather D V 1968 Nausea and vomiting in pregnancy. American Journal of Obstetrics and Gynecology 102(2): 137–175

Health Education Authority (HEA) 1994 The balance of good health. HEA, London

Health Education Authority (HEA) 1997 Eight guidelines for a healthy diet—a guide for nutrition educators. HEA, Abingdon

Helman A D, Darnton-Hill I 1987 Vitamin and iron status in new vegetarians. American Journal of Clinical Nutrition 45: 785–789

Kelsay J L, Frazier C W, Prather E S, Canary J J, Clark W M, Powell A S 1988 Impact of variation in carbohydrate intake on mineral utilization by vegetarians. American Journal of Clinical Nutrition 48: 875–879

Key TH, Thorogood M, Appleby PM, Burr MH, 1996 Dietary habits and mortality in 11 000 vegetarian and health conscious people: results of a 17 year follow-up. British Medical Journal 313: 775–779

Kramer M 1987 Determinants of low birthweight: methodological assessment and meta-analysis. Bulletin of the World Health Organization 65(5): 663–737

Ministry of Agriculture, Fisheries and Food (MAFF) 1993 Household food consumption and expenditure 1992. Annual report of the National Food Survey Committee. HMSO, London

Naeye R L 1979 Weight gain and the outcome of pregnancy. American Journal of Obstetrics and Gynecology 135: 3–9

National Advisory Committee on Nutrition Education (NACNE) 1983 Proposals for nutritional guidelines for health education in Britain. Health Education Council, London

Office of Population, Censuses and Surveys (OPCS) 1988 Congenital malformation statistics 1981–1985: notifications, England and Wales. Series MB3 No. 2. HMSO, London

Pike J T 1988 Alternative nutritional therapies—where is the evidence? AIDS Patient Care February: 31–33

Roberts I F, West R J, Ogilvie D, Dillon M J 1979 Malnutrition in infants receiving cult diets: a form of child abuse. British Medical Journal 1: 296–298

Stein Z, Susser M, Saenger G et al 1975 Famine and human development: the Dutch hunger winter of 1944–45. Oxford University Press, New York

Sulaiman N D, Florey C D, Taylor D J, Ogston S A 1988 Alcohol consumption in Dundee primagravidas and its effects on outcome of pregnancy. British Medical Journal 296: 1500–1503

Thorogood M, Mann J, Appleby P, McPherson K et al 1994 Risk of death from cancer and ischaemic heart disease in meat and non-meat eaters. British Medical Journal 308: 1667–1671

Wald N, Sneddon J, Densem J, Frost C, Stone R 1991 Prevention of neural tube defects: results of the Medical Research Council vitamin study. Lancet 338: 131–137

Wynn A, Wynn M 1990 The need for nutritional assessment in the treatment of the infertile patient. Journal of Nutritional Medicine 1: 315–324

FURTHER READING

American Dietetic Association 1997 Vegetarian Diets—Position of the American Dietetic Association. Journal of the American Dietetic Association 97: 1317–1321

Bond A (for the Vegetarian Society) 1995 Vegetarian vitality: a report on the health benefits of the vegetarian diet and the nutritional requirements of vegetarians. The Vegetarian Society, Altrincham, Cheshire

British Nutrition Foundation 1992 Unsaturated fatty acids: nutritional and physiological significance: the report of the British Nutrition Foundation's task force. Chapman & Hall for the British Nutrition Foundation, London

Department of Health (DoH) 1994 Children. In: Nutritional aspects of cardiovascular disease. Report of the Cardiovascular Review Group of the Committee on Medical Aspects of Food Policy (COMA) (Report on Health and Social Subjects 46). HMSO, London: 145–148

Department of Health (DoH) Nutrition Task Force 1995 Eat Well 2. HMSO, London

Doyle W 1994 Teach yourself healthy eating. Hodder & Stoughton, Sevenoaks

National Heart Forum 1997 At least five a day.

National Research Council Committee on Diet, Nutrition and Cancer 1982 Diet, nutrition and cancer. National Academy Press, Washington DC

Stockley L (for the Health Education Authority) 1993 The promotion of healthier eating: a basis for action. HEA, London

World Health Organization. Study Group on Diet, Nutrition and Prevention of Noncommunicable Diseases 1990 Diet, nutrition and prevention of chronic diseases: report of a WHO study group (Technical Report Series 797). WHO, Geneva

USEFUL ADDRESSES

The Vegan Society
7 Battle Road
St Leonards on Sea
East Sussex TN37 7AA
Tel: 01424 427393
Website: www.vegansociety.com

The Vegetarian Society
Parkdale
Dunham Road
Altrincham
Cheshire WA14 4QG
Tel: 0161 928 0793
Website: www.vegsoc.org

The Vegetarian Society is a registered charity with a main aim of promoting vegetarianism. It produces a range of information of interest to health professionals and the public.

15

Diet in infancy, childhood and adolescence

LEARNING OBJECTIVES

After studying this chapter you should be able to:

- explain the nutritional advantages of breast-feeding and its importance for child health
- describe the process of weaning and the foods that should be included in a weaning diet to prevent the development of deficiency disorders
- plan diets for healthy children of all ages to ensure that their nutritional needs are met
- discuss the causes and prevention of childhood obesity.

BREAST-FEEDING

All mammals produce milk with which to feed their young. Each species of mammal produces a milk of a specific composition which is the ideal food for the young of that species. Human breast-milk is the best food for a young human. The infant formulae on the market are substitutes for human breast-milk. Their composition is carefully controlled to ensure they are as near human milk as possible. However, breast-feeding should be encouraged wherever possible.

Establishing breast-feeding

Breast-feeding is still not the most usual form of infant feeding, so health professionals need to be aware of its nutritional and immunological benefits, so that they can promote it. In the UK, the mothers who are most likely to breast-feed are those who:

- live in the South and West of England
- have their first baby after the age of 25
- were educated beyond the age of 18 (Martin & White 1988).

Important factors in establishing successful breast-feeding are:

- good antenatal advice
- good postnatal advice/support
- early mother–baby contact
- frequent breast-feeding
- maternal diet
- culture.

A survey of the infant feeding practices among Asian Families (Thomas & Avery 1997) showed that while 38% of white babies were only ever bottle-fed, the figures were much lower among Asian mothers with only 10% of Bangladeshi babies, 18% of Indian babies and 24% of Pakistani babies being only bottle-fed.

Antenatal advice

Pregnant women at antenatal classes should have the advantages and disadvantages of breast-feeding explained to them, and be able to discuss them in a relaxed atmosphere with their midwife and their partner if they wish. Expectant mothers also need to understand the basic physiology of breast-feeding. The book published by the Health Education Authority, *Feeding Your Child From Birth To Three* (Welford 1994), explains this clearly.

In a study to investigate how first-time mothers belonging to a socioeconomic group with low rates of breast-feeding make the decision whether or not to initiate breast-feeding (Hoddinott & Pill 1999), it was concluded that the decision was based more on her having seen someone breast-feeding rather than her theoretical knowledge. Encouraging the development of an antenatal apprenticeship with a breast-feeding mother from the same social network was recommended as a way to encourage more people to initiate breast-feeding.

Postnatal advice/support

New mothers frequently find their baby both physically and emotionally exhausting. At this time, they are particularly liable to abandon breast-feeding. A survey of infant feeding practice (White et al 1992) showed that only 63% of women tried to breast-feed, and that by the time the baby was 6 weeks old, 37% of this group had stopped. Women who stop breast-feeding do so for a variety of reasons; inadequate milk supply was the most commonly stated (DHSS 1988).

The milk supply is affected by anxiety and tiredness, so while lactation is becoming established, women need support with their domestic tasks and emotional support to encourage them not to abandon breast-feeding.

There are national and local support groups for breast-feeding women. These offer the support of local meetings and some provide breast-feeding counsellors and lists of shops, restaurants and public places where there are facilities for breast-feeding. The addresses of national organisations are at the end of the chapter.

Early mother–baby contact

It is now common practice to put the baby to the breast as soon after delivery as possible. This helps in the development of the suckling reflex, which is particularly strong straight after delivery (Righard & Alade 1990). As well as encouraging the suckling response, this also helps to establish the mother–child bond, and the hormonal response to suckling stimulates lactation. This early suckling needs sympathetic and competent help to ensure correct positioning of the baby at the breast, thus encouraging the suckling reflex and giving the new mother confidence. During this early period no other fluids such as water or infant formula should be given to the infant. The policy of 'rooming-in', now common in most maternity units, where babies are kept beside their mothers rather than in nurseries, and can be fed on demand, does much to help establish this early contact.

Frequent feeding

The traditional idea of 4-hourly feeds is not appropriate to breast-feeding the newborn. They need to be fed as frequently as mother and baby want. Frequent suckling of the newborn baby:

- stimulates milk production
- increases the mother's confidence in being able to feed her child
- reduces discomfort from breast engorgement as the milk comes in
- reduces the likelihood of sore nipples.

The length of a feed and whether it is from one or both breasts depends on the baby.

Babies should stay on the first side for as long as they seem to want and then be offered the second side. Some babies only take one side at a feed, others take both sides and a third group chop and change, feeding from one breast at one feed and then both breasts at the next feed (Welford 1994).

Maternal diet

During pregnancy, deposits of fat are laid down to be used as an energy store for breast-feeding. However, most mothers need an extra 1680–2520 kJ (400–600 kcal) per day, depending on the stage of breast-feeding (DoH 1991) and an increased fluid intake. There is an additional protein requirement of 11 g, but as most women's normal intake exceeds the reference nutrient intake (RNI) plus 11 g, there is no need to increase the dietary protein intake during lactation. Most women find that lactation increases their hunger and thirst. They should be encouraged to drink to quench their thirst and to establish a routine of having a drink before, after or while they feed their baby, and to prepare a drink they can have during the night while feeding the baby. This extra fluid should come from a variety of sources—tea, coffee, fruit juice, milk drinks and water are all suitable. Alcohol, caffeine and some drugs pass into the breast-milk. High intakes of strong coffee and tea should be discouraged (Clement 1989), as these may cause sleeplessness in some babies. Continuing to drink 500 ml of milk a day will provide extra calcium, riboflavin, protein and energy.

The extra energy requirement should be filled from a variety of sources. High-energy, high-salt or sugary snacks such as crisps and sweets should be discouraged, because, although they provide calories and take no time to prepare, they contain few other nutrients such as vitamins or minerals. Snacks such as wholemeal sandwiches, toast, fruit or biscuits and cheese are better and take little time to prepare.

The maternal diet influences the composition of breast-milk. This is why there are worldwide differences in its composition (WHO 1985). There is much folklore but little scientific evidence about which foods lactating women should or should not eat because they pass into their milk and affect the baby, causing fractiousness, wind or colic. The response to foods is very individual: some mothers need to avoid spicy foods and onions and others cannot tolerate fruit, whereas others find that they can eat almost anything. Mothers should not gorge on any one food because large quantities will pass through into the milk and this may upset the baby. Breast-feeding is the method of choice for feeding babies in families where there is a history of allergy, as there is evidence that it delays the onset and reduces the severity of allergies (Broadbent & Sampson 1988). Some breast-fed infants are sensitive to the cow's milk in their mother's diet (Cant et al 1986). If a mother is advised to exclude cow's milk and cow's milk products from her diet, she needs an alternative source of calcium in the diet and calcium supplements may be necessary.

Advantages of breast-feeding

1. Breast-milk has the ideal composition for the infant's needs, provided in a safe clean form at the right temperature.
2. The feeds need no preparation and there is no equipment to sterilise.
3. Breast-milk contains anti-infective factors which cannot be manufactured and added to infant formulae. This has considerable health benefits for the infant both in childhood and later life (Wilson et al 1998). The promotion of breast-feeding has been highlighted as a way to assist improvements in health and reduce health inequalities of mothers and children in the UK.

The *disadvantage* is that it is a time-consuming process which can only be done by the mother. It can be difficult to continue breast-feeding when the mother returns to work. This can be overcome by the child's carer giving infant formula or expressed breast-milk during the day and the mother continuing to breast-feed in the morning and evening.

Composition of breast-milk

Colostrum

This is the first milk produced and its composition is very different from the mature milk which is being produced by the end of the first week of lactation.

Protein. Colostrum contains five times more protein than mature milk, 20% of which is casein. The majority of the other 80% of protein is secretory immunoglobulin A (IgA); the rest is other whey proteins, the most important of which are lactoferrin and lysozyme. Lactoferrin is an iron-binding protein which helps iron absorption from the gut. Lysozyme inhibits bacterial growth in the gut.

Fat and carbohydrate. There is less fat and carbohydrate in colostrum than in mature milk; the nature of these components is described below in the section on mature milk.

Vitamins and minerals. Colostrum contains all of the known vitamins. It has a higher sodium concentration than mature milk. The trace elements present are bound to proteins to form parts of enzymes.

Mature milk

There is considerable variation in the composition of human breast-milk depending on maternal diet, the frequency with which the infant is fed and the duration of the feed. The average value for the energy content of mature human milk is 70 kcal (290 kJ) per 100 ml (see Table 15.1).

Protein. The protein content is less than colostrum. It is predominantly soluble whey proteins and contains immunoglobulins A, G and M (IgA, IgG and IgM), as well as lysozyme and lactoferrin.

Fat. The hind milk (produced towards the end of the feed) has a greater fat concentration than the fore milk (produced at the beginning of the feed). This means that the hind milk has a greater energy content and increased satiety value. 50% of the energy content of mature milk of women in the UK is provided by fat (Holland et al 1991). The actual fatty acid composition is affected by the fatty acid composition of the maternal diet. Breast-milk contains adequate amounts of the essential fatty acids, linoleic acid and alpha-linolenic acid, and the long-chain polyunsaturated fatty acids which are incorporated into the brain and retina (DoH 1994a).

Carbohydrate. As in all mammalian milks, lactose is the principal carbohydrate in human breast-milk. Lactose provides about 37% of the energy of human milk and the lactose level is higher than in cow's milk (see Table 15.1). Lactose is digested to glucose and galactose.

Vitamins and minerals. The vitamin content of human milk reflects the nutritional status of the mother. If the maternal diet is adequate, then the vitamin content of the milk will supply all the baby's needs. Thus breast-fed infants under the age of 6 months do not require vitamin supplements if the mother had, and continues to have while lactating, an adequate diet during her pregnancy (DoH 1994a).

Iron, copper, zinc, manganese, chromium, molybdenum, cobalt, selenium, iodine and fluorine are all present in breast-milk, however, the concentration in breast-milk is not sufficient to fulfil the requirements of infants once they have reached 6 months.

Anti-infective factors

These are immunoglobulins, maternal antibodies, lymphocytes and macrophages, which limit the multiplication of bacterial and viral pathogens in the gastrointestinal tract of the infant. Other factors are the enzyme lysozyme, and the iron-binding protein lactoferrin, both of which have a non-specific inhibitory action on bacterial growth. Human milk contains a growth factor which facilitates the colonisation of the infant's gastrointestinal tract with *Lactobacillus bifidis*. These bacteria are protective and help to maintain a low pH, which inhibits bacterial growth in the gut. So breast-feeding is not only nutritionally the best, it also protects the baby against infection. Howie et al (1990) showed that babies who were breast-fed for the first 13 weeks of their life had a reduced incidence of respiratory and gastrointestinal infections and that this protection lasted for their first year of life, even if breast-feeding had finished.

Inadequate milk supply

A regular check on the newborn's weight gain must be made, however the infant is being fed, to ensure that breast-feeding is successful and that the baby is receiving adequate milk. Babies respond to hunger in different ways. Some babies who are receiving inadequate milk are restless, unhappy and difficult to soothe, while others appear very calm and sleep a lot. Weight gain is the only certain way of checking that a baby is receiving enough milk.

If the milk supply is inadequate it can often be increased by feeding the baby more often, which increases nipple and breast stimulation and so increases milk production. Other factors, such as the mother's diet, and whether she is receiving sufficient rest or is anxious, should also be discussed. In most cases the problem can be overcome, but sometimes it is necessary

Table 15.1 Comparison of the composition of human milk, cow's milk, infant formula and follow-on milks (per 100 ml) (from DoH 1994a, with permission).

		Mean values for mature human milk	Mean values for whole cow's milk	Infant formula*	Follow-on formula*
Energy	kJ	293	284	250–315	250–335
	kcal	70	68	60–75	60–80
Protein	g	1.3†	3.3	1.2–1.95	1.5–2.9
Carbohydrate	g	7	4.9	4.6–9.1	4.6–9.1
Fat	g	4.2	4.0	2.1–4.2	2.1–4.2

*The acceptable range under EC Directive (EC1991)
† Including non-protein nitrogen

to combine breast- and bottle-feeding and in other cases it is necessary to abandon breast-feeding and bottle-feed the baby. If this is the case, it should be handled tactfully so that the mother feels neither guilty nor a failure.

Expected weight gain for infants

When estimating body weight, it is customary to allow for some weight loss immediately after birth. This loss is usually made good by about the 10th day. Normal birth-weights for infants in the UK are between 3.3 and 3.5 kg for both sexes. Box 15.1 gives average weekly weight gains for the first year of life. During this time, infants increase in length by 25 cm.

Variations from the figures are to be expected. Babies do not gain weight at a constant rate. Many healthy babies show a more rapid weight gain than these figures indicate.

Food requirements of healthy infants

Fluid. A figure of 150 ml/kg body-weight per day may be taken as a guide to fluid requirements. Additional fluid may be required in hot climates or during hot summer weather.

Protein. A breast-fed infant obtains approximately 2 to 2.5 g protein per kg body-weight daily. Cow's milk and breast-milk proteins are equally effective in supplying the amino acids needed by the infant. Nevertheless, an intake of approximately 3 g cow's milk protein per kg body-weight daily has been recommended. The total daily RNIs for protein at different ages up to 1 year are given in Table 15.2.

Energy. The estimated average requirements (EARs) for energy for the first 12 months of life are given in Table 15.3.

Contraindications to breast-feeding

In conditions where it is physically difficult for the baby to breast-feed (e.g. cleft palate) expressed milk should be used wherever possible. In some inborn errors of metabolism (e.g. galactosaemia) an infant cannot be breast-fed. In others (e.g. phenylketonuria) it is possible to combine breast-feeding with feeding a

---

Box 15.1 Average weight gains from birth to 1 year (Shaw & Lawson 1994)

- 200 g per week for first 3 months
- 150 g per week for second 3 months
- 100 g per week for third 3 months
- 50–75 g per week for fourth 3 months

Table 15.2 Reference nutrient intakes (RNIs) for protein for the first 12 months of life (from DoH 1991, with permission)

Age	RNI (g/day)
0–3 months	12.5
4–6 months	12.7
7–9 months	13.7
10–12 months	14.9

Table 15.3 The estimated average requirements (EARs) for energy for the first 12 months of life (from DoH 1991, with permission)

Age	Male MJ (kcal)	Female MJ (kcal)
0–3 months	2.28 (545)	2.16 (515)
4–6 months	2.89 (690)	2.69 (645)
7–9 months	3.44 (825)	3.20 (765)
10–17 months	3.85 (920)	3.61 (865)

specialised infant formula, but this needs expert dietetic supervision.

Breast-feeding and human immunodeficiency virus (HIV) infection

Breast-feeding mothers who are HIV-positive can transmit the infection to their infants in breast-milk (European Collaborative Study 1992). It is for this reason women in the UK who are HIV-positive are advised not to breast-feed their infants (DHSS 1988). However, in developing countries where there is a high mortality rate for non-breast-fed infants due to malnutrition and infectious diseases, mothers should be advised to breast-feed their infants (WHO 1992).

WELFARE FOOD SCHEME VITAMIN SUPPLEMENTS

In the UK, vitamin supplements are available for expectant mothers and children under 5 years of age. These are provided free for families receiving Income Support.

The daily-dose vitamin drops contain:

- 200 µg vitamin A (retinol equivalents)
- 20 mg vitamin C
- 7 µg vitamin D.

It is recommended (DoH 1994a) that all infants *except* the following groups receive this supplement:

1. Breast-fed babies up to the age of 6 months, *if* their mothers had a good diet throughout pregnancy. If there is doubt about the nutritional quality of the

mother's diet, then the vitamin drops should be started at 1 month.

2. Infants who are bottle-fed and receiving at least 500 ml of infant formula or follow-on milk. These infants do not require the supplement because the milk they are drinking is supplemented.

From the age of 1 year, all children should receive the vitamin supplement and this should be continued to the age of 5 years, unless the child eats a good varied diet. It is particularly important that children who are 'faddy' or difficult eaters and those who are on restricted diets, such as vegetarians, continue to receive this supplement.

FORMULA FEEDING

Most women find breast-feeding an enjoyable and satisfactory experience, but some do not and, for these, bottle-feeding with an approved infant formula is a satisfactory alternative.

Infant formula milks should always be used for artificial feeding of babies. The immature kidneys and liver enzyme systems of a baby cannot cope with the high solute and protein load of any type of unmodified cow's or goat's milk.

Choice of infant formula

In the UK a wide range of infant formula milks are on the market, all of which conform to the European Community Directive on composition of infant formulae (Commission of the European Community 1991). They are made from cow's milk which has been modified to more closely resemble human milk. Most mothers continue to feed their babies the formula they used in the maternity unit.

The infant formula milks available in this country can be divided into two groups: whey-dominant milks and casein-dominant milks.

Whey-dominant milks. Cow's milk has been modified so that there is a ratio of the two proteins casein:whey of 40:60. This is similar to that of human milk.

Casein-dominant milks. The ratio of casein:whey is 80:20 in these milks, which is similar to that of cow's milk.

Whey-dominant milks are generally considered to be the most suitable for babies under 3 months-of-age (Thomas 1994). Although it is believed by many that casein-dominant milks are the more satisfying for hungry babies, there is no scientific proof of this (Taitz & Scholey 1989).

The carbohydrate content of infant feeds is designed to reflect that of mature breast-milk, and lactose, maltodextrins and glucose syrups are used. The content of some micronutrients is higher than in breast-milk—this is to compensate for the reduced bioavailability of some minerals in infant formulae.

Whichever infant formula the parent or carer decides to use, education in how to sterilise all equipment and how to make up the feed to the correct dilution is necessary. Like breast-fed babies, bottle-fed babies should be demand-fed. If the baby's weight gain is inadequate or the baby appears hungry, then the frequency or volume of the feed should be increased but not the concentration of the feed. It is usual to allow 150–200 ml/kg body-weight per day, which is normally divided into feeds at 3- to 4-hourly intervals. In hot weather, the baby may require extra cool boiled water to drink between feeds.

In the UK there is a voluntary code of practice covering the marketing of infant formulae. It is intended to promote breast-feeding and ensure that infant formulae are used properly. It states that:

- All infant formula packaging should state that breast-feeding is best for babies.
- Breast-feeding mothers should not be given free samples of infant formula.
- Maternity hospitals should not use promotional material, such as cot labels or posters.
- Infant formulae should only be advertised in professional journals.

There are also European Economic Community (EEC) directives on the export, advertising, labelling and composition of infant formula.

The 1994 Committee on Medical Aspects of Food Policy (COMA) report (DoH 1994a) covers all aspects of infant feeding and the recommendations for infant feeding and drinks are summarised in Box 15.2.

WEANING

Weaning is the process of expanding the diet to include foods and drinks other than breast-milk or infant formula. It is a gradual process—the age at which it is started and the rate at which it progresses vary between babies. Weaning should occur between 4 and 6 months (DoH 1994a), although a minority of babies will be ready for weaning at 3 months (DHSS 1988).

Babies are not ready to be weaned at an earlier age for several reasons:

- they do not have the neuromuscular coordination needed to move food from the tip of the tongue to the back of the mouth

- their gastrointestinal tract is too immature to digest and absorb the food
- their kidneys cannot regulate the high solute load.

Box 15.2   COMA recommendations for infant feeding and drinks (from DoH 1994a, with permission)

- Breast-milk supplies the best source of nourishment for the early months of life. Mothers should be encouraged and supported in breast-feeding for at least 4 months and may choose to continue to breast-feed as the weaning diet becomes increasingly varied.
- An infant who is not breast-fed should receive infant formula or follow-on milk. Follow-on milk is not recommended as replacement for breast-milk or infant formula before 6 months.
- Pasteurised whole cow's milk should only be used as a main milk drink after the age of 1 year. Intakes of iron and zinc and vitamins A and D should be ensured from other dietary sources or supplements. Semi-skimmed cow's milk is not suitable as a drink before the age of 2 years, but thereafter it may be introduced gradually if the child's energy and nutrient intake is otherwise adequate and if growth remains satisfactory. Fully skimmed cow's milk should not normally be introduced before the age of 5 years.
- Goat's and sheep's milks should not be given to infants, and if used after this age the milk must be pasteurised or boiled.
- Milk (also including breast-milk, infant formula, follow-on formula) or water should constitute the majority of the total drinks given. Other drinks should usually be confined to meal times and, because of the risk to dental health, they should not be given in a feeding bottle or at bedtime.

At birth the gastric, intestinal and pancreatic enzymes are not fully developed (Milla 1988), so foods other than breast-milk and infant formulae cannot be digested and absorbed properly.

The developmental changes which make weaning appropriate for the infant are listed in Box 15.3. The absorption of all nutrients from the gut becomes more efficient with age.

If the mother is well nourished, a breast-fed baby receives all the required nutrients in breast-milk for the first 4 months. By the age of 6 months, a diet of breast-milk only is likely to be supplying the infant with inadequate amounts of one or more of energy, protein, vitamins A and D, iron and zinc.

Delayed weaning. If weaning does not start until the child is older than 6 months the child risks suffering from nutritional deficiencies and may find developing the ability to chew difficult (Stephenson & Allaire 1991).

Box 15.3   Changes occurring between the ages of 4 and 7 months that make weaning appropriate

4 months

The infant can maintain posture if supported in a seat. The kidney has matured and is better able to conserve water and compensate for the varying solute concentration of weaning foods.

5 months

The infant can form a bolus of soft puréed food in the mouth and then move it to the back of the mouth and swallow it.

6 months

The infant begins to chew.

7 months

The infant begins to shut the mouth and turn away from food that is not liked, rather than spit or dribble it out.

Iron deficiency anaemia

Iron deficiency anaemia is a nutritional problem in infants and toddlers throughout the world (McPhail & Bothwell 1989) and a high incidence has been reported in the UK by Gregory et al (1995). Preliminary results from their National Diet and Nutrition Survey indicated that 12% of the 18-to 30-month age-group they studied were anaemic. This survey was of a nationally representative sample. Other workers have found a higher incidence among Asian communities, e.g. 20% in Bradford among lower socioeconomic groups (Ehrhardt 1986).

Infants and toddlers with an iron deficiency are usually apathetic and subdued. They have a poor appetite and are easily tired by exercise. Iron deficiency can also cause delay in psychomotor development, which may be permanent. This topic is discussed in much greater detail by Walter (1992).

Stages of weaning

For ease, weaning can be divided into three stages:

Stage 1	4–6 months
Stage 2	6–9 months
Stage 3	9–12 months

However, it must be remembered that these are guidelines and babies seldom conform to rules.

Stage 1

The choice of the first weaning food depends on the local diet and food availability. In the UK a non-wheat cereal such as baby rice or fruit or vegetable purée is usually used. These are chosen because they are less likely to cause an allergic food sensitivity. It is usual for the solid food to be introduced before a morning feed, although it does not matter which feed it is, as long as the parent or carer has time to be relaxed and the baby is alert and hungry. Sometimes babies are too hungry to try a new food. If this is the case, carers will find their infants more cooperative if the new food is given after a small feed, so that the infant is no longer too hungry.

If a cereal is used, it should be reconstituted with expressed breast-milk, infant formula or boiled water. This is mixed to a fluid consistency. If puréed fruits and vegetables are used, they should be prepared without the addition of salt and sugar (sugar should only be added to very sour fruits to make them palatable). Initially, one to two teaspoonfuls of food is adequate, but this quantity increases as the baby's appetite increases. As more solids are eaten, the amount of breast-milk or infant formula drunk will reduce. If the baby appears at first to spit the food out, this does not necessarily mean that the food is disliked, but rather that the baby has not yet developed the skill of using the tongue to propel the food to the back of the mouth. As the baby becomes accustomed to taking food from a spoon, the consistency of the food should become thicker.

Later, when the first food is well accepted, another food should be given before another feed, and then before a third feed, so that the baby becomes used to a varied diet of cereal, fruit and vegetables, meat, fish and pulses. At this stage, all food must be sieved, puréed or very finely minced. It is important that iron-rich foods such as fortified cereals, meat, offal, pulses and green vegetables are introduced, to prevent the development of iron deficiency.

Stage 2

By the age of 6 to 9 months the child should be able to chew, and consequently minced and mashed food that includes small soft lumps can be given. Some of the food that the rest of the family is eating can be mashed with a fork and used (see below on choice of weaning foods). During this stage, as the infant becomes more proficient at chewing, they should be encouraged to feed themselves. Foods like soft cooked vegetables, for example carrots, and chopped soft fruit such as pear and banana, and finger foods such as toast, should be introduced.

At this stage, babies must never be left alone while feeding because of the risk of choking, and babies or toddlers must not be given small hard sweets or nuts because of the risk of accidental inhalation.

Stage 3

By the end of this stage the baby should be eating similar foods to the rest of the family, as three main meals with either drinks of milk or snacks between them.

Food no longer needs to be mashed; it can now be chopped and the infant should be encouraged to feed themselves, with supervision.

By degrees, meals begin to follow the pattern of the rest of the family, with the first feed becoming breakfast, the next the midday meal and the third tea. The early morning milk feed is replaced by a drink of water or diluted fruit juice, if the child wakes early. The bedtime breast- or bottle-feed is usually the last feed to be dispensed with. Box 15.4 gives an example of a suitable menu for a 1-year-old child.

Choice of weaning foods

It is not necessary to buy commercially produced weaning foods. However, many mothers find them easy to prepare and use, especially when they are away from home. Most mothers choose commercial products as first weaning foods (White et al 1992). They are available in jars, tins and dehydrated in packets. The dehydrated foods are particularly useful in the early stages because they can be reconstituted in small amounts. It is important that the instructions on the packaging are followed carefully so that the food is stored correctly, prepared hygienically and the correct quantities fed to babies of the appropriate age. Stage One or puréed foods are followed by Stage Two or junior foods, which contain soft lumps.

All of these commercial products taste bland to the adult palate, but not to the baby, whose taste sensation is more sensitive. Salt and sugar should never be added to these products. It is obviously cheaper if the infant can be fed a portion of the family meal, particularly as his or her appetite increases. If the food is cooked without salt or seasoning, and these are added after the baby's portion has been taken out, the family's potatoes, vegetables and main dish (casseroles, stews, fish, egg or pulse dishes) are all suitable, as long as they can be sieved or very finely minced or chopped.

Constipation can be common during weaning. This can be cured by giving extra fruit juice or fruit.

Box 15.4 Menu suitable for a child aged 1 year

Waking

Water, fruit juice or milk if desired

Breakfast

Fruit juice
Cereal such as Weetabix, puffed wheat or porridge with milk
Wholemeal toast fingers with butter or margarine

Mid-morning

Piece of fruit or cup of milk

Midday meal

1 to 2 tablespoons flaked fish, meat finely chopped or minced, or finely grated cheese
2 tablespoons mashed potato
Vegetable, chopped
Milk pudding, fruit and custard or yoghurt, or fresh fruit
Diluted fruit juice

Mid-afternoon

Diluted fruit juice or milk and biscuit or fruit
(A mid-afternoon snack may not always be necessary depending on the length of time between meals and whether or not the child has a sleep)

Evening meal

Wholemeal bread sandwich with savoury filling such as egg or cheese, tinned fish or meat, or
Savoury snack such as baked beans with toast
Fresh fruit
Milk to drink

Bedtime

Some children still require a milk feed

Wholemeal bread and wholegrain cereals such as Weetabix can be included in the diet from about 8 months. These provide non-starch polysaccharides (NSP) and will prevent constipation from developing. Bran should never be given because it causes gastro-intestinal discomfort and inhibits the absorption of minerals from the gut.

Appendix 6 should be consulted for a comprehensive list of which foods can be included in the weaning diet. The MAFF (1997) publication *Healthy Diets for Infants and Young Children* is a useful practical guide.

Stopping breast-feeding

It is not necessary to change a breast-fed baby on to a bottle, as a teaspoon, cup or training beaker are all suitable. By the age of 10 to 12 months most babies can drink from a cup. The amount of milk drunk needs to be reduced gradually as more solid food is eaten, so that a 1-year-old who is eating a mixed diet receives approximately 500 ml of milk a day. Carers should be encouraged to continue giving breast-milk or infant formula for the first year of life. Breast-feeding can be continued for as long as the mother wishes. If it is stopped before the age of 6 months, the baby should be given an infant formula. Babies should be discouraged from using a feeding bottle once they reach 1 year. Ordinary cow's milk can be included in foods in the first year of life—for example as yoghurt, custard and cheese from 4 months, and cow's milk can be used to mix cereals from 6 months—but it should not be given as a drink until the infant is 1 year old (DoH 1994a).

Follow-on milks. Follow-on milks are not suitable for young infants and are not intended for use until the age of 6 months, as they generally have a higher protein content than infant formulae. They contain high levels of iron and vitamin D and are intended to be used as a nutritious drink once weaning is established.

Goat's and sheep's milk. These milks should not be used for infants but can be used from 1 year if they have been pasteurised. When compared with cow's milk, goat's milk has a lower iron, folic acid, vitamin A and vitamin D content. Sheep's milk has a higher vitamin A concentration than cow's milk but contains less iron, vitamin D and folate (DoH 1994a). If these milks are used, vitamin and mineral supplements are necessary.

Drinks for infants

Water. Infants need to be given drinks that are microbiologically safe. All water used to make up infant formula feeds and for giving to infants less than 6 months old should be boiled and cooled. Fizzy water is not suitable for infants, nor is bottled water labelled 'natural mineral water' as it may contain higher concentrations of sodium, fluoride, nitrate and sulphate than the immature kidneys are able to cope with. These recommendations are for waters available within the UK—in other areas it may be necessary to boil water until the infant is older.

'Baby' fruit juices and drinks. These are available in a variety of forms: as granules, concentrated liquids or ready-to-feed. They are flavoured with herbal extracts or fruit juice and contain sugars such as glucose, sucrose or fructose and usually have vitamin C added to them. The range of allowed additives is far less than for the fruit squashes and soft drinks intended for adults. Care should be exercised when giving infants these drinks because the sugars in the drink and the acid in fruit juice can cause dental caries and erosion of the teeth enamel (see Chapter 16). These drinks and fruit juices should be well diluted if they are given to infants and young children and given as part of a meal. Fizzy drinks are not suitable for use in a weaning diet.

THE TODDLER AND THE PRE-SCHOOL CHILD

At this stage, the diet should follow the adult pattern. As teeth develop, the child should be encouraged to use them and should be given such foods as raw apples, raw carrots, crusts, toast, vegetables and other foods in a form which requires more chewing. Children's appetites show great variation from day to day, both between individuals and at different ages. Quantities should be adjusted in accordance with appetite and it must be remembered that eating is a social occasion and that young children copy their elders and enjoy sitting with the rest of the family and sharing their meal.

Where the feeding of young children is concerned, certain points require special mention. These are listed below.

Milk. This is still a very important part of the diet of the toddler and pre-school child, approximately 500 ml per day should be drunk. If too much milk is drunk, it will reduce the appetite so that less of other foods is eaten. Full-cream pasteurised milk should be used, or semi-skimmed. 500 ml of whole (silver-top) milk provides a 2-year-old with all the calcium and riboflavin needed, half the protein and a quarter of the energy requirements.

Because milk is such an important food, if it is excluded from the child's diet for any reason, special attention needs to be paid to the diet to ensure adequate supplies of these nutrients are included. Soya-based formula milks are a suitable substitute for cow's milk. The actual choice depends on the reason why cow's milk has been excluded, and dietetic advice should be sought. Some commercially produced soya milks are not fortified with vitamins and are therefore not suitable.

Welfare Milk. In the UK children attending nursery sessions are eligible to receive 1/3 of a pint of milk a day, each day that they attend nursery, and children under 5 years whose parents receive income support or job-seekers allowance are eligible to receive 1 pint of milk a day. For up-to-date information on eligibility for welfare milk see the National Dairy Council website: www.milk.co.uk.

Variety. Emphasis should be on a varied diet containing fruit and vegetables, meat, offal, fish, cheese and eggs. If a wide range of food is introduced during the first year, there is less likelihood of food refusal later. The best way of introducing a child, 1-year-old or younger, to a varied diet is to encourage sitting at the table for the family meals. The child is then likely to want a share of what he or she sees everyone else having, especially if the child has not been given too many between-meal snacks.

Appetite. It should be appreciated that appetite will vary from meal to meal and day to day, and that a healthy child should not be forced to eat when he or she is not hungry. Sweets, biscuits and similar titbits should not be used routinely as rewards or snacks, and the appetite should be permitted to regulate the quantity of food taken at meal times.

Food refusal. Every effort should be made to keep meal times relaxed and stress-free. The food refusal should not be discussed within the child's hearing— instead the refused meal should be removed. However, it is not appropriate to replace the meal with a favourite food. It is unrealistic of parents and carers to expect a child to enjoy all foods, many adults have food preferences and avoid some foods. A study by Gillman et al (2000) has shown that the quality of the diet is better in older children and adolescents when children are encouraged to eat with the rest of the family. Encouraging this at an early age is helpful in preventing food refusal.

Vitamin D. In infancy, almost the only dietary sources of vitamin D are the proprietary milks and precooked cereal foods fortified with this vitamin. When these foods are discontinued, vitamin D intake can be extremely low. A vitamin D supplement, e.g. Welfare Food Scheme vitamin drops, should therefore be continued during the second year of life at least. It is particularly important that breast-fed babies receive this supplement if their mother's diet is poor (Train et al 1995).

Teeth. The remains of sugary and starchy foods lodging between the teeth provide a medium for the growth of bacteria which produce acids capable of eroding dental enamel (see Chapter 16). Biscuits and sweets should not be eaten between meals.

Drinks for toddlers

Diet squashes and fizzy drinks are not suitable for toddlers because of their high levels of artificial sweeteners. They should receive a range of drinks. Cow's milk is still an important contributor of nutrients. Surveys show that water is infrequently given to children to drink. Its use should be encouraged. If they are given, squashes and juices should be well diluted and given in cups at meal times, rather than between meals, to reduce the risk of caries.

Tea. Although tea is given to many young children, it should not be encouraged as the main drink, i.e. at all meals, because the tannins in it reduce the absorption of minerals, particularly iron, and if it is sweetened with sugar it will contribute to the development of dental caries.

SCHOOL CHILDREN AND ADOLESCENTS

Once the age of 5 years is reached, skimmed milk can be included in the diet. Regular meals are important and the child should be taught not to miss meals, particularly breakfast, and not to substitute snacks of sweets, biscuits, cakes and crisps for meals. The guidelines in Chapter 14, to encourage the increased consumption of starchy foods, fruit and vegetables and decrease fat and salt, are appropriate to this age-group (DoH 1994b). It must be remembered that if the fat and sugar content of a diet is reduced, then the energy content of the diet must be increased to replace that which was provided by the fat and sugar, otherwise weight loss will occur. Box 15.5 gives a sample menu for a 7-year-old child.

As children become older, they become involved in the purchasing and preparation of food and so gain more control over the type of food that they eat. If care is taken throughout childhood and adolescence to ensure that children understand the importance of a healthy diet and public health initiatives ensure that it is available, the health of the population will improve.

School meals

The 1980 Education Act abolished national nutritional standards for school meals and allowed local authorities to establish their own form, pricing and nutritional content of meals. The range of types of meals includes a set-price meal (the most usual in primary schools) and a cash cafeteria system (common in secondary schools). Some schools combine systems, while others only provide a service for those receiving free school meals, and this may only be a sandwich-type lunch. Although school meals only make a contribution to the overall nutrition of children, their impact can be considerable. The COMA report (DoH 1989) showed that the dominant foods in children's weekday lunches were chips, pastries and buns and that chips eaten as part of a school meal accounted for 50% of the chips eaten by children on weekdays.

Box 15.5 Menu suitable for a child aged 7 years

Breakfast

Cereal with milk
Wholemeal toast with butter or margarine
Fruit juice, milk, tea or coffee

Lunch

School meal or packed lunch:
Wholemeal bread sandwiches with a filling of egg, cheese, meat or fish
Raw carrot or salad and/or a piece of fresh fruit
Piece of cake or biscuit or fruit loaf or yoghurt
Drink of milk, fruit juice or water

Teatime

Because many children now take a packed lunch to school, it is normal for them to have a main meal with the rest of the family in the evening

Home from school

Milk, fruit or wholemeal toast or bread with butter or margarine, jam, honey, peanut butter or savoury spread

Evening meal

Meat, fish, cheese, egg or pulse dish
2 potatoes
Vegetable
Pudding or fresh fruit
Drink of milk, water or fruit juice

A survey of school meals and packed lunches by the Consumer Association (1992) showed that children tend to choose the fattier snack foods and that lunches eaten by secondary school children were low in fibre, iron and folate and high in fat and sugar. This same report showed that packed lunches were now taken by almost half of the children and only one in four packed lunches included any fruit. The usual content of a packed lunch was sandwiches, crisps, a chocolate bar and a sweet drink (compare the packed lunch suggested in Box 15.6).

Children over the age of 5 years should be encouraged to have a fat intake that does not exceed 35% of their energy intake (DoH 1991). 75% of children surveyed in 1983 (DoH 1989) had a dietary fat intake that was higher than this. As children favour the fattier foods and snacks at lunch time, steps taken to influence their lunch-time choice must be potentially beneficial. Many schools offer healthy choices of lunch, but not all of the children choose to eat them. The school nurse, teachers, school meal staff and community dietitian have key roles in promoting healthy eating

> **Box 15.6** Components of a good packed lunch
>
> - Sandwiches or filled rolls (quantity depends on a child's age and appetite)
> - A piece of fruit and/or raw salad vegetables
> - A 'treat', e.g. yoghurt, fromage frais, currant bun, biscuit or cake (not the same item every day)
> - Drink—water, fruit juice, low-calorie squash
>
> The 'treat' component of the lunch could consist of low-fat yoghurt, fruit jelly, fruit bun or fruit bread. Biscuit, cake or crisps should be varied so that the child does not have a particular item, e.g. crisps, every day, but alternate foods of higher and lower fat content.

within the school. This can be done in a variety of ways, including inviting parents to special healthy eating events, healthy eating clubs and encouraging cross-curricular activities so that knowledge gained in the classroom is not seen in isolation but used to influence the choice of food.

Nutritional standards for school meals

New nutritional standards for school meals are to be introduced, and up-to-date information can be obtained from the Department of Education and Skills. The consultation document, 'Ingredients for success' (DFEE 1998) proposed that:

1. Nursery schools which provide lunch should offer at least one item from each of the main food groups (protein, starchy carbohydrates, dairy products and fruit and vegetables) every day.
2. Primary schools, where set meals are the norm, should offer lunches containing portions of different foods weighing a certain amount.
3. Secondary schools, where cafeterias are popular, should offer at least one item from each of the four main food groups.

As part of the 'Health-promoting Schools Initiative' (DoH 1999), pilot schemes of providing free fruit for primary schools were introduced in 2001. Further information is available from the DFES (www.dfes.gov.uk).

Adolescence

It is important to remember when influencing the dietary habits of adolescents that a normal part of their change from child to adulthood is to want to make their own choices and exert their independence. This may show itself by adoption of unconventional patterns of eating or unusual diets. This is often the age at which a vegetarian diet is adopted. Children who become vegetarian should have an understanding of a healthy diet as the basis for making choices and they need to understand how to modify their diet so that it is nutritionally adequate (see Chapter 14).

The national diet and nutrition survey of the diets of British schoolchildren aged 4–18 years (Gregory 2000) showed that the most commonly consumed foods were white bread, savoury snacks, biscuits, potatoes and chocolate confectionary. While the average intake of vitamins was adequate and the average intake of minerals was also adequate, in the older age-groups—11–14 years and 15–18 years—low mineral intakes were common, in particular zinc, iron, magnesium and potassium.

Many adolescents, particularly girls, are unhappy about their weight and shape and adopt eating habits which they hope will change these features. This makes them particularly vulnerable to developing an eating disorder. A study by Bull (1988) showed that 5% of girls were dieting to lose weight, 15% were watching what they ate in an attempt to lose weight and 35% of the total sample considered themselves to be overweight. Low dietary intakes of iron, calcium, thiamin and riboflavin were found in the groups who were restricting their dietary intakes in an attempt to lose weight (the advice later in this chapter on dietary treatment for childhood obesity is also appropriate for adolescents). Adolescent boys are generally less concerned about their weight, although a few boys do develop anorexia nervosa.

Because of their growth spurt, teenage boys, particularly if they are active, will appear to have an insatiable appetite, consuming in excess of 3000 kcal a day. They should be encouraged to increase their consumption of starchy foods, such as bread and potatoes, to supply this extra energy rather than eat sugary, fatty snacks. However, since they do not generally have a weight problem and foods such as bread and potatoes are not always readily available, this advice might seem irrelevant to them. They need to understand the impact that a high-fat diet will have on their future health.

INFANT AND CHILDHOOD OBESITY

The study by Bundred et al (2001) has shown that the prevalence of overweight and obesity in children aged under 4 years is increasing and the increasing prevalence of obesity in older children is well documented (Troiano & Flegal 1998).

It is general practice to consider as obese a child whose weight for height index is greater than 120% or whose weight is two or more centiles above their height centile (Shaw & Lawson 1994). Adult body mass index (BMI) charts are not suitable for using with children. BMI changes with age in childhood, the median at birth being 13 kg/m^2 which increases to 15.5 kg/m^2 at the age of 6 years and continues to increase to a median of 21 kg/m^2 at 20 years (Cole et al 2000). Further information about the use and interpretation of BMI can be obtained from the Child Growth Foundation (address at end of this chapter). Every attempt should be made to prevent obesity developing by encouraging physical exercise, regular meals and sensible eating.

At the same time an interest in and enjoyment of food should be encouraged, rather than creating an obsession with calorie content of foods and fear of weight gain. The overweight child is likely to be unhappy because of: possible teasing by family and friends, poor achievement at competitive games, tiring easily or embarrassment about his/her size.

Overweight children are also more likely to suffer from degenerative diseases in later life (Mossberg 1989).

Infant obesity

Infant obesity is now less prevalent than it was, as mothers and health professionals have become more aware of it and the steps that they should take to prevent it developing. It is associated with over-feeding of bottle-fed babies, either because the feed was made up incorrectly or the babies were encouraged to drink more than they required. A breast-fed baby can reject the breast when enough has been drunk, but if there is milk left in a bottle an infant will be encouraged to drink it. Early weaning has also been associated with infant obesity.

Most carers are very anxious when they realise their infant is overweight. They need to be reassured that the aim of nutritional advice is to slow the infant's weight gain rather than to encourage weight loss. The advice given will depend on the infant and circumstances, but should include discussion of the following topics.

Hunger. An explanation should be given that babies do not cry only when they are hungry. They also cry because they are tired, bored or uncomfortable. So, feeding an infant should not always be the immediate response to crying.

Infant formula. Infant formula must be made up correctly and no extra food, such as cereal or sugar, should be added to the bottle. Infants do not need to be encouraged to finish a bottle-feed if they appear satisfied and have had enough.

Weaning. Puréed fruits and vegetables should be encouraged as weaning foods rather than relying solely on cereals and desserts.

Between-meal drinks. As the dietary intake of solids increases, the amount of milk or infant formula taken should decrease, with between-meal milk feeds becoming unnecessary. Encouraging a child to change from a feeding bottle to a cup often helps with this, as a smaller volume is drunk from a cup.

Childhood obesity

Obesity does not develop in children because of any one factor, but rather as a result of a combination of factors. The most common factors are listed in Box 15.7.

Childhood obesity is a risk factor for adult obesity (Charney et al 1976), but not all babies who gain weight rapidly become obese children and adults. Surveys in the UK have shown 35% of infants to be overweight. This declines to 7% in the 6- to 11-year-old

---

Box 15.7   Causes of childhood obesity

Dietary

- Large amounts of infant formula or cow's milk consumed as well as an adequate diet.
- Increase in availability of high-fat/high-sugar convenience foods and snacks.
- Excessive consumption of fatty, sugary foods.

Social

- Less physical activity, increase in television viewing and playing of computer games, etc.
- Pressures to eat certain types of food by peers, family, advertisements,
- Changing family eating patterns.

Genetic

It is always difficult to differentiate between familial overfeeding and an inherited tendency to obesity. However, there are those who are very efficient users of energy and as such gain weight on a relatively modest calorie intake. If one parent is overweight, the child has an increased likelihood of obesity. This is further increased if both parents are overweight (Stunkard 1986).

Psychosocial

- Association between food and affection.
- Desire to please by eating.

age-group, and only half of this group can be expected to become overweight adults. It is more difficult to diagnose obesity in children than in adults because of the growth spurts to which they are subject. However, once a child has reached 6 years and his/her weight is 20% over his/her weight for height, this is a good indication. A child who is suspected of being overweight should have his/her height and weight plotted regularly on the centile lines of a paediatric growth chart.

Dietary treatment

The use of a paediatric growth chart shows where growth spurts can be expected and also ensures that excessive weight loss does not occur. The dietary treatment of childhood obesity should be aimed at encouraging a very gradual weight loss, or slowing down of the rate of weight gain, and a modification of eating habits to prevent further excessive weight gain and to ensure health in the future.

Rapid weight loss should *never* be encouraged in children because a nutritionally adequate diet is required at all times for normal healthy growth and development.

It is very important to help overweight children and their families assess their dietary intake and explore why the obesity has developed. The following questions will help in identifying the causes:

- Does the child's diet include a lot of highly refined, high-energy convenience foods?
- Does it include between-meals snacks, such as sweets, crisps, milk drinks or fizzy drinks?
- What does the child do in his/her free time? Is the child very active or is free time spent playing computer games and watching television?
- Does the child eat out of boredom?

Often, it is a combination of these factors that are responsible; once the child becomes overweight more food is eaten for comfort and to overcome the loneliness and boredom that result from the physical and social limitations imposed by obesity.

A sensible weight-reducing diet for a child should be suitable as a healthy diet for all the family. This avoids the problems of overemphasis on low-calorie foods, the feeling of being different, and the need for the child to eat different meals from the rest of the family. Simple measures which can be taken include:

1. Eliminating extra sugar from the diet by substituting low-calorie squashes and fizzy drinks or diluted fruit juice for ordinary squashes and fizzy drinks.
2. Not adding sugar to drinks and breakfast cereals.
3. Changing to a higher-fibre breakfast cereal which does not contain sugar.
4. Restricting the number and types of between-meal snacks.
5. Having fresh fruit as an alternative snack and dessert.
6. Encouraging the consumption of more fruit and vegetables.
7. Establishing a routine of regular meals including breakfast.
8. Restricting the number of times fatty food and chips are eaten and substituting higher-fibre, lower-fat foods such as pasta, rice and potatoes, and grilling foods instead of frying them.
9. Encouraging regular exercise (Robinson 1999).
10. Changing to skimmed or semi-skimmed milk.

If the child is over 5 years old, the fat content of the diet can be reduced by substituting skimmed for semi-skimmed milk or whole-cream milk. Low-fat cheeses, yoghurts and spreads should be used rather than the full-fat versions.

This does not mean that the child is never allowed sweets, crisps, chips and ice-cream, but that they are thought of as treats and included in a sensible, well-balanced diet. In this way, the child will learn to enjoy a healthy diet and have the right attitudes towards food.

If the obesity is severe, it may be necessary to restrict the energy intake, but if this is done the diet must still contain adequate protein, minerals and vitamins for growth. If an energy restriction is to be imposed, it should provide at least 60% of the theoretical EAR for a child of that age (Bentley & Lawson 1988) and growth should be carefully monitored. If the child only eats a limited range of foods, it may be necessary to provide a multivitamin supplement or mineral supplements.

VEGETARIAN AND VEGAN DIETS FOR CHILDREN

Lactovegetarian and lactoovovegetarian diets can be nutritionally adequate for infants during the weaning period and throughout childhood, as long as parents and carers are aware of the child's nutritional needs and how best they can be met.

Infants being weaned on diets restricted in animal protein should particularly be offered a variety of foods at each meal. Protein sources should be mixed. Each meal should provide vitamin C, and an energy supplement from a fat source should be considered if there are doubts about the adequacy of energy intake.

(DoH 1994a).

> **Box 15.8**   A day's sample menu for a vegetarian or vegan child
>
> **Breakfast**
>
> Cereal with milk or fortified soya substitute
> Bread with margarine or butter and yeast extract
> Diluted fruit juice
>
> **Dinner**
>
> Nut rissoles or vegi-burgers, boiled rice or mashed potato and peas
> Milk pudding made with cow or soya milk, or fruit
>
> **Tea**
>
> Beans on toast or cheese sandwich
> Raw tomato, grated carrot
> Milk or soya-based yoghurt and banana
>
> **Between-meal snacks**
>
> Nuts, dried fruit, bread, toast, biscuits, and occasional cakes and crisps
> NB: Whole nuts should not be given until the child is 2 years old because of the risk of choking. They should only be used finely ground.

British vegan infants who are breast-fed are reported to grow and develop normally. However, a study by Sanders (1988) has shown that the energy intake of vegan children is lower than that of non-vegetarian children and they tend to be smaller and lighter than the general population.

It is important to remember that many of the foods included in a vegetarian diet are bulky and not very nutrient-dense and a child with a poor appetite may not be able to consume an adequate quantity of food to provide a satisfactory energy or protein intake. If this occurs, mineral and vitamin deficiencies will also occur.

Weaning foods suitable for vegetarian babies

Stage 1. Pulse and lentil purées, vegetable and fruit purées, and milk puddings and custards using cow's milk or soya-based milk.

Stage 2. Bread, pasta, rice, finely ground nuts, cheese and soya products such as tofu.

If the parents rely on ready prepared weaning foods, they may need help in identifying those which are vegetarian or contain halal or kosher ingredients. If they are unable to do this, they will rely on desserts and puddings, which will have a detrimental effect on

the child's dental health and nutritional status (DoH 1994a).

Diets of vegetarian/vegan children should contain:

- Welfare Food Scheme vitamin drops to the age of 5 years
- a source of vitamin C at each meal (fruit, vegetables, diluted fruit juice)
- fortified breakfast cereals
- a portion of cheese, eggs, pulses, seeds or nuts at each dinner and tea time
- 500 ml cow's milk or fortified soya milk (NB: this does not have to be as milk, but can be incorporated into sauces, puddings, etc)
- a portion of starchy foods at each meal. This should be in a form that is not too bulky for the child and depends on the child's appetite, e.g. white bread or mashed potato may be more appropriate than wholemeal bread or a jacket potato.

Vegan children also need a vitamin B_{12}–fortified food, for example a fortified breakfast cereal or fortified soya milk.

An example of a day's menu for a vegetarian or vegan child is given in Box 15.8.

Vegetarian teenagers

Vegetarian teenagers are at particular risk of receiving an inadequate diet for the following reasons:

- increased requirements for nutrients during the growth spurt
- unconventional eating habits
- isolation within their family and peer group.

Vegetarian diets are more common among adolescents with eating disorders than the general adolescent population (O'Connor et al 1987).

Teenagers who are the only vegetarians in meat-eating families are at particular risk of dietary deficiency. They need to know how to be able to prepare pulses, nuts and seeds and include them in their diet. Otherwise their diet will rely too heavily on cheese and cheese-containing ready prepared foods which have a high saturated fat content or, if cheese is not eaten, their diet will be deficient in protein, vitamins and minerals. *The Teenage Vegetarian Survival Guide* (Grose 1993) is useful for this age-group.

Iron deficiency can be a problem for teenage girls who become vegetarian, as the adaptation of increased absorption of iron from the diet takes time to develop.

REFERENCES

Bentley D, Lawson M 1988 Clinical nutrition in paediatric disorders. Baillière Tindall, London: 191

Broadbent J B, Sampson H A 1988 Food hypersensitivity and atopic dermatitis. Paediatric Allergic Diseases 35: 1115

Bull N L 1988 Studies of the dietary habits, food consumption and nutrient intakes of adolescents and young adults. World Review of Nutrition and Dietetics 57: 24–74

Bundred P, Kitchiner D, Buchan I 2001 Prevalence of overweight and obese children between 1989 and 1998: population based series of cross sectional studies. British Medical Journal 322: 326–341

Cant A J, Bailes J A, Marsden R A, Hewitt D 1986 Effect of maternal dietary exclusion on breast-fed infants with eczema. British Medical Journal 293: 231–233

Charney E, Goodman H C, McBride M, Lyon B, Pratt R 1976 childhood antecedents of adult obesity. New England Journal of Medicine 295: 6–9

Clement M I 1989 Personal view—caffeine and babies. British Medical Journal 298: 1461

Cole T J, Bellizzi, Flegae K M, Dietz W M 2000 Establishing a standard definition for child overweight and obesity worldwide: international survey. British Medical Journal 320: 1240–1243

Commission of the European Community (CEC) 1991 Directive on infant formulae and follow-on formulae (91/321/EEC). Official Journal of the European Community L175: 35–49

Consumer Association 1992 School dinners—are they worth having? Which? September: 502–504

Department for Education and Employment (DFEE) 1998 Consultation: Ingredients for Success. HMSO, London

Department of Health (DoH) 1989 The diets of British school children. Sub-committee on Nutritional Surveillance, Committee on Medical Aspects of Food Policy (COMA) (Report on Health and Social Subjects 36). HMSO, London

Department of Health (DoH) 1991 Dietary reference values for food energy and nutrients for the United Kingdom. Report of the Panel on Dietary Reference Values of the Committee on Medical Aspects of Food Policy (COMA) (Report on Health and Social Subjects 41). HMSO, London

Department of Health (DoH) 1994a Weaning and the weaning diet. Report of the Working Group on the Weaning Diet of the Committee on Medical Aspects of Food Policy (COMA) (Report on Health and Social Subjects 45). HMSO, London

Department of Health (DoH) 1994b Nutritional aspects of cardiovascular disease. Report of the Cardiovascular Review Group of the Committee on Medical Aspects of Food Policy (COMA) (Report on Health and Social Subjects 46). HMSO, London

Department of Health 1999 Our healthier nation: saving lives. HMSO, London

Department of Health and Social Security (DHSS) 1988 Present day practice in infant feeding (Report on Health and Social Subjects 32). HMSO, London

Ehrhardt P 1986 Iron deficiency in young Bradford children from different ethnic groups. British Medical Journal 292: 90–93

European Collaborative Study 1992 Risk factors for mother to child transmission of HIV. Lancet 339: 1007–1012

Gillman M W, Rifas-Shiman S L, Frazier A L et al 2000 Family dinner and diet quality among older children and adolescents. Archives of Family Medicine 9: 235–240

Gregory J R, Collins D L, Davies P S W, Clarke P C, Hughes J M 1995 National diet and nutrition survey of children aged $1\frac{1}{2}$ to $4\frac{1}{2}$ years. HMSO, London

Gregory J 2000 National diet and nutrition survey: young people aged 4–18 years. Vol. 1. Report of the National Diet and Nutrition Survey. HMSO, London

Grose A 1993 The teenage survival guide. The Vegetarian Society, Altrincham, Cheshire

Hoddinott P, Pill R 1999 Qualitative study of decisions about infant feeding among women in East End of London. British Medical Journal 318: 30–34

Holland B, Welch A A, Unwin I D, Buss D H, Paul A A, Southgate D A T 1991 McCance and Widdowson's composition of foods, 5th Edn. Royal Society of Chemistry, Cambridge

Howie P W, Forsyth J S, Ogston S A, Clark A, Florey C du V 1990 Protective effect of breastfeeding against infection. British Medical Journal 300: 11–16

Ministry of Agriculture, Fisheries and Food (MAFF) 1997 Healthy diets for infants and young children. A guide for health professionals. HMSO, London

Martin J, White A 1988 Infant feeding 1985 Office of Population Censuses and Surveys, Social Surveys Division. HMSO, London

McPhail A P, Bothwell T H 1989 Fortification of a diet as a strategy for preventing iron deficiency. Acta Paediatrica Scandanavica Supplement 361: 114–124

Milla P J 1988 Intestinal absorption and digestion of nutrients. In: Cockburn F (ed) Fetal and neonatal growth. John Wiley, Chichester: 93–103

Mossberg H O 1989 40-year follow-up of overweight children. Lancet ii: 491–493

O'Connor M A, Touyz S W, Dunn S M, Beaumont P J V 1987 Vegetarianism in anorexia nervosa? A review of 116 consecutive cases. Medical Journal of Australia 147: 540–542

Righard L, Alade M 1990 Effects of delivery room routines on success of first breast feed. Lancet 336: 1105–1107

Robinson T N 1999 Reducing children's television viewing to prevent obesity: a randomised trial. Journal of the American Medical Association 282: 1561–1567

Sanders T A 1988 Growth and development of British vegan children. American Journal of Clinical Nutrition 48: 822–825

Shaw M, Lawson V (eds) (for the Paediatric Group of the British Dietetic Association) 1994 Clinical paediatric dietetics. Blackwell Scientific Publications, Oxford

Stephenson R D, Allaire J H 1991 The development of normal feeding and swallowing. Pediatric Clinics of North America 38(6): 1439–1453

Stunkard A J et al 1986 An adoption study of human obesity. New England Journal of Medicine 314: 193–198

Taitz L S, Scholey E 1989 Are babies more satisfied by casein-based formulas? Archives of Disease in Childhood 64: 619–621

Thomas B (ed.) 1994 Manual of dietetic practice, 2nd Edn. Blackwell Scientific Publications, Oxford

Thomas M, Avery V 1997 Infant Feeding in Asian Families. HMSO, London

Train J J A, Yates R W, Sury M R J 1995 Lesson of the week: Hypocalcaemic stridor and infantile nutritional rickets. British Medical Journal 310: 48–49

Troiano R P and Flegal A M 1998 Overweight children and adolescents: description, epidemiology and demographics. Paediatrics 101: 497–504

Walter T 1992 Early and long-term effect of iron deficiency anaemia on child development. In: Foomon S J, Zlotkins S (eds) Nutritional anaemias. Raven Press, New York: 81–92

Welford H 1994 Feeding your child from birth to three. Health Education Authority, London

White A, Freeth S, O'Brien M 1992 Infant feeding 1990. HMSO, London

Wilson A C, Forsyth S J, Greene S A, Irvine L, Han C, Howie P 1998 Relation of infant diet to childhood health: seven year follow up of cohort of children in Dundee infant feeding study. British Medical Journal 316: 21–25

World Health Organization (WHO) 1985 The quality of breast-milk. Report on the WHO collaborative study of breast-feeding. WHO, Geneva

World Health Organization (WHO) 1992 Consensus statement from WHO/UNICEF consultation on HIV transmission and breast feeding (30 April–1 May 1992). WHO, Geneva

FURTHER READING

Bond A (for The Vegetarian Society) 1995 Vegetarian vitality: a report on the health benefits of the vegetarian diet and the nutritional requirements of vegetarians. The Vegetarian Society, Altrincham, Cheshire

Coles A, Turner S (for the HEA) 1993 Catering for healthy eating in schools. Health Education Authority, London

Deitz W H 2001 The obesity epidemic in young children. British Medical Journal 322: 313–314

Fairbank L, O'Meara S, Renfrew M J, Woolridge M, Sowden A J, Lister-Sharp D 2000 A systematic review to evaluate the effectiveness of interventions to promote the initiation of breast feeding. Health Technology Assessment 4: 25

Office of Population Censuses and Surveys and the MRC Dunn Nutrition Unit 1995 National Diet and Nutrition Survey for the Ministry of Agriculture, Fisheries and Food and the Departments of Health: Children aged $1\frac{1}{2}$ to $4\frac{1}{2}$ years—Volume 1: Report of the diet and nutrition survey. HMSO, London

Royal College of Midwives 1991 Successful breastfeeding, 2nd Edn. Churchill Livingstone, Edinburgh

Sharp I (for the Expert Working Group) 1992 Nutritional guidelines for school meals: report of an expert working group. The Caroline Walker Trust, London

USEFUL ADDRESSES

British Heart Foundation
14 Fitzhardinge Street
London W1H 6DH
Tel: 020 7935 0185
Website: www.bhf.org.uk

Child Growth Foundation
2 Mayfield Avenue
Chiswick
London W4 1PW
Tel: 020 8995 0527

La Lech League
27 Old Gloucester Street
London WC1W 3XX
Tel: 0207 242 1278

Maternity Alliance
5th Floor
45 Beech Street
London EC2P 2LX
Tel: 0207 588 8583 or 0207 588 8582

National Childbirth Trust
Alexandra House
Oldam Terrace
Acton
London W3 6NH
Tel: 0208 992 8637
Website: www.nctpregnancyandbabycare.com

National Dairy Council
5–7 John Princes Street
London W1M 0AP
Tel: 020 7499 7822
Website: www.milk.co.uk

Vegetarian Society
Parkdale
Dunham Road
Altrincham
Cheshire WA14 4QG
Tel: 0161 928 0793
Website: www.vegsoc.org

16

Diet and dental disease

LEARNING OBJECTIVES

After studying this chapter you should be able to:

- describe the normal formation and structure of teeth
- explain the processes involved in dental disease
- evaluate the contribution of diet to the development of dental disease
- critically review the advantages and disadvantages of fluoridation of the water supply
- provide dietary advice that would ensure good dental health.

Healthy teeth and gums are part of good general health. They are essential for good nutrition, understandable speech and an attractive appearance.

TEETH

Humankind has two natural sets of teeth. The first is the milk teeth.

Milk teeth. There are 20 milk teeth, which erupt between the ages of 6 months and 2 years and, by the age of 12, have all been replaced by a set of 32 permanent teeth.

Permanent teeth. There are four types of permanent teeth. Each type has a characteristic shape which enables it to be used for a specific function (Table 16.1). The front teeth are the incisors; next to them are the canines, then the premolars and lastly the molars.

Tooth structure

All teeth have the same basic structure as that shown in Figure 16.1. The part which projects above the gum is the crown; the part which is embedded in the jaw is the root.

Table 16.1   Permanent teeth: form and function

Type	Number	Shape	Function of tooth in mouth
Incisor	8	Chisel-edged	Act as scissors for biting food
Canine	4	Conical	Tear off food
Premolar	8	Square, the chewing edge	Act as mill-stones, food is ground
Molar	12	has cusps	between the cusps

Box 16.1   Stages of development of adult teeth

Birth to 3 years

At birth, the jaws are already filled with developing teeth. The organic framework for enamel and dentine is deposited and calcification of the teeth starts. Teething begins on average at the age of 6 months and is usually accompanied by flushed cheeks, discomfort and dribbling.

3 years

The crown of the tooth is still buried in the jaw. It has reached its adult size but is not completely calcified.

6–7 years

Milk teeth start to be lost. Crown of tooth erupts into the oral cavity.

9–11 years

The development of the root of the tooth is completed.

Enamel. The entire crown is covered with enamel. Enamel is the hardest material in the body. Its complex, dense, crystalline structure contains the minerals calcium, phosphate and fluoride. The covering of enamel protects the biting and grinding surfaces of the tooth.

Dentine and cement. The structure of these two layers is similar. It is like dense bone without any blood vessels. The dentine layer is harder than the cement.

Pulp. This is the core which contains the blood vessels and the nerve.

Root. The root of the tooth is embedded in a socket in the jaw and fastened by the periodontal ligaments, which link the cement to the bone.

Tooth development

Permanent teeth take a long time to develop (see Box 16.1). They begin to develop at 32 weeks in utero and are complete by 9–12 years of age, even if not fully erupted.

Saliva

Saliva contains glycoproteins, buffers, antibacterial substances, calcium, phosphates, fluoride and other mineral ions. It functions not only as a lubricant to aid chewing but also to protect teeth from demineralisation. Saliva washes away some of the food debris and acid surrounding the teeth and dilutes and buffers the acids produced by oral bacteria.

DENTAL DISEASE

The two types of preventable dental disease are dental caries and periodontal disease. Both begin early in life. The highest incidence of caries formation is during childhood and adolescence. It is rare for new caries to be formed after the age of 25 although existing sites will be enlarged. Periodontal disease occurs mainly in adults and is their most common cause of tooth loss.

Dental caries

This is the progressive destruction of the enamel, dentine and cement of a tooth. Studies have shown a higher incidence of caries among children from lower

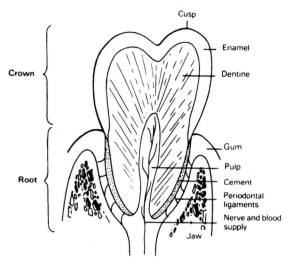

Figure 16.1   Cross-section of a molar tooth.

socioeconomic groups (Cushing & Gelbier 1988). 28% of inner-city 3-year-olds had caries, whereas in Bishop's Stortford, where there was a greater proportion of children in higher social classes, there was an incidence of 14% (Silver 1992).

The incidence of dental caries is higher in:

- single-parent families
- families where no one is in paid employment
- families of Asian origin
- families where the parents speak little English.

In medieval times it was thought that caries were caused by worms in the teeth. It has been known since 1890 that caries only develop if three factors are present:

1. susceptible teeth
2. substrate for cariogenic bacteria
3. cariogenic bacteria.

Susceptible teeth

The availability of fluoride and good overall nutrition during the period of tooth development make a tooth less susceptible to caries. Where there is severe malnutrition, teeth will be more susceptible to caries. Genetically, the teeth of some people are more resistant to caries than those of others.

1 Streptococcus mutans + sucrose + susceptible tooth
↓
2 Streptococcus mutans metabolises sucrose to produce lactic acid
↓
3 Lactic acid lowers pH below 5.5
↓
4 Calcium leaves the enamel of the tooth
↓
5 Enamel structure damaged
↓
6 Lactic acid reaches dentine and cement
↓
7 Calcium leaves dentine and cement
↓
8 Dentine and cement damaged
↓
9 Bacteria enter pulp of tooth
↓
10 Root becomes infected and abscess forms

Figure 16.2 The 10 steps of development of dental caries.

Substrate

Cariogenic bacteria metabolise carbohydrates as an energy source. Different bacteria are adapted to metabolise different carbohydrates. Sucrose, glucose, fructose and maltose are used, of which sucrose is the most important substrate, but it is only marginally more cariogenic than the other three (DoH 1989).

Cariogenic bacteria

Certain strains of streptococci, lactobacilli and actinomyces are cariogenic. These bacteria metabolise carbohydrates to produce acids. *Streptococcus mutans* is the most important of the cariogenic bacteria. It metabolises sucrose to produce lactic acid, which lowers the pH surrounding the teeth. Once the pH falls below 5.5, calcium ions start leaving the tooth enamel. This process is called demineralisation.

The 10 steps of development of dental caries are illustrated in Figure 16.2.

Dental plaque

This is the sticky whitish material that accumulates on the teeth. It consists of bacteria in a matrix of salts, proteins and polysaccharides. The polysaccharides are synthesised by the bacteria and act as a reserve substrate if sugar is not available.

Plaque starts to form at the junction of the teeth and gums. It thickens and spreads over the entire tooth surface as the bacteria multiply and synthesise more polysaccharides. Plaque encourages caries formation by:

- enabling bacteria to stick to the teeth
- allowing acids to accumulate around the teeth
- preventing saliva from reaching the teeth, so stopping it from washing them and neutralising the acid
- providing the cariogenic bacteria with a reserve energy supply—the polysaccharides—which can be used in the absence of sugars.

Periodontal (gum) disease

This is disease of the tissues around the teeth and occurs where plaque and gums meet. Bacteria in the plaque produce toxins and enzymes which diffuse out of the plaque into the gums. Here they cause irritation, inflammation and tissue damage. These sites of tissue damage are then invaded by other bacteria which infect the root and destroy the periodontal ligaments. The result of destruction of these is looseness of teeth and eventually tooth loss.

DIET AND DENTAL DISEASE

Nutrition and tooth development

Teeth start to develop before birth. At this stage the mother's general nutrition is important. There is no evidence to show that a diet high in calcium and vitamin D improves the strength of the developing teeth. However, the teeth of children of mothers who were poorly nourished in pregnancy are less resistant to caries formation later.

Certain drugs, including tetracyclines, taken during pregnancy will affect the calcification process of the tooth, causing the enamel to be pitted and discoloured. This will only be noticed years later when the permanent teeth have erupted.

The calcification of the tooth is a long process occurring over many years. If dietary fluoride is available, it is incorporated into the enamel. The healthiest teeth develop when adequate supplies of all nutrients are available. However, two vitamins are particularly important. Vitamin A is needed for enamel development and vitamin D for dentine formation. Once the teeth are fully formed, vitamin deficiencies which cause gum damage, i.e. lack of vitamin C, will cause tooth loss.

Fluoride and tooth development

The World Health Organization lists fluoride as an essential nutrient because of its importance in the prevention of development of caries. If fluoride is available for the entire period of tooth development and maturation, it will provide the tooth with lifelong protection. Ensuring that UK drinking water contains fluoride at a level of 1 part per million is thought to be the best way to accomplish this (Murray et al 1991). The importance of water fluoridation in reducing inequalities in dental health has been emphasised recently by the UK Government in the white paper *Saving Lives: Our Healthier Nation* (DoH 1999). When fluoride is incorporated into the tooth, the enamel is strengthened and made more resistant to demineralisation. The shape of the tooth is also changed. It is smaller and has fewer fissures. This is important because it is in these fissures that plaque and food debris can collect.

In a systematic review of water fluoridation (McDonagh et al 2000), the effectiveness of fluoridation in reducing the incidence of caries was confirmed. Concern has been expressed about the adverse effects of water fluoridation; fluorosis (mottling) of the teeth, bone fractures, problems with bone development, cancer and senile dementia have all been suggested. This systematic review only found evidence to support the increased prevalence of dental fluorosis as an adverse effect.

Fluoride in the diet

Water and soil contain fluoride in small and varied amounts. This means that most foods contain some fluoride but the amount will be very variable. If the water supply is not fluoridated, fluoride tablets can be taken. However, there is the risk of overdosage if they are used with a fluoride-containing toothpaste and fluoridated water. Fluoride-containing toothpastes have a beneficial effect, but this is not as great as fluoride in the water or fluoride tablets.

Diet and dental caries

Aristotle was one of the first to link carbohydrates with tooth decay. He noted that the sugar in figs caused teeth to rot. A normal diet contains a variety of carbohydrate-containing foods but not all of them are cariogenic. The cariogenicity of a food depends on:

- the physical form of the food
- the type of carbohydrate in the food
- the frequency of consumption of the food.

Physical form

Sticky foods which contain non-milk extrinsic sugars (see Chapter 2) that adhere to the tooth surface and become stuck between the teeth are the worst. This is because the bacteria are able to metabolise them for longer, resulting in a prolonged period of low pH, so allowing longer for demineralisation of teeth. Chewing stimulates the flow of saliva which washes the teeth and dilutes and buffers any acids present. Fibrous foods have a slight abrasive effect and do not adhere to teeth. It used to be thought that finishing a meal with a fibrous food such as an apple or celery would clean the teeth. This is not true, since only superficial food particles are removed. However, these foods are still valuable as sugar-free snack foods.

Drinks which contain non-milk extrinsic sugars are harmful, as they coat the teeth and act as a substrate for cariogenic bacteria. Acid drinks, such as fruit juices and soft drinks, are also harmful because their acidity lowers the mouth pH and encourages demineralisation of the teeth.

A survey by the Office of Population Censuses and Surveys (OPCS 1994) on children's dental health in the UK in 1993 reported that soft drinks were causing erosion of milk teeth in 50% of 6-year-olds.

Type of carbohydrate

Complex carbohydrates (starches) are large molecules. Large molecules cannot diffuse into the plaque so they cannot be metabolised by the bacteria in the plaque. Smaller molecules such as sucrose, glucose and fructose diffuse freely and so are available as an energy source.

Sucrose in the diet is without doubt the major cause of dental caries. It is the sugar most commonly eaten and is rapidly metabolised to produce acids. Sweets and the addition of sugar to drinks are not the only sources of sucrose in the diet. Sucrose is contained in many manufactured foods. Epidemiological evidence links increasing sugar consumption with increased incidence of caries in many countries. In the UK, the incidence of caries increased with the availability of sucrose in the 19th century. Wartime periods of sugar rationing have been accompanied by a reduction in the incidence of caries.

The acidity of some fruits can cause demineralisation when sucked and will lead to eventual destruction of the front teeth. This is a particular problem if grapefruit and lemons are sucked, a habit common in some Asian communities.

Frequency of intake

The pH of the mouth drops 2.5 minutes after eating a sucrose-containing food and stays low for up to 1 hour. This means that if sucrose is consumed three times a day, pH will remain below 5.5 for about 3 hours. The demineralisation which occurs during this time is sufficient to destroy the enamel progressively. If low concentrations of sucrose are consumed infrequently, the demineralisation is slight and, once the pH has returned to normal, remineralisation will occur. It is not only the amount of sucrose present in a food that is harmful but the frequency with which sucrose is eaten. Sugar-containing drinks and between-meals snacks are particularly harmful.

The site of dental caries can be used to identify the probable food which caused the caries (Table 16.2)

Table 16.2 Relationship of type of food to site of dental caries

Caries site	Type of food
Front teeth	Sweet drinks in infant feeders
Smooth surfaces of teeth near gums	Boiled sweets
Between the teeth, particularly the molars and premolars	Biscuits, cakes and toffees

Nursing bottle caries

Although dental caries are slow to progress in some situations, in others the tooth can be destroyed within months of erupting. Winter et al (1966) identified the link between feeding sweetened drinks in bottles at bedtimes and sleep times and using sweetened dummies as comforters, with a higher incidence of dental caries.

These practices persist and, to help overcome them, the COMA panel (DoH 1994) recommends that infants over 1 year should not use a feeding bottle. It is particularly important that cups are used for fruit juices, sugar-containing drinks and milk substitutes. Soya milk substitutes used instead of cow's milk contain sugars which can be cariogenic, so these too should be drunk from a cup.

Dental disease in sick children

Special attention must be paid to preventing dental decay in children who are unwell or have a disability. This is because it is difficult to provide these children with dental treatment. Both dental procedures which cause the gums to bleed and those which require a general anaesthetic are potentially more hazardous for sick children and some children with disabilities are particularly difficult for dentists to treat.

Children in hospital are at greater risk of developing dental caries because they usually have free access to sugar-containing drinks and sweets. It is easy to understand how this arises but if this continues for a long time or new habits developed in hospital are continued at home, tooth damage occurs.

Another reason why children who are unwell are more likely to develop caries is the addition of sugar to children's medicines in an attempt to make them more palatable. This is a particular problem if medicines are taken between meals and last thing at night over a long period of time. If the child is confined to bed, dental hygiene often suffers and, when the medical condition or treatment causes a dry mouth, saliva will not wash the teeth or buffer the acids produced.

PREVENTION OF DENTAL CARIES

There are four important factors in the prevention of dental caries:

- incorporation of fluoride to strengthen teeth
- efficient tooth brushing to remove plaque
- dietary changes
- regular dental treatment.

Dietary changes

The overall aims of changes in diet are to reduce both the amount and frequency of sucrose consumption.

- Always choose the sugar-free alternative if one is available, e.g. puffed wheat instead of sugar puffs; cream crackers instead of custard creams.
- Do not add sugar to drinks.
- Do not add extra sugar to infant and baby foods.
- Eat fresh fruit or starchy foods such as bread between meals. The sugars present in them have negligible effect (DoH 1994).
- Avoid sticky foods.
- If sugary foods and sweets are eaten, they should be eaten as part of, or at the end of, a meal.

The food and pharmaceutical industries could also reduce the incidence of caries by making the following changes:

- Stop adding sugars to infant and baby foods, fruit juices, vitamin preparations and paediatric medicines.
- Reduce the amount of sugar added to manufactured goods.
- Produce more savoury, sugar-free snack foods.

Good dental care and correct diet are important for all age-groups as effective, attractive, disease-free mouths contribute to overall wellbeing and are vital for the consumption of a healthy diet.

REFERENCES

Cushing A, Gelbier S 1988 The dental health of children attending day nurseries in three inner London boroughs. Journal of Paediatric Dentistry 4: 77–83

Department of Health (DoH) 1989 Sugars and dental caries. In: Dietary sugars and human disease (Report on Health and Social Subjects 37). HMSO, London: 16–20

Department of Health (DoH) 1994 Weaning and the weaning diet. Report of the Working Group on the Weaning Diet of the Committee on Medical Aspects of Food Policy (COMA) (Report on Health and Social Subjects 45). HMSO, London

Department of Health (DoH) 1999 Saving lives: Our healthier nation. HMSO, London

McDonagh M S, Whiting P F, Wilson P M et al 2000 Systematic review of water fluoridation. British Medical Journal 321: 855–859

Murray J J, Rugg-Gunn A J, Jenkins G N 1991 Fluoride in caries prevention, 3rd Edn. Wright, London

Office of Population, Censuses and Surveys (OPCS) 1994 Children's dental health in the UK. HMSO, London

Silver D H 1992 A comparison of 3-year-old's caries experience in 1973, 1981 and 1989 in a Hertfordshire town, related to family behaviour and social class. British Dental Journal 172: 191–197

Winter G B, Rule D C, Mailer G P, James P M C, Gordon P H 1966 Role of the comforter as an etiological factor in rampant caries of the deciduous dentition. Archives of Disease in Childhood 41: 207–212

FURTHER READING

Department of Health (DoH) 1989 Sugars and dental caries. In: dietary sugars and human disease (Report on Health and Social Subjects 37). HMSO, London: 16–20

Health Education Authority (HEA) 1990 A handbook of dental health for health visitors. HEA, London

Health Education Authority (HEA) 1999 Nutrition and oral health guidelines for pre-schools. HEA, London

Holt R, Roberts G, Scully C. 2000 Oral health and disease. British Medical Journal 320: 1652–1655

Office of Population Censuses and Surveys 1995 National diet and nutrition survey for the departments of health: Children aged $1\frac{1}{2}$ to $4\frac{1}{2}$ years—Volume 2: Report of the dental survey. HMSO, London

17

Nutrition and older people

Good Nutrition contributes to the health of elderly people and to their ability to recover from illness (DoH 1992a).

LEARNING OBJECTIVES

After studying this chapter you should have a better understanding of the:

- causes and consequences of malnutrition for older people
- prevention of malnutrition in older people
- particular nutritional needs of older people in residential care
- practical planning and serving of food for older people in residential care.

Although many long for retirement, few look forward to old age. Many people see it as a time when, with failing faculties, they will no longer be able to live useful, independent lives. With appropriate support, however, most people are perfectly able to live satisfactory lives until they are well into their 9th decade. Ensuring that they are well nourished is an essential part of this support.

THE OLDER POPULATION

Infection, disease and accidents, combined with the gradual degenerative processes, are the main causes of death for most of the population. The maximum age for humans is said to be 110 years. Very few people approach this age. As medical treatment improves and death as a result of infection, disease and accidents becomes less likely, the population lives longer. The figures for the number of people over retirement age in this country show the dramatic effect of improved medical services and better standards of living. In 1901 there were 2.4 million people over retirement age (male 65 years, female 60 years), this being 6% of the total population. By 1991 this figure had increased to 18.4% of the population of the UK and it is predicted that by the year 2031 it will have increased to 25.9% (OPCS 1993). This inevitably places increasing demands on health and social services.

The age distribution within the group is also changing, since more people now live longer.

The ageing process

This process starts once growth is complete at the age of 25. Few people are aware that it has started and it causes no problems. Later on, these processes speed up and physiological changes become apparent. It is not always easy to distinguish between the frailty caused by physiological changes and the physical decline which accompanies malnutrition. The degenerative changes which accompany ageing include:

- loss of sensations of smell and taste
- deafness
- failing sight
- osteoarthritis
- osteoporosis
- arterial disease
- reduction of glucose tolerance
- decline in muscle bulk and strength.

The study to estimate numbers of cognitively impaired and physically disabled elderly people estimated that 11% of men and 19% of women over 65 years, totalling 1.3 million elderly people in England and Wales, were classified as disabled and that 38% of disabled elderly people have cognitive impairment (Medical Research Council 1999):

- 28% reported moderate to severe disabilities
- 38% reported mild disabilities
- the incidence of disability increased with age
- for the group aged 80 years and over the reported incidence of moderate to severe disability had increased to 56%.

Much can be done to prevent or ameliorate disability and to encourage productive aging and enhance quality of life. Kerschner & Pegues (1998) have identified the importance of the enjoyment of food in contributing to the quality of life of older people and the links between health, independence, diet and wellbeing for older people. The position paper on nutrition, aging and continuum of care (ADA 2000) has identified that not only do older people benefit from their receiving good nutrition, but so does society. By improving health, reducing dependence and decreasing the length of hospital stays, the utilisation of health care resources is contained.

NUTRITIONAL REQUIREMENTS OF OLDER PEOPLE

The nutritional requirements for most nutrients for older people are the same as those of the younger population. The only exceptions to this are a fall in energy requirement with age and an increased requirement for vitamin D in the housebound. However, it can be extremely difficult for older people to have a diet that is nutritionally adequate when their appetite is poor, they are in pain or have a disability. This is discussed further, later in this chapter.

Energy requirements

Reduction in energy requirements occurs because:

- activity declines with age, so less energy is expended
- changes in body composition and function lead to a reduction in basal metabolic rate.

Figure 17.1 shows the changes in energy requirement that occur with age and reduction in activity, for men. There is a similar change for women; their energy

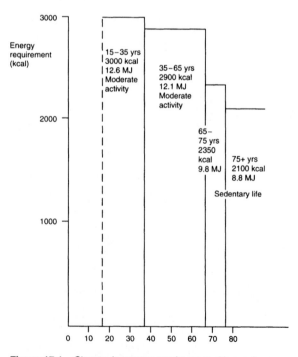

Figure 17.1 Change in energy requirement with age for men.

requirement drops from 2200 kcal (9.2 MJ) at the age of 18, to 1810 kcal (7.6 MJ) at the age of 75 years.

This reduction means that the diet has to be of a high nutritional quality to ensure that the requirements for all other nutrients are met, while the energy intake (total amount of food) eaten is reduced.

The practical implications of this reduction in energy requirements are not, as might be assumed, that older people should eat less, although this tends to accompany the decrease in appetite, but rather that emphasis should be placed on improving the quality of the food and its nutrient density.

Underweight older people

There are health benefits for older people who are not underweight. Campbell et al (1990) showed that a low body-weight in old age is associated with increased risk of morbidity and mortality. A study of acute medical admissions and geriatric outpatients showed that, when their body mass was lower than the local average, underweight older people lacked the metabolic reserves they require for responding to infection and, if they have been underweight for a long time, they may have been eating a diet that was inadequate in many nutrients.

To ensure an adequate energy intake the Committee on Medical Aspects of Food Policy (COMA) report (DoH 1992a) recommends that all elderly people have their energy requirement calculated using a PAL of 1.5 (see Chapter 7) irrespective of their activity level.

Overweight in elderly people does occur but is more common in the young elderly (DHSS 1979) and is associated with a high incidence of osteoarthritis in the knee (Felson 1988). Older people should be encouraged to maintain their correct body-weight to prevent the problems associated with underweight and overweight.

Certain individuals in the older population will have increased requirements of certain nutrients. For example, older people who are housebound, who live in institutions or who eat no meat or only fish were identified as being at risk of vitamin D deficiency. The Department of Health (1998) recommended that they receive a dietary supplement of 10 µg per day (see Chapter 6).

Those older people who are immobilised, have bed sores or prolonged fevers, will have an increased nitrogen requirement and require more protein to prevent a negative nitrogen balance (see Chapter 4).

As age increases, so does the incidence of disease and disability. Both of these factors reduce appetite and food intake (see Fig. 17.1), thus making the quality and nutrient-density of the diet that is eaten increasingly important.

MALNUTRITION

A survey of elderly people conducted by the DHSS and published in 1979 showed that 3% of the subjects in the study were suffering from clinical malnutrition (DHSS 1979). If this figure, which does not include those subjects who were obese, is applied to the entire elderly population, it means that over 300 000 people have inadequate diets, which inevitably has a detrimental effect on their health and quality of life. The commonest nutritional disorders found in the survey were obesity, and low intakes of folic acid, vitamin C, vitamin D, B vitamins, iron and calcium. The symptoms of some of these deficiencies are summarised in Table 17.1.

Malnourished older people can be divided into two categories:

1. *Generalised malnutrition.* The diet contains inadequate supplies of several nutrients. This is due to generalised self-neglect, and can be caused by a wide variety of circumstances, such as illness, disability, depression and bereavement.

2. *Deficiency of a particular nutrient.* This occurs when a particular food or group of foods is excluded from the diet. Two examples are:
  a. iron deficiency in those with poor teeth who avoid meat because it needs chewing, or for

Table 17.1 Nutritional deficiencies which can occur in some older people

Nutrient	Symptoms of deficiency	Easy dietary sources
Vitamin C	Weakness and tiredness Sore, bleeding gums Poor wound healing	Fruit juice
Vitamin D	Osteomalacia Bone pain Spontaneous fractures Low serum calcium	(Sunshine) Fortified margarines, fortified milk products and fortified cereals
Folic acid	Megaloblastic anaemia Tiredness and lassitude Inflamed red tongue	Green vegetables Yeast extracts

Iron	Hypochromic
	  anaemia
	Tiredness
	Headaches
	Brittle, spoon-shaped
	  nails
	Sore tongue
		Meat

whom its cost or difficulty of preparation excludes it from the diet

b. low vitamin C intake in those who have very little fruit and vegetables in their diet because of cost, difficulty with shopping or because they feel they 'disagree' with them.

Subclinical malnutrition

A large group of older people are thought to suffer from subclinical malnutrition. This means that their diet is not so poor that they show the clinical features of malnutrition, but their body stores of nutrients are depleted. If exposed to any sort of stress that reduces their dietary intake or increases their requirements, this group is likely to become clinically malnourished. They are inevitably a group at higher risk of developing other diseases.

Causes of malnutrition in older people

Malnutrition is rarely the only problem of an older person. Malnutrition does not usually occur in isolation but is precipitated by other social, physical or medical problems (see Box 17.1).

Extreme age

The increasing frailty of extreme old age increases the risks of malnutrition.

Social isolation and loneliness

14% of elderly people live alone. As life-expectancy increases, this percentage will also increase. Whereas 34% of elderly people under 80 years reported loneliness in a survey, 49% of those over 80 years did so (Jones & Cranston 1993).

It is easy to understand why people living alone cannot be bothered to cook for themselves. Meal times are particularly lonely for the recently bereaved. The importance of social contact to the wellbeing of older people must never be underestimated. The practical problems of catering for one are also difficult. It is hard to find small portions of fresh food, especially meat. Single people will often avoid eating meat rather than be embarrassed in the butcher's shop by asking for a small amount. Pre-retirement courses (considered towards the end of the chapter) are a very successful way of introducing new methods of cooking and types of food that are suitable for a single person. They also provide an opportunity to discuss the changing dietary requirements of retirement and later life. Luncheon clubs also provide social contact in addition to food.

Widowers are a particularly vulnerable group. They are frequently unaware of the value of a well-balanced diet to health and often find shopping, planning and preparing their own meals difficult. The plight of men in this group has led to the term 'widower's disease' being applied to vitamin C deficiency. A man aged 75 years and living alone is four times more likely to have a low dietary intake of vitamin C than a man of the same age who lives with his wife or family.

Loss of appetite

Enjoyment of and appetite for food are dependent on the visual appearance, taste and smell of a food. It is easy to appreciate how a decrease in appetite and loss of interest in the preparation of meals accompanies a reduction in the senses of taste and smell, particularly if this is also accompanied by a physical disability which makes the actual preparation of food difficult.

During the 10-year period between the ages of 74 and 85 years there is a 65% reduction in the sense of taste. It is the perceptions of salt and sweetness that decrease the most; the perception of bitterness remaining relatively unchanged. This reduction that accompanies age cannot be overcome. However, other causes such as poor oral hygiene, smoking and side-effects of some drugs can be reduced.

Salivary secretion also decreases in older people. This contributes to the loss of taste and makes chewing and swallowing more difficult, as saliva acts as a lubricant. This can be overcome in part by ensuring that foods are moist and drinks are served with meals.

Ways of compensating for loss of taste and smell

Older people in particular need encouragment to take an interest in food and their appetite needs to be stimulated to help overcome the reduction in taste and smell.

Box 17.1 Causes of malnutrition in older people

- Therapeutic diets
- Loneliness and isolation
- Mental illness
- Physical disability
- Dysphagia
- Illness
- Digestive disturbances
- Accident
- Poverty

This can be done by:

- Discussing a meal before it is served:
  — involve customers/clients in menu planning
  — display the menu
  — plan special seasonal events and theme menus such as a strawberry tea or Bonfire Night supper.
- Enhancing the flavour of dishes:
  — increase the sweetness of some dishes; this is not appropriate for diabetics or those who are overweight but is a useful way of increasing calories for those who are underweight
  — provide a range of sauces and pickles which can be eaten with the food, so enhancing the flavour
  — use more strongly flavoured foods such as mature cheese and smoked fish
  — note: be careful when using salt because many elderly people are taking diuretics.
- Taking care with presentation:
  — make sure food looks appetising
  — serve appropriately sized portions, not too large or too small, and extra helpings.
- Paying attention to oral hygiene—use of a mouth wash will help prevent particles of food from collecting in the mouth.
- Reviewing drug treatment.

Mental disturbances

Senile dementia affects 5% of the post-retirement population. People in this group often forget to prepare or eat meals. Older people who are isolated often become depressed and demotivated. They cannot summon up enthusiasm to shop for, prepare or eat meals. The local services of lunch clubs, day centres and meals on wheels are very important in improving the nutrition of this group.

Even when being cared for, this group of older people is at particular risk of becoming malnourished. Techniques for overcoming some of the feeding problems associated with dementia are described in Chapter 19 (p. 180). Morley & Kraenzle (1995) have identified that successful treatment of depression among older people stops and reverses weight loss.

Physical disability

10% of elderly people are housebound because of physical disabilities. In elderly people these include hemiplegia, arthritis, Parkinson's disease and injuries from accidents. An enthusiastic multidisciplinary team can do much to encourage their clients to regain interest in food and make its preparation as easy as pos-

sible. The provision of specially adapted utensils, perhaps instruction in use of a microwave oven, provision of practical meal ideas and recipes, and ensuring someone gets the shopping are all facets of this team approach.

Examples of convenience foods which may usefully be included in the diet of older people are:

- frozen vegetables
- 'boil in the bag meals', e.g. fish in sauce
- instant mashed potato
- tinned milk puddings
- frozen ready-prepared meals.

Therapeutic diets

It is not always realised that some therapeutic diets cause malnutrition in older people, for example:

- keeping to a strict weight-reduction diet long after the ideal (target) weight has been reached
- self-imposed exclusion of carbohydrate in a well-intentioned attempt to control diabetes.

Older people who are prescribed special diets should see a dietitian regularly to check that they are still eating a well-balanced diet. Morley & Kraenzle (1994) identified being on a special diet as a cause of malnutrition and weight loss for older people in a nursing home.

Teeth

Healthy teeth and gums are essential for comfortable eating and effective chewing. The daily energy intake of older people with ill-fitting dentures is 200 to 300 kcal less than for those with adequate dentition. This is because eating is uncomfortable, and these people gradually adopt a soft, bland diet. Poor chewing of food is sometimes the cause of indigestion. Regular dental care to check that dentures are well-fitting, that there are no decaying teeth and that gums are healthy is important for older people.

Dysphagia

Dysphagia is a condition in which the action of swallowing is either difficult or painful. It has a variety of causes. Whatever the cause, it results in a reduction in dietary intake which can lead to dehydration and malnutrition.

Some of the causes of dysphagia are:

- cerebrovascular attack
- multiple sclerosis

- motor neurone disease
- malignant disease of the oesophagus or oropharynx
- benign disease
- radiotherapy
- result of surgery
- confusion.

It is more likely that dysphagia will be identified and treated if its onset is rapid, for example following a cerebrovascular accident (CVA), than if it develops slowly, for example accompanying a benign stricture of the oesophagus.

A range of strategies can be used to ensure that a dysphagic client receives adequate nutrition (see Box 17.2). It is essential for these to be used in a range of combinations depending on an individual's needs. Layne (1990) recommends that clients with dysphagia have individual care plans which include their feeding strategies.

The swallowing team. Many health care units for older people now have teams which specialise in treating dysphagic clients. The team members all have a specific interest in swallowing difficulties and are aware of the special problems that dysphagic clients have.

Dysphagia is very distressing for older people, making meal times both tiring and depressing. It is the aim of the swallowing team to restore as much enjoyment and dignity to meal times as possible, as well as to ensure that the client is well nourished.

The swallowing team should include a speech therapist, a physiotherapist, an occupational therapist, a dietitian and a member of the nursing or care staff. Although the multidisciplinary members of this team all have specific roles (see Box 17.3), they all work together to ensure the client receives adequate nutrition (Wyatt et al 1992).

Assisted feeding

It may be the case that, because of the severity of an individual's disabilities, he or she requires help in feeding. Everything possible should be done to maintain

---

Box 17.3 A brief outline of roles of members of the swallowing team

Speech therapist
- Assess swallowing
- Provide exercises/treatment to optimise swallow
- Advise on suitable textures and forms of foods
- Liaise with other staff

Physiotherapist
- Advise on correct seating/positioning of client during meal times
- Advise on breathing exercises to help client regain swallow

Occupational therapist
- Advise on correct seating and use of specially adapted utensils—this is particularly important for CVA clients and those who have a physical disability in addition to dysphagia. As the incidence of multiple disabilities increases with age, the occupational therapist has a particularly important role.

Dietitian
- Nutritional assessment of client
- Ensure nutrient requirements of individual fulfilled
- Encourage appetite
- Liaise with speech therapist and catering staff about texture and form of food

Nursing/care staff
- Provide pleasant dignified meal times
- Monitor food and drink intake
- Feed client if necessary
- Minimise client distress at meal times

All members of the team need to meet regularly to review the progress of their clients and plan their care.

---

independence, because being fed can be unpleasant and undignified.

An individual who is being fed has no control over:

- what is eaten
- the rate at which it is eaten
- the temperature of the food
- the amount put into the mouth on each occasion.

Some of these problems can be overcome by discussion with the client and relatives to establish, for example:

- which foods are disliked
- whether a drink is usually taken with the meal or after it
- whether the client has always been a slow eater or usually finishes a meal quickly.

If a client requires to be fed, then the carer should always be seated at or below the eye level of the per-

---

Box 17.2 Feeding strategies in dysphagia

- Intravenous fluids
- Supplementary feeding } See Chapter 23
- Gastrostomy feeding
- Modified texture and consistency diets:
  — whole range from excluding difficult-to-chew foods to completely puréed diet
  — fluid thickeners for drinks

son who is being fed. Only one person should be fed at a time and feeding should be a relaxed, unhurried process.

There are particular problems associated with feeding a stroke client. These are summarised below and are well reviewed in Cockcroft & Ray (1985).

Ataxia and dyspraxia. These result in poorly controlled, shaky movements. The client may find it difficult to get food on to the utensil and then get the utensil to the mouth.

Perceptual disorders. The client may not be aware of all the food on the plate or appreciate the spatial relationships between food, utensils and plate.

Comprehension problems. The client may no longer understand how to use implements or follow instructions.

Paralysis. This results in difficulties in using utensils.

Food textures

Clients who find chewing and swallowing difficult, uncomfortable and painful, but who are not at risk of choking, require food that is soft and easily broken-up in the mouth, but rarely require liquidised or puréed meals. If the mouth is sore due to oral surgery, infection or radiotherapy, then the client requires foods that are bland. Sharp flavours, acid-tasting foods and salty foods such as citrus fruits and juices, vinegar and yeast extracts are best avoided.

Generally foods that are difficult to chew and swallow are:

- hard foods—toast, crackers, raw vegetables
- chewy foods—some meats, poorly cooked vegetables
- sticky foods—mashed potato and bananas, although soft foods, can be particularly sticky and difficult to swallow
- crumbly foods such as fruit cake or dry sponge cake.

Because eating and drinking is difficult, all food that is consumed should be nutritious—drinks should be milky, or fruit juice or squash, perhaps with a glucose polymer added, and meals should be as nutrient-dense as possible. If meals need extra fluid added to be satisfactorily puréed, then milk, gravy, soup, sauce, fruit or vegetables (these have a high water content) or nutritional supplement drinks should be used. Water should not be used because it dilutes the nutrient content of the meal.

Clients with swallowing difficulties usually find liquids the most difficult things to swallow. Several special products are available for adding to not and cold liquids to thicken them.

Once the initial reservations about the strangeness of a thick drink have been overcome, these can be used very successfully.

As CVA clients regain their swallow, food textures are reintroduced in the following order:

1. semi-solid food, e.g. ice-cream, mousse
2. thick liquids, e.g. custard, thick yoghurt or thick, sieved soup
3. soft foods, e.g. mashed potato, puréed vegetables, mince, milk puddings
4. thin liquids, e.g. tea or fruit juice.

It must be remembered that not all clients regain their swallow fully and many remain on a diet with a texture modified in some form and may also require additional feeding, perhaps by gastrostomy. The dietary intake of these clients requires monitoring and reviewing.

Prevention of malnutrition

Much malnutrition could be prevented if all the people who care for older people were aware of the risks and the contributory factors.

The recommendations of the COMA Report (DoH 1992a) for maintaining good nutritional status in elderly people are in Appendix 7. They include the following recommendations:

- Health professionals should be made aware of the impact of nutritional status on the development of and recovery from illness.
- Health professionals should be aware of the often inadequate food intake of older people in institutions.
- Assessment of nutritional status should be a routine aspect of history taking and clinical examination when an older person is admitted to hospital.

Nutritional assessment

See Chapter 23.

Many units now have a standardised nutritional assessment procedure which is used for all older people on admission to hospital. Charles (1998) has identified the features essential for good nutritional assessment of the older person (see Box 17.4).

- *Height and weight measurement and calculation of the body mass index*. If it is impossible to obtain an accurate height measurement, which is often the case for a disabled or confused client, then measuring the demispan may be easier (Bassey 1986). Demispan is the measurement from the web of the outstretched

---

Box 17.4 Hallmarks of good nutritional assessment for the older adult (Charles 1998)

Nutritional assessment should:
- be specific for over 65-year-olds
- not take longer than 5–10 minutes to perform and record
- be reliable and accurate
- not require extensive complicated equipment
- be non-invasive
- give a useful and/or meaningful result
- be easily repeatable over time

---

fingers of an outstretched arm to the sternal notch, and is related to height. There are limitations to the use of anthropometry for the assessment of older adults, so it is important that anthropometry is not used in isolation (WHO 1995).

- *History*:
  — Discuss client's current weight—is it steady or has weight been gained or lost recently?
  — Discuss client's appetite—is it good or is it declining?
  — Discuss client's meals—who usually provides them; does the client usually eat alone; is the client able to shop and prepare their own food?
  — Does the client suffer from a sore mouth, diarrhoea, constipation, vomiting or chewing and swallowing problems?
- *Physical appearance*:
  — Does the client look fat or thin; do the client's clothes fit or do they look as if there has recently been a loss of weight?
  — Does the client wear dentures—if so, do they fit? If the client has his/her own teeth does he/she receive dental treatment?
  — Does the client's skin look healthy?

Serum albumin, serum transferrin and serum haemoglobin are all important biochemical parameters for assessing nutritional status.

Dehydration

Care must be taken to ensure that older people receive an adequate fluid intake. They need 6–8 cups of fluid a day and this should be incorporated into the daily routine. If fluid is spilt, this must be taken into consideration and more given to compensate (see p. 180 on improving nutritional intake for clients with dementia).

Insufficient fluid leads to:

- raised urea—causing nausea
- headache

- constipation
- urinary tract infections
- confusion.

A survey by Seymour et al (1980) showed that many older clients admitted to hospital with an acute confusional state were dehydrated and their condition improved when they were rehydrated.

Constipation

In a systematic review of the effectiveness of laxatives in the elderly it was recommended that the use of laxatives was not appropriate for all elderly people (Pettigrew et al 1997). They recommend a stepped-care approach which used advice on how to improve diet as the first step, then if this was unsuccessful the use of laxatives. Constipation affects the quality of life of many people. Older people should be encouraged to eat a diet which contains a high-fibre breakfast cereal, wholemeal bread, fruit and vegetables and adequate fluid to prevent constipation (see Chapter 24).

Health education programmes

Health education programmes aimed at all older people including pre-retirement groups and those who work with older people are of great value and should be encouraged (DoH 1992a).

Pre-retirement courses. These courses are run by many organisations for their employees who are approaching retirement age. These courses should include several sessions in which nutrition is discussed, and should include easy cooking methods, ideas for menu planning for one and the emergency food store (see Box 17.5).

Box 17.5 The emergency food store

There are times when, because of illness or bad weather, older people are unable to go shopping. To ensure that this does not mean that they have nothing to eat, they should keep a store cupboard. Some suggestions for such an emergency store include:

Tinned soup
Dried fruit
Long-life milk
Tinned fish
Instant mashed potato
Instant fruit juices
Breakfast cereals
Tinned meat
Crispbread or biscuits

Box 17.6 lists topics in nutrition which should be included in a pre-retirement course.

Nutrition education. Older people are willing to make changes to their diets in order to improve their health when they have the benefits of the changes explained (Kumanyika et al 1999). Even the frail 75+ years age-group can benefit from nutrition education. This is based on a few simple dietary changes which will improve their diet (Box 17.7).

Home care assistants

Home care assistants give invaluable support to frail and housebound older people. They frequently do the shopping as well as preparing the only cooked meal of the day. Home care organisers often hold nutrition seminars for their staff to ensure that home helps are aware of the potential risk of malnutrition in older people and understand the dietary restrictions that some of their clients have, e.g. a sugar-free diet for some people with diabetes.

Meals on wheels

The number of meals each individual receives in a week depends both on the individual's infirmity and the local resources. Although this service has been run-

---

Box 17.6 Topics for nutrition sessions of a pre-retirement course

1. Basic good nutrition—the younger group of older people should be encouraged to reduce their fat intake and increase their intake of fruit, vegetables and starchy foods (DoH 1992a, 1992b)
2. Identify ideal body-weight—discuss problems associated with underweight and overweight
3. Role of fibre in the diet—its importance along with an adequate fluid intake in preventing constipation
4. Look after your teeth
5. Fluid intake—should be 7–8 cups a day
6. Meal planning
7. Use of convenience foods
8. The emergency food store (see Box 17.5)

Box 17.7 Simple changes to improve the diet of older people

- Have a glass of fruit juice every day.
- Have a fortified wholegrain cereal (e.g. Weetabix) with milk for breakfast.
- Try to eat meat or fish once every day.
- Have a milk drink at bedtime.
- Eat at least one serving of vegetables every day.

---

ning for many years, there are some problems associated with it.

Portability. Not all meals travel well; some arrive at their destination tepid and unappetising.

Loss of nutrients. The nutritional value of a meal which is served and kept warm deteriorates. A survey carried out in Reading showed that after the meal had been kept warm for 1 hour, it had lost half of its vitamin C content and half of its thiamin content. Another survey has shown that for some recipients of meals on wheels, their diet contained less vitamin C on the day that the meal was provided than on the days when they catered for themselves!

Punctuality. It is impossible to provide all recipients of meals with a lunch at 12.45 pm. Older people will have created their own routines and prefer to keep to them, so they do not like their lunch to arrive at 11.15 am or 1.45 pm.

Food will only improve nutritional status if it is eaten. The meal which is shared or of which half is kept for tomorrow will obviously not be as beneficial as the meal which is completely consumed. The contribution of the social contact of the meal being delivered is important, although limited. When new methods of improving this service are being considered, this, as well as the nutritional value of the food, must be taken into account.

Lunch clubs

If transport is available, this is the ideal service. The meal does not have to travel, so a wider variety of dishes can be served and there is less deterioration of the vitamin content. The club also provides social contact and a pleasant dining environment which helps to stimulate appetite.

NUTRITIONAL INTAKE OF OLDER PEOPLE IN INSTITUTIONS

The nutritional intake of older people in institutions is influenced by a range of social, environmental and physical factors including:

- monotonous menu
- poor presentation of food
- rushed meals
- no help in feeding frail residents
- lack of non-starch polysaccharides (NSP)-rich foods in menu
- lack of foods containing vitamin D
- lack of foods containing vitamin C and poor cooking methods leading to its destruction
- no involvement of residents in menu planning.

Davies & Holdsworth (1979) identified 26 factors which make an elderly person at risk of malnutrition. Many of them have already been mentioned in this chapter. These risk factors are listed in Thomas (1994), which should be consulted if greater detail is required.

Institutional catering for older people

All residents, whether in a hospital ward or residential home, should look forward to and enjoy their meals. This can be accomplished by:

• *Careful planning of menus.* Residents should be involved in this and if possible, a menu card should be available beforehand showing the choice of dishes. Puréed meals must only be served as a last resort as they look unappetising and if the senses of taste and

smell have deteriorated, they will all taste the same. Puréed meals should be served as individual components—i.e. individual small dishes of puréed meat, vegetable and potatoes—not a large dish of thick-looking soup.

• *Careful laying of tables.* As many people as are able should eat at a table which is attractively laid. Those who are able to should pour their own tea, serve their own vegetables, etc. People should not be forced to eat seated with people they do not like or whose eating habits they find distressing.

• *Allowing time for meals.* Time should be allowed for the meal to be eaten in a relaxed, leisurely manner.

• *Taking care over portion size.* Serve small attractive portions and have second helpings available and offered.

REFERENCES

American Dietetic Association (ADA) 2000 Nutrition, aging and the continuum of care. American Journal of the American Dietetic Association 100: 580–595

Bassey E J 1986 Demispan as a measure of skeletal size. Annals of Human Biology 13: 499–502

Campbell A J, Spears G F S, Brown J S, Busby W J, Borrie M J 1990 Anthropometric measurements as predictors of mortality in a community population aged 70 years and over. Age and Ageing 19: 131–135

Charles R 1998 Nutritional assessment methods for the older Irish adult in the clinical and community settings. Proceedings of the Nutritional Society 57: 599–602

Cockcroft G, Ray M 1985 Feeding problems in stroke. Nursing Mirror 160(9) Davies L, Holdsworth M D 1979 A technique for assessing nutritional `at risk' factors in residential homes for the elderly. Journal of Human Nutrition 33: 165–169

Department of Health (DoH) 1992a The nutrition of elderly people. Report of the Working Group on the Nutrition of Elderly People of the Committee on Medical Aspects of Food Policy (COMA) (Report on Health and Social Subjects 43). HMSO, London

Department of Health (DoH) 1992b The health of the nation: a strategy for health in England. HMSO, London

Department of Health 1998 Nutrition and bone health: with particular reference to calcium and vitamin D. Report of the sub group on bone health, working group on the nutritional status of the population of the committee on medical aspects of food and nutrition policy (Report on Health and Social Subjects 49). HMSO, London

Department of Health and Social Security (DHSS) 1979 Nutrition and health in old age. (Report on Health and Social Subjects 19). HMSO, London

Felson D T 1988 Epidemiology of hip and knee osteoarthritis. Epidemiology Review 10: 1–28

Jones D, Cranton S 1993 Health survey of a random sample of elderly people. In: Robins D (ed) (for Department of Health) Community care—findings from Department of Health funded research 1988–1992. HMSO, London

Kerschner H, Pegues J M 1998 Productive Aging: a quality of life agenda. Journal of the American Dietetic Association 98: 1445–1448

Kumanyika S K, Adams-Campbell L, Van Horn B et al 1999 Outcomes of a cardiovascular nutrition counseling program in African-Americans with elevated blood pressure or cholesterol level. Journal of the American Dietetic Association 99: 1380–1391

Layne K A 1990 Feeding strategies for the dysphagic patient: a nursing perspective. Dysphagia 5: 84–88

Medical Research Council 1999 Profile of disability in elderly people: estimates from a longitudinal population study. Medical Research Council cognitive function and aging study and resource implications study. British Medical Journal 318: 1108–1111

Morley J E, Kraenzle D 1994 Causes of weight loss in a community nursing home. Journal of the American Geriatrics Society 42: 583–585

Morley J E, Kraenzle D 1995 Weight loss. Journal of the American Geriatrics Society 43: 82–83

Office of Population, Censuses and Surveys (OPCS) 1993 1991-based national population projections. HMSO, London

Pettigrew M, Watt I, Sheldon T 1997 Systematic review of the effectiveness of laxatives in the elderly. Health Technology Assessment 1: 13

Seymour D, Cape R, Campbell A 1980 Acute confusional states and dementia in the elderly: the role of hydration, volume depletion, physical illness and age. Age and Ageing 9: 137–146

Thomas B (ed) 1994 Manual of dietetic practice, 2nd Edn. Blackwell Scientific Publications, Oxford

World Health Organization 1995 Physical status: the use and interpretation of anthropometry. Report of a WHO Expert Committee (World Health Organization Technical Report Series No. 854). WHO, Geneva

Wyatt R, O'Neil P, Bodey S 1992 The management of dysphagia. Care of the Elderly October: 388–392

FURTHER READING

Barratt J 2000 A client with Alzheimer's disease, fed via percutaneous endoscopic gastrostomy, with personal reflections on some of the ethical issues arising from this case. Journal of Human Nutrition and Dietetics 13 (1): 51–54

Campbell J 1993 The mechanics of eating and drinking. Nursing Times 89(21): 32–33

Cockcroft G, Ray M 1985 Feeding problems in stroke. Nursing Mirror 160(9)

Copeman J 1999, Nutritional care for older people. Age Concern, London

Expert Working Group for the Caroline Walker Trust 1995 Eating well for older people: practical and nutritional guidelines for food in residential and nursing homes and for community meals: report of an expert working group. The Caroline Walker Trust, London

Health Visitors' Association and National Dairy Council 1992 Good nutrition for older people: a practical interpretation of the Department of Health's report on `the nutrition of elderly people'. National Dairy Council, London

Nutrition Advisory Group for the Elderly, British Dietetic Association (NAGE) 1989 Eating a way into the `90s. Ellesmere Press, Skipton

Webb G P, Copeman J 1996 The nutrition of older adults. Arnold and Age Concern, London

Weinberg A D, Menaker K L 1995 Dehydration: evaluation and management in older adults. Journal of the American Medical Association 274: 1552–1556

USEFUL ADDRESSES

Age Concern Cymru
1 Cathedral Road
Cardiff
Tel: 0292 031 7566

Age Concern England
Astral House
London SW16 4ER
Tel: 0208 679 8000
Website: www.ace.org.uk

Age Concern Scotland
113 Rose Street
Edinburgh EH2 3DT
Tel: 0131 220 3345

Disabled Living Foundation
380–384 Harrow Road
London W9 2HU
Tel: 0870 603 9177
Website: www.dlf.org.uk

Help the Aged
St James's Walk
London EC1R 0BE
Tel: 0207 253 0253
Website: www.helptheaged.org.uk

Royal College of Speech and Language Therapists
2 White Hart Yard
London SE1 1NX
Tel: 020 7378 1200
Website: www.rcslt.org

The Stroke Association
Stroke House
123–127 Whitecross Street
London EC1Y 8JJ
Tel: 020 7490 7999
Website: www.stroke.org.uk

18

Nutrition, culture and ethnicity

LEARNING OBJECTIVES

After studying this chapter you should be able to:

- describe how religion, ethnic origin and culture influence the diet of different ethnic groups
- apply the knowledge of different religious dietary laws to ensure that nutrition advice provided is culturally appropriate.

Towns and cities in the UK are cosmopolitan, with residents from all over the world, including India, Pakistan, Vietnam, China, the West Indies, Europe, Australia and Canada. All bring with them their own traditions and cultures. When providing dietary advice, it is important to ask these individuals about their diets and never to make assumptions, as the effect of religion and culture on diet has different significance for different individuals. This is influenced by the length of time the individual has been in the new country, their age, and their cultural background and religious beliefs.

Historically immigrants have settled in the same area as their relatives and friends, who can help them to find work and accommodation, and to adjust to the new culture. Consequently communities develop which retain much of the immigrants' traditional culture and diet. An important part of any culture is food, whether it is the fast-food of North America or the curry of India. Food choice is governed by food availability, cost, personal preference, tradition and upbringing and, for some people, by religious laws. Religious food laws developed for a variety of moral and practical reasons, which include an abhorrence of killing, ensuring food hygiene and safety and as a method of giving a group its own cultural identity.

When unwell and in the strange surroundings of a hospital, everybody likes to eat familiar food, this applies to the entire population, and every attempt should be made to provide patients in hospital with food that is familiar and does not offend their beliefs, as well as being nutritionally adequate. The extent to which western-style dietary habits are adopted varies and tends to be greater among the younger generations and those who have been in the UK for some time (HEA 1991).

ETHNIC GROUPS OF ASIAN ORIGIN

These include people whose families originate from India, Pakistan and Bangladesh. Their traditional diets are well understood in the UK. The traditional diet is based on cereals and vegetables. It is wrong to assume that all ethnic groups from the vast Indian subcontinent have the same diet. There are many regional variations. These are due to differences in religion, climate, food availability, agriculture and tradition.

Climate

The diet is based on locally produced foods and the type of food grown depends on the local climate (see Fig. 18.1 for geographical locations).

Northwest India and Pakistan have a temperate climate.
- Wheat is grown as the staple cereal and is made into chapattis. These are flat cakes which are either cooked on a griddle or shallow fried and are eaten at every meal.

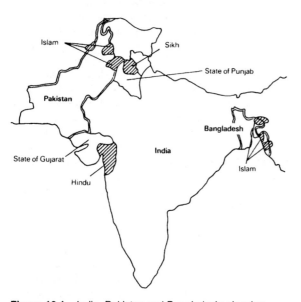

Figure 18.1 India, Pakistan and Bangladesh: showing areas from which people have emigrated to the UK, and the majority religions.

- Grazing is available for cows, so milk and milk products are included in the diet and ghee (clarified butter) is used for cooking.
- The vegetables grown include potatoes, carrots, cauliflowers and cucumbers.

Gujarat is an arid state.
- Millet is grown and ground into chapatti flour. Gujaratis in Britain usually use wheat chapatti flour because it is easier to obtain and cheaper than millet flour.
- There is less grazing available for cows, so the diet contains less milk and yoghurt, and groundnut and mustard seed oils are used instead of ghee for cooking.
- The vegetables grown are members of the gourd family. Gujaratis are unfamiliar with most of the vegetables cheaply available in Britain, so are far more familiar with aubergines and okra than with the traditional UK vegetables carrots and cabbage.

Bangladesh has a tropical climate.
- In the monsoon season much of this area, which is a fertile alluvial plain, is flooded. Rice is grown as the staple cereal on the flooded plains.
- Being so close to water, a lot of fish, both sea and fresh water varieties, is eaten.
- Very little dairy produce is available.

Asian religions

Many people of Asian origin adhere devoutly to their religions and the restrictions they impose. The three major religions are Islam, Hinduism and Sikhism (see Fig. 18.1). The dietary laws are summarised in Table 18.1.

Hinduism

This is the historic faith of the entire subcontinent. Many of the Hindu beliefs and customs have been incorporated into the Islamic and Sikh religions. In the UK, it is the immigrants from Gujarat and East Africa who are Hindu, those from Gujarat being likely to speak Gujarati as their first language.

Hindu dietary laws:

1. All life is sacred. No food that involves the taking of life can be eaten.
2. The cow is a sacred animal, though milk and milk products can be eaten.

Fasting. Devout Hindus believe that fasting influences events, so they fast frequently; for example, a woman will fast when her husband or child is ill. Fast days are decided on by the individual, after discussion with the priest, and are not predetermined. Some women may regularly fast for 1 or 2 days a week.

Table 18.1 Summary of the foods eaten by different religious groups

	Strict Hindus and Sikhs	Hindus	Sikhs	Muslims
Milk, yoghurt, ghee	Yes	Yes	Yes	Yes
Cheese (if not made with rennet)	Yes	Yes	Yes	Yes
Eggs	No	Rarely	Sometimes	Yes
Beef	No	No	No	Halal
Chicken	No	Rarely	Sometimes	Halal
Lamb	No	Rarely	Sometimes	Halal
Pork	No	No	Rarely	No
Fish	No	No	Yes	If it has fins and scales
Fruit	Yes	Yes	Yes	Yes
Vegetables	Yes	Yes	Yes	Yes
Pulses	Yes	Yes	Yes	Yes

Hindus do not fast by abstaining from all food and drink, but by restricting the amounts and types of foods they eat. Some people only eat foods that are considered pure on a fast day. These foods include fruit, nuts and potatoes. However, less strict Hindus eat lamb, chicken and white fish.

In addition, there are specific fast days:

- Mahashivrati—in March
- Ramu Nuami—in April
- Jan Mash Tami—in late August.

Diet. Most Hindus are vegetarian and some are vegan. This should be discussed with individuals to identify the most suitable nutritional advice to give them. Sweetmeats are particularly popular with Hindus. Box 18.1 provides an example of a day's menu for a Hindu.

Sweetmeats. These sweets, cakes and puddings are very high in calories (a small portion may contain 450 kcal, 1.75 MJ) and are made from sugar, ghee, full-cream milk powder and sweetened condensed milk (Govindji 1991).

These sweetmeats are eaten in particularly large quantities at times of celebration and during religious festivals. Examples of sweet meats are ladoo, jelabi and burfi.

Hindu religious festivals:

- Holi—lasts for 3 days in February/March
- Diwali—October/November

Sikhism

This is a reformist sect of Hinduism which rejects the caste system. Even though Sikhs are one of the smallest religious groups in India, in the UK they are a large group and some are likely to speak Punjabi as their first language. Like Hindus, the Sikhs believe that the cow is a sacred animal. Some Sikhs eat meat, but none eat beef. Like Hindus, some, but not all, fast once or twice a week.

Unlike Hindus, who worship mostly at home, devout Sikhs go to the temple, the gurudwaka, on a Sunday. The gurudwaka has a very important place in the Sikh community and serves up to three free meals a day. Most devout Sikhs will eat one meal a day, which consists of vegetable curry, chapattis and a dessert at the temple.

Box 18.2 gives an example of a day's menu for a Sikh.

Sikh religious festivals:

- Baisakhi—Sikh new year, April
- Diwali—October/November

Islam

This is the religion of Muslims. They believe in one God, unlike Hindus, who believe in many gods. The

---

Box 18.1 Example of a day's menu for a Hindu

Breakfast

Cereal and milk *or*
Vegetable curry with rice cakes
Tea made by boiling milk, tea and sugar together

Midday

Rice and lentils

Evening

Curried vegetables
Thin chapattis—the size and thickness of a chapatti depends on the local tradition. In general, chapattis made by Gujaratis are thin and small whereas those made by Punjabis are thick and large
Pickles—these are home-made and those which contain sugar are usually made with unprocessed sugar, *gurr.* Most contain a lot of oil
Fresh fruit

> **Box 18.2** Example of a day's menu for a Sikh
>
> **Breakfast**
>
> Chapattis or toast or bread
> Egg—boiled or fried
> Tea—made by the traditional UK method
>
> **Midday**
>
> Chicken curry
> Thin chapattis
> Side salad
>
> **Evening**
>
> Boiled rice or chapattis
> Channa dahl (pulse curry)
> Vegetable dish such as onion bhaji

Muslim holy day is Friday. Muslims come to the UK from Pakistan, Bangladesh, the Middle East, Malaysia and Africa. Muslims:

- are forbidden to eat pork and pork products
- must not drink alcohol, because it leads to loss of self-control
- are not vegetarian, but must eat meat killed in a special way—this is called halal meat.

Examples of a day's menu for Muslims are given in Box 18.3.

Muslim festivals. Eids—festivals—occur four to five times a year. *Ramadan* (Ramazan) is the ninth month of the Islamic (lunar) year. The lunar year has 355 days, so Ramadan occurs 10 days earlier in the western calendar each year. Muslims are expected to fast during the daylight hours of Ramadan. Everyone over the age of 12, except those who are ill, travelling, pregnant or breast-

feeding, is expected to fast. A person who is exempt from fasting during Ramadan is expected to make up the fast time at a later date. When Ramadan occurs in the summer, the period of fasting is much longer than when it falls in winter, so it is of far greater nutritional significance to those people who are unwell.

During the period of fasting, a large breakfast (sehri) is eaten before sunrise and another large meal (iftar) is eaten after sunset. Ramadan makes the management of diabetes more difficult (see Chapter 27, 'Diet and Diabetes Mellitus').

Cooking methods and traditional foods

Many of the foods included in the western diet are not excluded from the Asian diet because of religious reasons, but simply because the flavour is unfamiliar or there is uncertainty about how they should be cooked.

Meals are based on a pulse curry, rice or chapattis and relish or chutney. The tastes differ because of the numerous spice combinations used.

Along with the rest of the UK population, many Asians suffer from overweight and raised lipids. It is important that the dietary advice that they receive to overcome these problems is acceptable to their beliefs and practices. The major differences are summarised below.

Vegetables

- These are not served as a plain boiled accompaniment to a meal as is customary in the UK.
- They are fried in ghee or oil with spices and then served, or fried and stewed with other vegetables, meat or pulses and then served as the main dish with rice or chapattis.
- Raw vegetables, such as tomato and onion, are frequently served as a side-salad dressed with lemon juice and spices.

Spices

- Over 100 spices are used in Indian cookery.
- Different amounts of a variety of spices are added to each dish to give it its characteristic flavour.
- Many people find a hospital diet very bland. One way of overcoming this is to season the food with chilli powder or bottled chilli sauce instead of salt and pepper.

> **Box 18.3** Examples of a day's menu for a Muslim
>
> **From Pakistan**
> **Breakfast**
> Cereal or
> Bread/toast and boiled egg
> Tea made by boiling milk,
> sugar and tea together
>
> **From Bangladesh**
> **Breakfast**
> Cereal or
> Bread and jam
>
> **Midday**
> Chapatti
> Meat or vegetable curry
> Side salad
>
> **Midday**
> White rice
> Vegetable curry
> Dahl curry
>
> **Evening**
> As midday
>
> **Evening**
> White rice or chapatti
> Fish or vegetable curry
> Vegetable samosa

Meat

- Meat is not eaten at every meal; it is usual for small amounts of meat to be cooked with vegetables and served three or four times a week.
- The most commonly eaten meats are chicken and lamb.
- Pulses, such as lentils, are used instead of, or with small amounts of, meat in curries and stews.

Cheese

The cheese that is traditionally eaten is paneer, this is a soft curd cheese which has a mild flavour similar to that of cottage cheese. Cheeses available in the UK may be unpopular because of their texture.

The foods eaten by different religious groups of immigrants are summarised in Table 18.1.

Box 18.4 summarizes the dietary advice suitable for the treatment of overweight, diabetes and raised blood lipids.

'Hot' and 'cold' foods

Foods are traditionally classified as 'hot' or 'cold'. Whether a food is hot or cold depends on religion, and local or family tradition. In general, foods that taste sweet, bitter or sour are classified as cold and foods that taste salty or are high in animal protein are hot. Hot foods are believed to raise the body temperature and excite the emotions. Cold foods are thought to lower the body temperature, calm the emotions and make a person cheerful and strong. This food classification becomes important during illness, pregnancy and lactation, e.g. someone with a fever will eat 'cold' foods.

However, as the allocation of foods into hot or cold categories shows some local variation, it is best to consult patients about whether they are currently avoiding any foods or trying to eat more of a particular food.

Nutritional deficiencies

A traditional Indian diet as eaten in India is nutritionally adequate. However, in some situations deficiencies of iron, folic acid, vitamin B_{12} and vitamin D occur.

Vitamin D deficiency. (see Chapter 6). There is an increased incidence of rickets and osteomalacia among residents of Asian origin in the UK. Reasons for this include:

- The diet is low in vitamin D and high in fibre and phytate which bind calcium, making it unavailable.

> **Box 18.4** Dietary advice for Asian diabetic or overweight patients (Govindji 1991)
>
> **Practical advice on reducing fat**
>
> - Use less ghee or oil during cooking and in spreading.
> - Measure the amount of fat added with a tablespoon and gradually reduce the total amount used.
> - Choose polyunsaturated oils (corn, sunflower or safflower oil), monounsaturated oils (olive oil, rapeseed or peanut oil) and polyunsaturated margarine or low-fat spread wherever possible.
> - Try making ghee with a mixture of butter and polyunsaturated margarine.
> - Save fried snacks for special occasions only.
> - Buy lean meat, trimming off any visible fat before cooking.
> - Eat boiled rice routinely, and fried rice only occasionally.
> - Choose low-fat dairy products.
>
> **Practical advice on reducing sugar**
>
> - Try to eat sweetmeats on special occasions only.
> - Do not add gur to curries and pickles.
> - Replace sugar and gur with artificial sweeteners, e.g. aspartame.
> - Choose low-calorie and diet drinks in preference to sugared fizzy drinks.
>
> **Practical advice on increasing fibre intake**
>
> - Revert to traditional eating habits by including dahls, vegetarian dishes and wholemeal chapattis in meals as often as possible.
> - Choose wholemeal or granary bread, high-fibre breakfast cereals and brown rice in preference to the more refined low-fibre varieties.
> - Eat more vegetables, particularly with their skins (e.g. jacket potatoes).
> - Choose fresh fruit instead of fruit juice.

- The traditional clothing and behaviour of the women and children prevent them from being exposed to sunshine.

Henderson et al (1987) and Clements (1989) showed that there was no definite single cause for this deficiency and that it is probably due to a combination of environmental, genetic, cultural and dietary factors. Increasing the dietary intake of vitamin D and increasing the amount of time spent in the sunshine are beneficial.

Foods rich in vitamin D which should be incorporated into the diet are margarine and breakfast cereals that have been fortified with vitamin D. Yoghurt, cottage cheese, eggs, tinned oily fish and cheese are also useful.

Iron and vitamin B$_{12}$ deficiencies. These can occur in any population where meat and animal products are not eaten. Iron-rich foods which should be included in the diet are pulses, fortified breakfast cereals, oats, dried fruit and wholewheat products. Foods containing vitamin B$_{12}$ are milk, yoghurt and cottage cheese.

Folic acid deficiency. This occurs for two reasons:

• The traditional vegetables are expensive, so smaller portions are eaten.
• The less-familiar UK vegetables are over-cooked and the folic acid is leached into the cooking water and thrown away.

Foods rich in folic acid are raw fruit and vegetables, green vegetables, dried fruit, nuts and fortified breakfast cereals. The folic acid content of the diet is particularly important for women of child-bearing age.

Weaning

Asian infants are usually weaned at a later age than their white counterparts. Their traditional weaning diet is the family food which has had some of the spices rinsed off. Many mothers now feed their children on commercially produced foods, sweet foods are often chosen to ensure that the children are receiving a meat-free diet. This can cause problems as the children develop a sweet tooth and do not become accustomed to the traditional spicy flavours; it also encourages the development of dental caries (DoH 1988). Because of the lack of iron-rich foods in the diet, particularly meat, the incidence of anaemia is high (Duggan et al 1991).

JUDAISM

Orthodox Jews are strict observers of their laws, ceremonies and traditions. They adhere to dietary laws (the Laws of Kashrut) as an act of self-discipline. These laws govern both the types of food eaten and its preparation, and are summarised below.

The Laws of Kashrut

1. Meat must come from animals which chew the cud, are cloven hoofed and have been killed ritually.
2. Milk or milk products must not be eaten at the same meal as meat. They must also be prepared and stored separately.
3. Fish must have fins and scales. The eating of eels and shellfish is forbidden.

4. No cooking or preparation of food should be done on the Sabbath. Food which was prepared before the Sabbath can, however, be eaten on the Sabbath.

Food and meal times are important parts of Jewish family life and tradition.

Kosher meat

Many orthodox Jews live in well established Jewish communities where they are able to buy their meat from a kosher butcher. The orthodox method of slaughtering animals for meat is very quick and ensures maximum blood-loss. Once the animal has been killed, its carcass is salted and soaked in water. This process removes any remaining blood from the meat and is known as koshering. In areas where kosher meat is unavailable, halal meat from Muslim butchers is sometimes used.

Pork is the only commonly eaten meat in a mixed diet that comes from an animal that does not chew the cud. The pig is considered an unclean animal and serving pork and pork products is offensive. Hospitals can cater for the specific dietary needs of Jewish patients in two ways:

1. The first is suitable for liberal Jews who, when in hospital, stop eating meat and become vegetarian. By doing it this way they can be certain that milk and meat are not eaten together, and that pork is not eaten.
2. The first method is not acceptable to or suitable for more orthodox Jews, so frozen kosher meals are usually bought and re-heated in the hospital kitchen. A milk-free margarine should be available in hospital for this ethnic group.

A sample hospital menu suitable for a patient who adheres to the laws of Kashrut is shown in Box 18.5.

Festivals

Passover. This is an 8-day festival which occurs in spring. Leavened bread cannot be eaten during Passover and it is replaced by unleavened bread which does not contain yeast.

Rosh Hashanah. This is a 2-day festival occurring in September. Many traditional foods, for example honey cake, are eaten during this festival.

Yom Kippur. This occurs in the autumn, 10 days after Rosh Hashanah, and is accompanied by a 25-hour fast, during which no food or drink is consumed.

Box 18.5 Sample hospital menu for a Jewish patient

Breakfast

Cereal with milk
Toast, butter and marmalade

Midday

Grilled fish with lemon
Mixed vegetables
Baked jacket potato
Fresh fruit

Evening

Cheese salad
Boiled potatoes
Milk pudding

AFRICAN-CARIBBEAN DIETS

Afro-Caribbeans in the UK are familiar with the foods available and their choice of food is not generally governed by any dietary or religious taboos. They are unlikely to suffer from nutritional deficiency disorders. The use of oil for cooking most foods, and the popularity of sweet foods, does mean that in some situations the diet has a high energy content leading to obesity and conditions which are associated with obesity, such as hypertension and diabetes (Cruickshank & Beevers 1989). The starchy staple in the diet varies and includes tubers such as yam and sweet potato, rice and plantains. These are often cooked in a stew with other vegetables and small amounts of meat.

Rastafarianism

The Rastafarians are the one group of the West Indian population who may be malnourished. This religion is popular among young West Indians. Rastafarians believe that the Emperor Haile Selassie was their Messiah and that eventually all black people will return to Ethiopia, their promised land. Their dietary rules are a combination of the desire to eliminate all western influences from their life and the Old Testament food laws. Strict Rastafarians are vegetarian and some are vegan (see Chapter 14). The less strict Rastafarians who eat meat, never eat pork. Foods that are prohibited include all canned, preserved and convenience foods and alcohol. Traditional foods and cooking methods are used whenever possible. Salt is not added when cooking. Foods that are acceptable are called Ital foods. These foods are unrefined cereals and

organically grown vegetables and are expensive to buy. The vegetables that are eaten are usually cooked for a long time and the water, containing the folic acid, thrown away.

There has been very little research to investigate the nutritional status of this group. It is likely that some of the young women and children will have a diet that contains insufficient supplies of iron, vitamin B_{12} and folic acid. The exclusion of animal products from the diet restricts the intake of vitamin B_{12} and iron, and studies of children fed vegan products show that the diet is inadequate (Jacobs & Dwyer 1988). Few Rastafarians use pulses frequently as a substitute for meat. Babies are not fed commercially produced foods: they are breast-fed for a long time and weaned onto a high-carbohydrate diet based on cereals and starchy vegetables, which often may not be supplemented with the Welfare Foods Scheme vitamin drops and does not contain any of the vitamin-fortified baby foods.

CHINESE DIETS

Like the diets of other ethnic groups, there is considerable variation in the diets of people of Chinese origin. This is partly influenced by the area of origin. People of Chinese origin in the UK come mainly from southern China, Hong Kong, Malaysia and Singapore.

Southern China. Most immigrants to the UK originated from Southern China, so their traditional diet is based on rice, which is grown in this wetter region of China. Rice is eaten either boiled or made into rice noodles.

Northern China. The climate here is drier, so the cereals millet, sorghum and wheat are grown. Wheat is the most important and is used to make Chinese-style breads, noodles and dumplings.

Cooking methods. Traditional cooking methods involve cutting the food into small pieces which can be cooked quickly by stir-frying, deep frying or steaming. These cooking methods were developed because fuel was often in short supply.

Vegetables

- Salads are not usually eaten in China and it is rare that vegetables are eaten raw.
- Root vegetables are uncommon.
- Green vegetables and vegetables belonging to the gourd family are usually used.
- Vegetables are preserved by pickling, salting and drying.

Meat

Less meat is eaten than in the traditional UK diet. Vegetarian dishes are common and soya bean curd is used as a protein source in some. The most popular meats are chicken and pork, which are flavoured with sauces and dips which depend on the area of origin (Thomas 1994).

Flavourings

Soy sauce, chilli sauce, root ginger, garlic, onions and monosodium glutamate are all used to flavour foods.

Dim-sum

These are small filled dumplings which can be sweet or savoury, steamed or fried, are bought ready prepared and are a popular between-meals snack.

An example of a day's Chinese meals is given in Box 18.6.

Yin and Yang

The Chinese also have hot and cold food beliefs. Foods considered to be hot are Yang and foods considered to be cold are Yin. Good health depends on a balance of Yin and Yang. The classification of foods into Yin and Yang varies and cooking methods influence their category. Pregnancy is considered to be a Yang condition so fewer Yang foods, in particular red meats, may be eaten (Thomas 1994).

Information about foods which are available and culturally appropriate for the Chinese population in the UK can be found on the Chinese section of the British Nutrition Foundation web-site: www. nutrition.org.uk/chinese.htm

---

Box 18.6 Example of a day's Chinese meals

Breakfast

Egg and toast *or*
Breakfast cereal *or*
Congee (a rice porridge which is served on its own or with meat or fish)

Midday

Boiled rice *or* fried noodles, served with several main dishes which usually include a meat dish, a vegetable dish and a clear soup

Evening

As midday

Vietnamese diets

Many of the Vietnamese in the UK are of southern Chinese extraction and so their diet is similar to that of the southern Chinese in many ways (Goodburn et al 1987). The main differences are:

- Different flavourings are used—a fermented fish sauce called *nuoc mam* is used or dark soy sauce to season dishes at the table. Vinegar, chilli sauce, black pepper and monosodium glutamate are popular flavourings.
- Salads and raw vegetables are included in most meals.
- Dairy products are rarely eaten, fresh milk being unavailable in Vietnam, and cheese is uncommon.

Although few dairy products are eaten, calcium deficiency is uncommon in Vietnam because the rice and vegetables have a high calcium content. Calcium deficiency can occur in the Vietnamese in the UK because vegetables have a lower calcium content than those grown in Vietnam.

REFERENCES

Clements M R 1989 The problem of rickets in UK Asians. Journal of Human Nutrition and Dietetics 2: 105–116
Cruickshank J K, Beevers D G 1989 Ethnic factors in health and disease. Butterworth, London
Department of Health (DoH) 1988 Third report of the Sub-committee on nutritional surveillance (Report on Health and Social Subjects 33). HMSO, London
Duggan M B, Steel G, Elwys G, Harbottle L, Nobel C 1991 Iron status, energy intake and nutritional status of healthy young Asian children. Archives of Disease in Childhood 66: 1386–1389

Goodburn P, Falshaw M, Hughes H 1987 Chinese food and diet. National Extension College, Cambridge
Govindji A 1991 Dietary advice for the Asian diabetic. Practical Diabetes 8(5): 202–203
Health Education Authority (HEA) 1991 Nutrition in minority ethnic groups: Asians and Afro-Caribbeans in the United Kingdom. Health Education Authority, London
Henderson J B, Dunnigan M G, McIntosh W B, Abdul-Motaal A A, Gettinby G, Glekin B M 1987 The importance of limited exposure to ultraviolet radiation and dietary factors in the aetiology of Asian rickets: a

risk-factor model. Quarterly Journal of Medicine 63: 413–425

Jacobs C, Dwyer J 1988 Vegetarian children: appropriate and inappropriate diets. American Journal of Clinical Nutrition 48: S811–818

Thomas B (ed) (for the British Dietetic Association) 1994 Manual of dietetic practice, 2nd Edn. Blackwell Scientific Publications, Oxford

FURTHER READING

British Dietetic Association Nutrition Advisory Group for Elderly People 1996 2nd Edition. In the minority through the 90's: a handbook for those who provide meals for elderly people in a multi-cultural society, 2nd Edn. BDA Nutrition Advisory Group for Elderly People, Birmingham

Clements M R 1989 The problem of rickets in UK Asians. Journal of Human Nutrition and Dietetics 2: 105–116

Douglas J 1987 Caribbean food and diet. National Extension College, Cambridge

Health Education Authority (HEA) 1992 Nutrition in minority ethnic groups—briefing paper. Health Education Authority, London

Hill S E 1990 More than rice and peas—guidelines to improve provision for black and ethnic minorities in Britain. The Food Commission, London

Karmi G 1996 The ethnic health handbook: a fact file for health care professionals. Blackwell Science, Oxford

Mares P 1982 The Vietnamese in Britain: a handbook for health workers. National Extension College, Cambridge

Nicholson B E, Harrison S G, Masefield G B, Wallis M 1985 The illustrated book of food plans: a guide to the fruit, vegetables, herbs and spices of the world. Peerage Books, London

Squires A (ed) 1991 Multicultural health care and rehabilitation of older people. Edward Arnold and Age Concern, London

USEFUL ADDRESSES

SHAP Calendar of Religious Festivals
Website: www.support4learning.org.uk/shap/index.htm
Text version can be obtained from:
The Working Party on World Religions in Education
c/o The National Society's RE Centre
36 Causton Street
London SW1P 4AU
Tel: 020 7932 1194
Fax: 020 7932 1199
Email: nsrec@dial.pipex.com

19

Nutrition and mental health

LEARNING OBJECTIVES

After studying this chapter you should have an understanding of:

- how good nutritional care contributes to the health, wellbeing and quality of life of people with mental health problems
- the effects that the drugs commonly used for the treatment of mental illness have on dietary intake and nutritional status and strategies to prevent malnutrition
- how to ensure that clients with dementia are well nourished
- the different types of eating disorders, and their causes and treatment.

NUTRITION AND MENTAL HEALTH

The treatment of mental illness has undergone a radical change in the last 50 years. No longer are mentally ill people kept in long-stay hospitals for long periods of time, rather they are cared for in the community and encouraged to be as independent as possible.

Mental illness can be divided into three broad categories:

- *Psychoses*, which can be subdivided into organic and functional psychoses:
  - *Organic psychoses* can be permanent or temporary. They are caused by brain tumours, febrile illness, brain damage due to excessive alcohol or drug intake, severe nutritional deficiencies (particularly of the B vitamins), Alzheimer's disease, Parkinson's disease and Huntington's.
  - *Functional psychoses*: schizophrenia, mania and depression.

- *Neuroses*: anxiety, reactive depression, phobias, obsessions and psychosomatic illness.
- *Personality disorders*.

Meltzer et al (1995) have estimated that about one in six adults have some symptoms of mental illness, mainly neuroses, and that less than 1% suffer from a severe psychiatric disorder. Within these categories there is a wide range of severity, and the support and care provided should be planned around the needs of the individual.

MENTAL ILLNESS AND NUTRITIONAL REQUIREMENTS

People who are mentally ill have the same requirements for protein and energy as do healthy individuals. Some conditions or treatments increase the requirements for specific nutrients, for example:

- Suboticanec et al (1990) have identified that patients with schizophrenia have an increased vitamin C requirement
- high alcohol intakes reduce absorption of thiamin
- some anticonvulsants increase folate and vitamin D requirements.

Mental illness as a cause of malnutrition

The ability of clients who are mentally ill to provide themselves with a diet that is nutritionally adequate is reduced by a host of factors, which are environmental and social as well as disease-related. These factors include:

- confusion
- disorientation
- apathy
- poor concentration
- poor housing
- poverty
- isolation
- lack of social skills
- lack of catering and storage facilities
- the planning, shopping for and preparation of a meal is a complicated task which can be overwhelming for some mentally ill people.

The chapters on food choice should be consulted to understand why people make the food choices that they do. In working with mentally ill clients it has to be remembered that they are often among the most disadvantaged in society (Drever & Bunting 1997) and consequently they will not always have easy access to healthy food and good cooking facilities.

Mental illness affects nutritional status in two ways:

1. The effects on nutrient intake of the symptoms of the disease (Table 19.1).
2. The effects of treatment on the nutrient intake. Many of the drugs used in psychiatry have side-effects which influence nutrient intake.

Dietary treatment for the inpatient

It is important that nutritional status is considered at all stages of mental illness, and in doing this it must be remembered that apparently bizarre diets can be nutritionally adequate. However, it is more likely that clients will require a vitamin supplement.

When acutely ill people are admitted to hospital their nutritional status should be assessed. It is likely they will be dehydrated. In most situations it is inappropriate to try to obtain a traditional diet history.

Immediate treatment should include monitoring food and fluid intake to prevent dehydration. Treatment with vitamin and mineral supplements may be required to restore body vitamin and mineral stores to normal (Carney et al 1982, Mandal & Ray 1987).

Adequate nutrition should be provided to prevent further weight loss. This should be as food, but it may be more satisfactory to provide nutritional supplements.

Clients will not always see the relevance of discussing their diet or want to change their eating habits. The check list in Box 19.1 is a useful guide on how to proceed with the discussion.

Means of overcoming malnutrition

As the client's health improves, the intake of all nutrients will increase and it is to be hoped that the patient will be discharged well nourished. Preventing malnutrition from developing again is important.

As the client's condition improves, the dietitian should be involved in identifying any long-standing nutritional deficiencies and try to correct these. The diet may be deficient in one or more nutrients. The following are most likely: protein, energy, fluid, fibre, non-starch polysaccharides (NSP), vitamin C, folate, B vitamins and iron. However, if the client has previously been on a particularly bizarre diet, all nutrients and micronutrients should be considered, as the patient may have been consuming toxic amounts of a particular nutrient.

Protein and energy deficiencies. Poor protein and energy intake are often associated with difficulties in self-care including meal planning, budgeting and shopping. These may be partially overcome by attend-

Table 19.1 Summary of the effects of mental illness on nutritional status

Illness	Symptom	Effect
Depression	Food refusal Missed meals/drinks Fluid refusal	Reduced nutrient intake leading to weight loss, dehydration and constipation
	Carbohydrate craving	Can cause weight gain
Anxiety	Poor dietary intake Gastrointestinal symptoms such as nausea and diarrhoea Limited range of foods eaten	Reduced nutrient intake leading to weight loss
	Restlessness	Increased energy expenditure can result in weight loss
Mania	Increased appetite Increased activity–therefore increased energy requirements Missed meals Diarrhoea	Weight loss
Alcoholism	High intake of carbohydrate (from beer)	Weight gain
	Missed meals Poor food intake Gastritis Malabsorption of thiamin and folic acid	Weight loss Nutritional deficiencies
Drug abuse	Missed meals Poor food intake Chaotic eating pattern	Weight loss Nutritional deficiency
Schizophrenia	Inability to shop and prepare meals	Weight loss
Phobias	Agoraphobia, for example, can result in inability to go shopping	Limited nutrient intake Weight loss
Psychoses	Distorted idea of role of food and its nutritional value	Weight loss or gain Specific nutritional deficiency or excessive intake of a particular nutrient

ance at a drop-in or day centre and/or the support of a community care worker or psychiatric community nurse.

Lack of fluid. (See strategies for ensuring fluid intake in dementia, p. 180.) Try to encourage a routine which includes frequent drinks.

Lack of dietary fibre. Encourage the inclusion of a high-fibre breakfast cereal, wholemeal bread and fruit and vegetables in the diet.

Low vitamin C intake. This can be overcome by including fruit juice or fruit and vegetables in the diet regularly.

Box 19.1 Communication check list (Kenworthy et al 1992)

- Take time to listen.
- Give information in simple sentences.
- Keep questions to the point.
- Ask one question at a time.
- Avoid generalisations.
- Do not make judgements.
- Write things down for the patient if necessary.
- Treat each patient as an individual.

B vitamins, folate and iron deficiencies. These deficiencies are more difficult to prevent by improving the quality of the diet, although a well-balanced diet does include adequate amounts. It may be necessary to recommend a multi-vitamin supplement and iron supplement.

Drugs used in psychiatry and their side-effects

A large range of drugs have been developed for the treatment of mental illness.

Psychotropic drugs can be divided into five categories:

1. minor tranquillisers
2. major tranquillisers
3. monoamine oxidase inhibitors (MAOIs)
4. tricyclic antidepressants
5. lithium salts.

Minor tranquillisers

Benzodiazepines such as diazepam and nitrazepam are used as treatment for neurotic anxiety, as a sedative and as an anticonvulsant respectively. These drugs can cause changes in appetite, gastrointestinal upsets, weight changes and altered taste sensation.

Major tranquillisers

- Phenothiazines such as chlorpromazine. This group of drugs inhibit riboflavin metabolism, so a riboflavin supplement will be required if the dietary intake is poor. The phenothiazine drugs act by blocking the action of the neurotransmitter, dopamine, in the brain. Dopamine has a role in controlling hunger and therefore meal frequency. When dopamine levels are high, hunger decreases; if the action of dopamine is blocked, it does not have this appetite-suppressing effect. Clients taking chlorpromazine often gain weight because they are always hungry and so eat more.
- Thioxanthines cause weight gain.
- Butyrophenones cause nausea, dyspepsia and loss of appetite. Weight gain or loss can occur.
- Dibenzo-diazepines such as clozapine can cause gastrointestinal disturbances, polydipsia, dry mouth or hypersalivation and change in weight—either an increase or a decrease.

Monoamine oxidase inhibitors

Monoamine oxidase inhibitors (MAOI) are a group of drugs used to treat depression and include the drugs tranylcypromine, phenelzine and isocarboxazid. In depressed clients the levels of certain amines in the brain are lowered. MAOIs act to increase the levels of these amines by reducing the activity of the enzymes, monoamine oxidases, which occur in the tissues. These enzymes usually act by destroying tyramine, an amine of the amino acid tyrosine. If not destroyed, tyramine inhibits the metabolism of catecholamines, including noradrenaline, resulting in severe headache, nausea, dizziness, hypertension and, in severe cases, subarachnoid haemorrhage. For this reason, patients receiving MAOIs should avoid foods which contain tyramine.

Foods to be avoided during MAOI treatment are:

- alcoholic drinks
- cheese and cheese spreads
- yeast and meat extracts and processed foods which contain these extracts
- flavoured textured vegetable protein
- food which has been stored for a long time
- preserved foods, for example pickled herrings
- game

- broad bean pods.

The tyramine content of certain foods varies, depending on the age of the food and how much of the tyrosine present has been degraded to tyramine. Wherever possible, people on monoamine oxidase inhibiting drugs should have meals produced freshly from fresh, frozen or tinned foods.

Tricyclic antidepressants

- Imipramine and amitryptyline cause weight gain. These drugs act by increasing the levels of the neurotransmitter noradrenaline in the brain. Noradrenaline stimulates and increases food intake by delaying the onset of satiety and it can also cause carbohydrate craving. Other side-effects of this group of drugs include metallic taste, dry mouth and constipation.
- 5-HT re-uptake inhibitors cause weight loss. This group of drugs increase the level of the neurotransmitter 5-hydroxytryptamine (5-HT, serotonin) in the brain. Like noradrenaline, 5-HT affects the satiety centre of the brain, but it increases the sensation of satiety so less food is eaten and meals are taken less frequently.

Lithium salts

Examples are lithium carbonate and lithium citrate, which are used as mood stabilisers.

In common with other drugs, they can cause nausea, a metallic taste in the mouth and increased thirst. Weight gain and mild oedema are also associated with prolonged use. Clients taking lithium salts should not restrict their fluid intake but be advised to drink low-calorie drinks rather than large quantities of soft drinks and sweetened tea and coffee. The serum lithium levels need monitoring regularly to ensure that toxic levels are not reached. Toxic doses cause vomiting, diarrhoea and loss of appetite.

There is an inverse relationship between dietary sodium intake and serum lithium levels. This means that any significant change in dietary sodium intake (e.g. change to a salt substitute or sudden increase in intake of salty snacks and prepared foods) will result in a change in the serum lithium level. The therapeutic range of serum lithium levels is narrow and dosage will need to change if diet is changed permanently.

Some of the drugs have side-effects which are distressing to both clients and relatives. These side-effects can include slurred speech, blurred vision, loss of facial expression, stiffness of limbs and those which can affect nutrient intake:

- increased or decreased hunger associated with weight gain or loss
- altered taste perception, metallic taste in mouth
- dry mouth, increased thirst
- nausea, upper gastrointestinal tract disturbances
- constipation
- carbohydrate craving leading to weight gain.

Strategies for overcoming some of the problems associated with psychotropic drugs

Constipation

- Increase fluid intake—it may be necessary to monitor fluid intake to ensure that confused patients are drinking at least 8 cups of fluid a day
- Increase fibre intake—by including wholemeal bread and wholegrain breakfast cereals
- Increase fruit and vegetable intake—the diet provided should include generous portions of fruit and vegetables.

Weight gain

Identify causes. Weight gain is not always due to the side-effects of drugs. It can be due to boredom and lack of opportunity to exercise, or merely to overconsumption of food, and can occur after admission to hospital, when the diet may contain more energy than is required. If the weight gain is due to increased intake of food, caused as a side-effect of drugs, it is not appropriate to start using a very low-calorie restricted diet. Instead, the dietary intake should be based on the individual's energy requirement and designed to include between-meal snacks, which will help alleviate the intense hunger that may be experienced and encourage the client to cooperate in restricting energy intake. It is particularly important to allow snacks during the evening, which is often a period of intense hunger.

Advice needs to be given about suitable snacks and these should be available. Fruit, bread and sandwiches should be available instead of high-fat, high-sugar confectionery and crisps. Other useful snacks are low-calorie soups and sugar-free drinks.

Increased thirst

Increased thirst will lead to weight gain if the extra fluid drunk contains sugar or includes a lot of milk.

Skimmed milk, artificial sweeteners and low-calorie drinks should be available and encouraged.

Psychiatric illness caused by nutritional deficiency

The links between dehydration and confusion are well documented (Seymour et al 1980). However, deficiencies of other nutrients as the causes of mental illness can go unnoticed as their incidence is so low.

Vitamin C. Kinsman & Hood (1971) described personality changes in a study of five healthy volunteers who took part in a vitamin C depletion study, and Walker (1968) identified severe depression as a symptom in patients with chronic scurvy.

Thiamin. Wernicke–Korsakoff syndrome has symptoms including ataxia, nystagmus, loss of memory and confusion. The incidence is increasing, particularly among alcoholics, although it can occur in any situation where dietary intake of thiamin is low or absorption is reduced due to prolonged vomiting.

Nicotinic acid. In mild cases of nicotinic acid deficiency, symptoms include anxiety, depression and irritability. Dementia can occur in more extreme cases. Cranmer (1983) has reported that patients with nicotinic acid deficiency may be admitted to a psychiatric hospital because of the severity of their symptoms.

Folic acid and vitamin B$_{12}$. It has been hypothesised that low levels of either vitamin B$_{12}$ or folate cause a deficiency of neurotransmitters, in particular 5-HT (serotonin) (Scott & Weir 1981). Godfrey et al (1990) have been able to show that dietary supplementation with methyl folate may improve the mental state of those showing biochemical evidence of deficiency.

DEMENTIA

Dementia is a chronic disorder which has many causes. The patient with dementia suffers from:

- poor memory
- personality changes
- disorientation
- decreased reasoning ability
- inattention to personal care.

The condition is usually progressive, resulting in an extremely frail, vulnerable and confused individual who is totally reliant on others for all his/her care, particularly for ensuring that he or she receives an adequate fluid and nutrient intake. Dehydration and vitamin deficiencies can cause temporary dementia and will make existing dementia more extreme.

The most common cause of dementia is Alzheimer's disease and, because high levels of aluminium have been found in the cerebral cortex of some patients with Alzheimer's disease, great interest has been expressed in the links between dietary aluminium intake and the development of Alzheimer's disease (MacLachlan 1986).

Aluminium occurs in water, toothpaste, antacids and some foods, particularly those cooked in aluminium saucepans. There is currently insufficient evidence to recommend that the population reduce its aluminium intake.

Demented patients will show a range of symptoms which will affect their ability to provide themselves with an adequate diet. Initially they:

- are forgetful and absent minded
- are unable to shop and prepare food
- forget to eat
- eat a monotonous, inadequate diet.

These symptoms progress at different rates for different individuals. Sometimes a stage is reached where food is not chewed properly, causing choking, and the individual may be unable to remember how to use cutlery or recognise food items. The increase in activity and agitation, which also occurs, increases the energy requirement and it is often necessary to use dietary supplements (see Chapter 23), which may eventually provide the majority of the client's dietary needs.

Strategies for ensuring adequate nutrition in patients with dementia

1. *Provide frequent meals and snacks.* This increases the number of opportunities clients have to eat. It is particularly important to provide snacks in the middle of the afternoon and during the evening, as these are the times in the day when the longest periods between meals occur and the snacks are unlikely to reduce appetite for the next meal. Examples of suitable snacks are milky drinks, biscuits, sandwiches, crackers and cheese. Fresh fruit, although generally advised as a between-meals snack, is inappropriate because of its low energy content. The use of supplement drinks between meals may be beneficial (Suski & Nielson 1989).

2. *Avoid confusion.* This can be achieved by serving only one course of a meal at a time with only the appropriate cutlery. When as much of the main course has been eaten as is wanted, clear it away and then serve the dessert.

3. *Reduce distractions.* Turn off the television, remove other distractions and try to make meal times calm and orderly so that clients can concentrate on their meal.

4. *Provide correct utensils.* Independence can be well maintained and nutritional intake ensured by eating food which can be eaten without utensils, e.g. sandwiches. Non-slip mats and specially adapted utensils may be helpful for some clients, especially if they also have a physical disability, e.g. arthritis.

5. *Ensure fluid intake.* Adequate fluid intake is very important. Dehydration will make confusion worse:
   - include regular drinks in routine
   - do not overfill cups and glasses, as this makes spillage more likely and drinking more difficult. If the cups are not full initially, they will need refilling to ensure an adequate fluid intake
   - monitor fluid intake
   - provide foods with a high moisture content such as jellies, sauces and milk puddings

6. *Allow time for meals.* Do not clear away quickly after each course. Allow clients as much time as they need to eat their meals.

7. *Provide second helpings.* More food will be eaten if a small helping is followed by a second helping. Instead of serving one large portion, serve a small one and encourage the client to have a second helping.

8. *Treat clients as individuals.* Some clients will be distressed by the eating habits of others. These clients should be provided with an area which is more conducive to the enjoyment of their meal.

9. *Provide plenty of space.* Ensure that the dining area is as large as possible, so that clients who wish to can move around as they eat.

10. *Serve appropriate food* (see Chapter 17). Food should be familiar and easy to eat as well as nutritious.

Nutritional support may be necessary for some clients either as supplement drinks or nasogastric or percutaneous endoscopic gastrostomy (PEG) tube feeding (see Chapter 23).

EATING DISORDERS

The most commonly recognised eating disorders are:

- *anorexia nervosa*, characterised by a refusal to maintain normal body-weight and an intense fear of gaining weight and fatness
- *bulimia nervosa*, characterised by recurrent binge-eating and attempts to prevent weight gain by purging behaviour
- *binge-eating disorder*, characterised by recurrent binge eating and a feeling of loss of control during binges.

Anorexia nervosa

Anorexia nervosa is a condition where the ability to satisfy the desire for food is lost. Interest in food and appetite remain but the sufferer cannot satisfy the desire. *Anorexia nervosa is not a condition where the desire for food is lost, but rather a condition where the ability to satisfy this desire is lost.*

The term anorexia nervosa was first used to describe a recognised clinical condition in 1873 by two different workers—Lasegue in Paris and Gull in London. Although both workers identified the same physical symptoms of the condition including weight loss, it was Lasegue's description which included reference to an emotion which was 'avowed or concealed' and he regarded the condition as an intellectual perversion.

The incidence of anorexia nervosa is increasing (West 1994), although it is difficult to identify how much the incidence has increased and how much the increased incidence is due to an increased awareness of the condition and its diagnosis.

The condition occurs most commonly among young women aged 15–23 years, with the average age of onset being 17.2 years (Theander 1970, Touyz & Beumont 1984). The condition has been shown to occur in older women (Szmukler 1985) and among men (Fichter et al 1985). A study by Carlat et al (1997) reported on 135 male patients who were identified as having an eating disorder. In this group 46% were identified as having bulimia nervosa, 22% anorexia nervosa and 32% an eating disorder that could not be specified.

The condition is generally thought of as affecting middle-class white females but this assumption is now being challenged. The under-representation of other socioeconomic and ethnic groups may be due to their under-utilisation of medical facilities and the denial by individuals of all groups that they suffer from the condition.

Causes of anorexia nervosa

Different single-factor causal theories have been proposed, but the trend in recent years is to view the disorder as heterogeneous and multi-factorial, arising from the interplay of psychological, familial, cultural, and biological predisposing factors.

(Garner 1993)

This condition is caused by many complex factors which are interrelated and the idea, initially portrayed by the popular press, of over-enthusiastic dieting is too simplistic. However, a study by Patton et al (1999) has shown that adolescent females who diet are 18 times more likely to develop an eating disorder than those who do not diet.

There are three broad categories of factors thought to be involved in the causation of anorexia nervosa. These are:

1. emotional and psychological
2. familial
3. cultural (Garner 1993).

As most young people are exposed to some or all of the factors which have been associated with the development of anorexia nervosa and not all of them develop the condition, it would appear that some people are more susceptible to developing the condition than others.

Emotional and psychological factors. Depression and anxiety appear to be common among patients with anorexia nervosa.

The symptoms of depression may not be the cause of the condition, but rather a response to the lethargy caused by the self-starvation. Garfinkel & Garner (1982) identified the development of anorexia nervosa by some people as a way of coping with family problems. These include.

- parental divorce
- alcoholism within the family
- physical and sexual abuse
- feelings of loneliness and shyness
- adolescent anxieties about:
  — approaching adulthood
  — sexual maturity
  — leaving home.

Family factors. The presence of a person with anorexia nervosa within a family will inevitably cause conflict. This means it can be very difficult to identify factors which may have precipitated the condition. Factors that have been specifically identified are:

- overprotective family
- mother has a dominant role
- father's role within the family seems passive
- parents have very high expectations for their children
- children strive to fulfil parents' expectations.

Genetic inheritance. It has been proposed that eating disorders are genetically determined. A twin study by Fairburn et al (1999) was unable to confirm this.

Cultural factors. While healthy eating advice recommends 'eat the right amount to be a healthy weight', many people have a distorted view of what a healthy weight for themselves should be, basing it on their size and shape rather than body mass index (BMI).

Much has been written about the unnaturally slim role-models with which young people are confronted in magazines, films, television and shop windows. Rintala & Mustajoki (1992) have claimed that the dummies used in shop windows to display clothes are now so thin that, if human, they would probably never menstruate. In 2000 the British Medical Journal called for advertisers to have a more responsible attitude towards advertising (Morant 2000).

Symptoms of anorexia nervosa

Low body-weight. The body-weight is 15% below that which would be expected (APA 1987), i.e. a BMI of less than 17.

Poor growth. During adolescence the expected growth spurts will not occur if the energy intake is restricted.

Fear of weight gain. People who have anorexia nervosa believe themselves to be overweight, feel fat and are terrified of gaining weight.

Amenorrhoea. There is a close link between body fat content and oestrogens, the normal body fat composition for women being 18–30%. If this is reduced, then the oestrogen production will be decreased and amenorrhoea will develop.

Electrolyte disturbances. These can occur as a result of excessive vomiting, laxative abuse or as a metabolic consequence of starvation. The most serious of these disturbances is hypokalaemia and this may be the cause of hospital admission.

Lanugo. People with anorexia nervosa may develop a fine downy hair which can cover the entire body.

Sensitivity to cold. Loss of the subcutaneous fat layer causes greater sensitivity to cold, and circulatory failure caused by malnutrition means that feet and hands feel cold in particular.

Hyperactivity. Sufferers are restless and can be extremely active as they try to 'burn off' more calories and so reduce their weight further.

Treatment of anorexia nervosa

In the treatment of anorexia, the sufferer's disinterest in treatment and lack of desire for a 'cure' make all approaches difficult, and the development of a feeling of trust between patients and those people trying to help them is of vital importance in establishing a therapeutic alliance. To achieve this a degree of honesty is essential.

It is now usual to treat anorexia nervosa sufferers as outpatients with a mixture of family therapy, psychotherapy and behavioural therapy and nutritional counselling. These are outlined below. Ideally, each patient should have an individual programme because, while many of the causes may be similar, they are not the same or of the same significance for all individuals. There are situations when an inpatient admission is essential because the weight loss is so great that it is life-threatening. A successful outcome of treatment depends on long-term treatment. A study by Szmukler et al (1986) found that 14% of patients required more than 4 years of treatment.

Family therapy. This is an effective treatment for the group of sufferers whose illness started before the age of 19 years and was of less than 3 years' duration (Russell et al 1987).

During family therapy, the family's cooperation must be gained and an understanding achieved of the way in which all members of the family relate to each other and deal with issues. This includes brothers and sisters as well as parents and the individual with the condition. After this, strategies are introduced to help the family change in some way. These changes often include how the patient manages his or her symptoms and life and how family members react to this.

Psychotherapy. This can occur both on an individual basis and in group sessions. Psychotherapy is lengthy and is based on encouraging the patient(s) to identify and explore their own feelings towards their life, as well as their weight, to help them understand themselves and overcome their eating disorder.

Nutritional counselling. The involvement of the dietitian with the treatment of sufferers with anorexia nervosa is a key part of their re-education programme, in helping them to maintain a normal weight, correct misconceptions about food and have a more balanced attitude towards food and its role in their life. It is also an important part of the weight-restoration programme.

Dietetic advice for anorexia nervosa. The energy requirements for a patient with anorexia nervosa are not enormous because the combination of low body-weight and starvation induce a state of hypometabolism which enables weight gain to proceed on relatively low energy intakes (Vaismann et al 1988). In most situations an initial daily intake of 1600 kcal ensures satisfactory weight gain. A gain of 0.5 kg/week should be aimed for. However, the initial weight gain will be more rapid than this, due to correction of dehydration and repletion of glycogen stores in muscle and liver, and there must be reassurance that, after this initial larger gain, a gain of 0.5 kg/week is to be aimed for.

The dietary advice should be structured around regular meals and snacks. Some sort of exchange system is often useful as it provides a basis for deciding on meals and enabling the individual to maintain control of his or her eating habits.

Enteral feeding may be necessary after admission for some inpatients. This should be done to overcome the immediate life-threatening consequences of the disorder and not as a curative procedure.

A hospital admission will be of little long-term value if it is seen as a period of 'fattening up' to be achieved as quickly as possible so that the patient can return to his or her normal life. It will be quickly followed by loss of weight as soon as the patient is discharged.

As well as regular meals, supplements may be provided so that smaller meals can be eaten until the patient has become accustomed to the increased volume of food, while ensuring that an adequate energy intake is maintained.

A realistic range of body-weight should be set as a target, with the BMI set at the bottom of the normal range (20–25) as this is less frightening to contemplate than a BMI of 25 when you already consider yourself overweight. Monitoring of the patient's weight is an important part of therapy, not only to assess its success or otherwise, but to reassure the patient that the weight gain is not spiralling out of control.

Although weight gain can be achieved, the condition is only resolved if the abnormal behaviour surrounding food, meal times and weight control is also resolved and the distortion in body image is corrected. This abnormal behaviour can include:

- abnormal eating habits
- hiding of foods
- self-imposed isolation during meals
- laxative abuse
- self-induced vomiting
- excessive exercising.

Exercise addiction has been proposed as a similar condition to anorexia nervosa, particularly in males (Yates et al 1983).

People with anorexia nervosa are fascinated by, and usually very knowledgeable about food, often spending long periods reading recipe books, preparing food for other people and studying what other people eat. This can lead to the condition being self-propagating. Anorexia nervosa does in some cases lead to death. However, once treatment has started, if weight gain occurs, then the hormonal and metabolic changes will be reversed.

Treatment of anorexia nervosa is a lengthy process, most successfully carried out by a multidisciplinary team working within a specialist unit. The aims of treatment are to:

- restore patients to normal body-weight

- restore their confidence in their ability to maintain their weight
- establish their acceptance of a normal meal pattern and a normal range of foods in the diet
- help them to be happy with their new weight.

Nursing of patients with anorexia nervosa can be difficult because such patients are very skilful at hiding from other people how little they actually eat, and are very resourceful at disposing of food that they do not want to eat. Ensuring that the prescribed diet is eaten and not concealed within the ward or regurgitated is a time-consuming task, which demands a lot of patience from nursing staff.

Bulimia nervosa

The true incidence of bulimia is difficult to establish, partly because, unlike anorexia nervosa, bulimia is difficult to identify from physical symptoms. Bulimics may well have been caught in the vicious circle of binge-eating followed by vomiting, purging, excessive dieting, fasting or vigorous exercise as a method of weight control. They may have endured the condition for 20 years before treatment is sought. It is not surprising that bulimics are ashamed of their behaviour, rarely admit to it and generally have very low self-esteem. Unlike anorexia sufferers, however, they are aware of their problem and would like help to overcome it. The disorder occurs in women of all ages, and has been shown to occur in men (Carlat et al 1997). Because it is a relatively new condition, defined in 1979 (Russell 1979), there is less information about its causes than about those of anorexia nervosa, but it is thought that some of the causes are similar.

Sufferers are usually of average or slightly above average weight and have a distorted perception of body-weight and size.

The physical symptoms which do occur are:

- erosion of dental enamel caused by contact with the acidic stomach contents during vomiting
- abdominal distension and discomfort following a normal-sized meal, caused by the damaging of normal gut peristalsis due to frequent large doses of laxatives
- electrolyte disturbances caused by loss of fluid and potassium by purging
- vitamin A and D deficiencies—these fat-soluble vitamins will be malabsorbed if castor oil is used as a purgative
- swollen salivary glands.

It is important to understand that for people with bulimia nervosa a 'binge' is not the consumption of four bars of chocolate consecutively, but rather a period of eating during which their eating is totally out of control and immense quantities of food are eaten. Farley (1992) showed that sufferers could consume 15 000 kcal in a 1–2 hour period. These binges may be pre-planned; they often occur in secret with the food being eaten straight from the freezer or uncooked, and are not just an over-indulgence in favourite foods. This binge-eating is then followed by feelings of depression and guilt and attempts to compensate for this over-consumption.

The diagnostic criteria for bulimia nervosa are an average of more than two binge-eating episodes per week occurring for a period of at least 3 months (APA 1987). However, it is likely that some people will have a less severe form of the condition, although it will still reduce the quality of their life.

The aims and methods used for the treatment of bulimia are similar to those used for anorexia nervosa in trying to help sufferers regain control of their eating habits and diet. The exceptions are that dietary supplements are not necessary to restore the patient to normal body-weight and the energy content of the diet will need to be calculated from estimated average requirement (EAR) to ensure maintenance of a normal weight. Patients are unlikely to be admitted to hospital because of the condition as it is not as potentially life-threatening. However, the condition causes a severe reduction in an individual's quality of life.

In common with anorexia nervosa, the aim of treatment for a patient with bulimia must be regaining the ability to control weight and adhere to a regular meal pattern. The most successful treatment for this has been identified by Fairburn et al (1992) as a programme of cognitive therapy during which approaches to body-weight and weight control are explored and patients are enabled to reduce their obsession with dieting and to establish control over their eating and thus eliminate binge-eating.

It may be that health care workers are encouraged to establish support groups for people with eating disorders.

Binge-eating disorder

Binge-eating disorder was identified by Spitzer et al (1993) who used the term to describe the condition of a group of people who binge eat but do not try to compensate for it. Binge-eating occurs on average 2 days weekly for 6 weeks or longer (Berg 1994). During the period of binge-eating there is a feeling of loss of control. Episodes of binge-eating usually involve three of the following:

- eating more quickly than normal
- eating until uncomfortably full
- eating large amounts when not physically hungry
- eating large quantities of food alone
- feeling guilty, disgusted or depressed about the bingeing.

This condition is associated with obesity, a history of drug or alcohol abuse, treatment for emotional problems, impaired social functioning and difficulties in employment.

Treatment for the condition includes helping the client to identify the cause of bingeing and enabling them to eat a balanced diet which they are in control of. The use of *The Balance of Good Health* (Chapter 14) will be helpful in enabling the client to plan appropriate meals.

Patients with eating disorders will present in a range of situations. The aim of this chapter is to offer an overview of the conditions and how they can be overcome.

REFERENCES

American Psychiatric Association (APA) 1987 Diagnostic and statistical manual of mental disorders, 3rd Edn, revised. APA, Washington

Berg F 1994 Binge eating disorder: what's it all about? Obesity and Health 8(2): 26

Carlat DJ, Camargo CA Jnr, Herzog DB 1997 Eating disorders in males: a report on 135 patients. American Journal of Psychiatry 154(8): 1127–1132

Carney M W P, Ravindran M G, Williams D G 1982 Thiamin, riboflavin and pyridoxin deficiency in psychiatric in-patients. British Journal of Psychiatry 141: 271–272

Cranmer J L 1983 Mental disorders and somatic illness. In: Lader M H (ed) Handbook of psychiatry. Cambridge University Press, Cambridge: 48–49

Drever F, Bunting J (1997) Patterns and trends in male mortality. In: Drever F, Whitehead M (eds) Health inequalities: decennial supplement. HMSO, London

Fairburn C G, Agras W S, Wilson G T 1992 The research on the treatment of bulimia nervosa: practical and theoretical implications. In: Anderson G H, Kennedy S H (eds) The biology of feast and famine. Academic Press, San Diego

Fairburn C G, Cowen P J, Harrison P J 1999 Twin studies and the aetiology of eating disorders. International Journal of Eating Disorders 26(4): 349–358

Farley D 1992 Eating disorders require medical attention. FDA Consumer 26(2): 27–29

Fichter M M, Daser C, Postpischil F 1985 Anorexic syndromes in the male. Journal of Psychiatric Research 19: 305–313

Garfinkel P E, Garner D M 1982 Anorexia nervosa, a multidimensional perspective. Bruner Mazel, New York

Garner D M 1993 Pathogenesis of anorexia nervosa. Lancet 341: 1631–1635

Godfrey P S A, Toone B K, Carney M W P, et al 1990 Enhancement of recovery from psychiatric illness by methyl folate. Lancet 336: 392–395

Gull W W 1873 Anorexia nervosa (apepsia hysterica). British Medical Journal 2: 527–528

Kenworthy N, Snowley G, Gilling C (eds.) 1992 Common foundation studies in nursing. Churchill Livingstone, Edinburgh

Kinsman R A, Hood J 1971 Some behavioural effects of ascorbic acid deficiency. American Journal of Clinical Nutrition 24: 455–464

Lasegue C H 1873 De l'anorexie hysterique. Archives of General Medicine 1: 385

MacLachlan D R C 1986 Aluminium and Alzheimer's disease. Neurobiology of Ageing 7: 525–532

Mandal S K, Ray A K 1987 Vitamin C status of elderly patients on admission into an assessment geriatric ward. Journal of International Medical Research 15: 96–98

Meltzer H, Gill B, Pettigrew M, Hinds K 1995 The prevalence of psychiatric morbidity among adults living in private households. HMSO London

Morant H 2000 BMA demands more responsible media attitude on body image. British Medical Journal 320: 1495

Patton G C, Selzer R, Coffey C, Carlin J B, Wolfe R 1999 Onset of adolescent eating disorders: population based cohort study over 3 years. British Medical Journal 318: 765–768

Rintala M, Mustajoki P 1992 Could mannequins menstruate? British Medical Journal 305: 1575–1576

Russell G F M 1979 Bulimia nervosa: an ominous variant of anorexia nervosa. Psychological Medicine 9: 429–448

Russell G F M, Szmukler G I, Dare C, Eisler I 1987 An evaluation of family therapy in anorexia nervosa and bulimia nervosa. Archives of General Psychiatry 44: 1047–1056

Scott J M, Weir D G 1981 The methyl folate trap. Lancet 2: 337–340

Seymour D, Cape R, Campbell A 1980 Acute confusional states and dementia in the elderly: the role of hydration, volume depletion, physical illness and age. Age and Ageing 9: 137–146

Spitzer R L, Yanovski S, Wadden T et al 1993 Binge eating disorder: its further validation in a multisite study. International Journal of Eating Disorders 13: 137–153

Suboticanec K, Folnegovic-Small V, Korbar M, Mestrovic B, Buzina R 1990 Vitamin C status in chronic schizophrenia. Biological Psychiatry 28: 959–966

Suski N S, Nielson C C 1989 Factors affecting food intake of women with Alzheimer's type dementia in long-term care. Journal of the American Dietetic Association 89: 1770–1773

Szmukler G I 1985 The epidemiology of anorexia nervosa and bulimia. Journal of Psychiatric Research 129: 143–153

Szmukler G I, McCance C, McCrone L, Hunter D 1986 Anorexia nervosa: a psychiatric case register study from Aberdeen. Psychological Medicine 16: 49–58

Theander S 1970 Anorexia nervosa: a psychiatric investigation of 94 female patients. Acta Psychiatrica Scandanavica Supplementum 214: 1–194

Touyz S W, Beumont P J V 1984 Anorexia nervosa: a follow-up investigation. Medical Journal of Australia 141: 219–222

Vaismann N, Rossi M F, Goldberg E, Dibden L J, Wykes L J, Pencharz P B 1988 Energy expenditure and body composition in patients with anorexia nervosa. Journal of Paediatrics 113: 919–924

Walker A 1968 Chronic scurvy. British Journal of Dermatology 80: 625–630

West R 1994 Eating disorders: anorexia nervosa and bulimia nervosa. Office of Health Economics, London

Yates A, Leehey K, Shisslak C 1983 Running–an analogue of anorexia? New England Journal of Medicine 308: 251–255

FURTHER READING

Bruch H 1978 The golden cage: the enigma of anorexia nervosa. Open Books, London

Cooper P J 1993 Bulimia nervosa: a guide to recovery. Robinson, London

Crisp A H, Joughlin N, Halek C, Bowyer C 1989 Anorexia nervosa and the wish to change. St George's Hospital Medical School, London

Health Education Authority (HEA) 1993 Food and body image. In: Every woman's health: information and resources for group discussion. Health Education Authority, London: 141–198

Orbach S 1988 Fat is a feminist issue I. Arrow Books, London

Stunkard A 1997 Eating disorders: the last 25 years. Appetite 29(2): 181–190

USEFUL ADDRESSES

Eating Disorders Association
Sackville Place
44 Magdelen Street
Norwich NR3 1JU
Tel: 01603 621414
Youth Helpline, for 18 years and under: Tel: 01603 765050
Website: www.edauk.com

The Priory Centre
11 Priory Road
High Wycombe
Bucks.
Tel: 01494 521431

Anorexia and Bulimia Nervosa Association
Women's Health Centre
Tottenham Town Hall
London N15 4RB

20

Nutrition for people with learning disabilities

LEARNING OBJECTIVES

After studying this chapter you should be:

- aware of the causes of nutritional deficiency associated with learning disabilities
- able to describe how good nutrition contributes to the health, wellbeing and quality of life for people with learning disabilities
- familiar with therapeutic diets used to treat some conditions to prevent the development of intellectual impairment.

CAUSES OF LEARNING DISABILITIES

Learning disability is a lifelong condition which results from damage to the brain. A large number of causes of learning disability have been identified and can be grouped into four broad categories (see Box 20.1).

Those members of the population who have a learning disability will have different needs for care and support. Some will be able to live totally independently, while others will require help and support from carers for every task and aspect of personal care. Those individuals who also have a severe physical disability will require considerable support.

The aims of all those caring for a person with a learning disability must be to ensure that the individual integrates as fully as possible into the community and is enabled to utilise all of the facilities necessary to achieve equal opportunities with the rest of society.

In the UK part of this process has been the movement from long-stay institutions to community homes. One of the consequences of this is that some individuals receive care from a specialist team, while others are treated by their general practitioner and practice team.

Box 20.1 Categories of causation of learning disabilities

Genetic or chromosomal
- Chromosomal abnormality (e.g. Down's)
- Damaged genes
- Inherited metabolic disorder (e.g. phenylketonuria)

Prenatal
- Illness of mother during pregnancy (e.g. rubella, toxoplasmosis, sexually transmitted diseases)

Perinatal
- Premature birth
- Injury at birth

Post natal
- Physical injury
- Infection (e.g. meningitis, encephalitis)
- Exposure to toxins (e.g. carbon monoxide)

NUTRITIONAL NEEDS OF PEOPLE WITH LEARNING DISABILITIES

A healthy diet is essential for the good health and well-being of everyone, and those with learning disabilities should not be excluded from its benefits. As in any population group, there are those with specific nutritional needs (Box 20.2).

Advice given and action taken to help overcome a specific nutritional problem must take into consideration the individual's specific nutritional requirements and feeding difficulties. Problems that can exist include:

- difficulty chewing and swallowing
- only eating a limited range of textures of foods, e.g. only foods which do not need chewing
- only eating a very limited range of foods
- only eating in a specific place

Box 20.2 Nutritional needs of people with learning disability

- Overcoming underweight
- Weight reduction and maintenance of a healthy weight
- Correction and prevention of specific nutritional problems
- Specific medical condition requiring specific dietary treatment, e.g. diabetes, hyperlipidaemia
- Special diets for the treatment of inborn errors of metabolism, e.g. phenylketonuria, galactosaemia
- Help in overcoming feeding problems
- Specialist advice for treatment of Prader–Willi syndrome

- being unable to discriminate between edible and inedible objects.

Some of these problems are behavioural and a multi-disciplinary approach to overcoming or alleviating them is required.

Surveys of the nutritional status of residents with learning disabilities in long-stay institutions have shown that malnutrition does exist among them (Macdonald et al 1989). The problems identified included: underweight, overweight, constipation, dehydration, and specific nutrient deficiencies.

The causes of this malnutrition are the same as for any group of frail individuals or people living in an institution (see Chapter 17 on nutrition and older people) and include:

- lack of choice
- poor menu planning
- inadequate provision of food
- dysphagia
- lack of help with feeding.

Much has been done to overcome these problems and, as people move into smaller living units, their individual nutritional needs will usually be met, as care staff have usually received training in nutrition. The booklet produced by the Home Farm Trust (1993) is particularly useful for this training.

It is important that as individuals move out of institutions, their nutritional status is assessed and that those who care for them understand their special needs, the importance of a healthy diet and how best they can enable the client to achieve this. A study by Bryan et al (2000) has identified the need for continued nutritional assessment of clients in the community. This study observed that following the move from a long-stay institution to a community home, clients showed adverse changes in nutritional status. In particular, these were unintentional changes in the weight of normal-weight clients, with change from normal weight to both overweight and underweight occurring. Increase in weight occurred more often than decrease in weight. If the client has a specific dietary problem and needs a special diet, then the carer needs to understand why the diet is important and which foods the client should eat and which are restricted in some way. These specific conditions are considered further.

UNDERWEIGHT

Regular weighing of clients, ideally once a month, is very important. This should be done at the same time of day wearing similar clothes, preferably on the same set of scales. These records should not be discarded annually, but should be kept so that any gradual trends in weight gain or loss can be recognised, as well as rapid changes. It must be remembered that a gradual loss of weight of 250 g a month, if not checked, can result in a loss of 6 kg in 2 years.

People who are chronically underweight may mistakenly be considered to be at their ideal weight just because it has always been their weight. This is not so and the advantages of increasing the body mass index (BMI) to within the normal range include:

- improved wellbeing
- increased resistance to infection
- less likelihood of developing pressure sores.

High energy requirements

Some forms of challenging behaviour involve almost constant activity, which results in an increased energy expenditure. Some people, particularly adolescents (see Chapter 15), who already have a high energy requirement need an increased food intake to provide the extra energy for this hyperactivity. As it is not always possible to obtain accurate weights for people with challenging behaviour, carers must be aware of the individual's physical appearance—the tightness or looseness of waistbands is a useful tool if other anthropometric methods cannot be used.

When no underlying medical cause has been found for weight loss or persistent weight loss, the dietary intake should be increased to achieve an ideal body-weight (BMI 20–25), this is likely to be at the bottom end of the range. Provision of an appropriate dietary intake is usually easier in a small living unit, but it is vital that all those caring for the individual know that the client actually needs this amount of food and is not being greedy and that the extra energy is provided as part of a healthy diet, not just as sweets and biscuits.

This increased energy requirement will be met for many individuals by increasing the amount of starchy staple foods eaten at a meal and having between-meals snacks, whereas others, who are not able to consume large amounts of food, may require nutritional support (Chapter 23).

In some situations challenging behaviour may diminish, particularly at meal times, as the client is no longer hungry all the time.

In some situations the hyperactivity may be due to a food allergy. This topic is discussed in Chapter 28.

Poor nutritional intake

Poor nutritional intake can be caused by anorexia, poor meal-time care, dysphagia, feeding problems, vomiting and regurgitation.

Anorexia

This can have a variety of causes:

- dehydration—raised blood urea due to dehydration causes anorexia
- hiatus hernia
- depression—people with learning disabilities may also suffer from mental illness
- unhappiness—refusal of food is a way in which individuals who have difficulty in communicating can express themselves
- unfamiliar food—particularly if combined with a change of environment, e.g. an individual who moves into a residential home from his parent's home may find the food unfamiliar, as may a client from a different ethnic or cultural background (see Chapter 18).

Meal-time care

Poor staffing levels. Some clients may be unable to feed themselves or may need help to feed themselves. Poor staffing at meal times means that clients will be unable to eat enough.

Hurried meal times. This means a lack of time for clients to feed themselves and for staff to help clients feed (see p. 158 on feeding).

Inappropriate food. Food that is unattractive, unfamiliar, poorly presented or difficult to eat is less likely to be eaten than that which is easy to eat and attractively presented.

Unsuitable utensils. Independence should always be encouraged by providing the most suitable utensils. This is particularly the case if the client also has a physical disability. The occupational therapist should be consulted to help overcome this problem; there is a large range of modified utensils, plate guards, non-slip mats and drinking cups available and the occupational therapist's advice about the correct type will be invaluable.

The strategies used to overcome some of these problems are similar to those used for the care of a person with dementia (see Chapter 19).

Dysphagia and feeding problems

Dysphagia can be due to neurological, physical and behavioural causes and the strategies used to overcome it depend on the cause. The part played by a multi-disciplinary team is important in overcoming this problem. The aim of this team should be not only to maintain good nutritional status but also to ensure as good a quality of life as possible, so that meal times are pleasant experiences and food is enjoyed.

Where it is impossible to provide adequate nutrition through the oral route, long-term nutritional support should be considered—jejunostomy and gastrostomy feeding are often used (see Chapter 23).

Delay in weaning can mean that the swallowing reflex does not develop, so parents should always be encouraged to start weaning before the age of 6 months and to introduce as wide a range of tastes and textures as possible.

Vomiting and regurgitation

This can be a problem for clients with severe learning disabilities. Many of them have difficulties in communicating, which makes identifying the causes of vomiting and regurgitation hard. Nevertheless, attempts should be made to alleviate the condition, as vomiting and regurgitation are distressing for the individuals, their carers and their families.

Box 20.3 lists six causes which should be considered.

If the symptoms start suddenly, they should be investigated to see if there is a medical cause. It is important that people with a hiatus hernia remain sitting upright for 20 minutes after a meal, eat small frequent meals and avoid very spicy and very fatty foods (see Chapter 24). The physiotherapist will be able to advise on seating so that poor posture can be overcome as much as possible. Poor posture can make swallowing difficult and inhibit gastric emptying. If food is not chewed properly, it should be cut up well before it is given to the person, who should be encouraged to eat more slowly and chew the food. It may be helpful to give small portions of food and provide second helpings.

It is easy in a busy environment to rush around attending to clients' physical needs, for example taking them to the toilet or changing their incontinence pads immediately after a meal. Those people who suffer from vomiting and regurgitation should be left until last to allow them longer in an upright position.

Food intolerances are difficult to identify in anybody, but even more so in those who have difficulty in communicating. However, observation of the person may show that vomiting is more likely to occur after a meal of fried foods or perhaps a meal containing milk or onions. Discussion with family and carers may help to identify the foods. Comments such as `onions make him sick' should not be ignored, although they may not always be factual statements. It is not appropriate to try to find the cause of food intolerance by strict exclusion of particular foods without dietetic help, as this can lead to nutrient deficiencies.

If the vomiting or regurgitation is behavioural in origin, then the help and advice of a psychologist is needed (Rast et al 1985). The psychologist also has a key role in helping to overcome some of the behavioural anomalies that can develop around meals and meal times. Examples of these include only eating a very limited range of foods, perhaps only food of a particular colour or form, e.g. cut into squares or mashed, only eating in a specific place and only using certain utensils.

Special care is needed for those clients whose disability includes an inability to discriminate between things that are edible and things that are not. Mealtime supervision is important and clients should not be given confusing foods e.g. pies in foil cases, eggs in shells and meat portions which include bones.

OBESITY

The consequences of obesity for clients with a learning disability are an increased incidence of chronic disease, difficulties for carers and difficulties with social integration. The needs of clients with a learning disability for health promotion to prevent obesity was identified in the *The Health of the Nation: a Strategy for People with Learning Disabilities* (DoH 1995).

Obesity can have a variety of causes:

- poor diet
- specific medical conditions, e.g. Down's syndrome, Prader–Willi syndrome
- lack of exercise
- side-effect of some drugs
- reduced mobility.

Every attempt must be made to prevent obesity from developing—see Chapter 14 on healthy eating for adults or pages 140–142 for children.

Box 20.3 Possible causes of vomiting and regurgitation in clients with learning disability

- Hiatus hernia and gastrointestinal disease
- Poor posture during and after meal times
- Food eaten too quickly and not chewed properly
- Being moved or re-positioned too quickly after a meal

Factors which make obesity more likely to develop are:

- lack of exercise
- the use of food as a reward or to prevent challenging behaviour.
- the provision of an inappropriate diet.

It is easy to see how carers and relatives may come to use sweets, confectionery and food as a reward and treat. While they are of value in some training programmes, an over-reliance on them will inevitably lead to over-consumption and the development of obesity and dental caries.

Families need to know how they can show their affection without always giving food, particularly high-sugar, high-fat snack foods. They also need to understand how obesity will affect the quality of life of their relative with a learning disability.

Many clients with moderate learning disabilities are aware that they are overweight and would like help to lose weight. This can be done either by attending a local slimming group, perhaps run by a practice nurse or at their social education/training centre, or it may be more appropriate for them to have an individual consultation with a dietitian. It should not be assumed that people cannot manage their own diet because of a learning disability (Cole 1990).

CONSTIPATION

Constipation is a common problem which is exacerbated by:

- low dietary fibre intake
- poor fluid intake
- reduced physical activity
- side-effects of drugs, particularly major tranquillisers and some anticonvulsants
- routine use of laxatives—an over-reliance on laxatives for a long period of time will mean that the colon will stop functioning normally (Moriaty & Silk 1988).

Constipation can be prevented by ensuring an adequate fluid intake of at least eight cups a day. This can be incorporated into the daily routine. It is important to make allowance for the amounts spilt and dribbled by those clients who are less able to hold a cup.

The fibre intake can be increased by providing a wholegrain breakfast cereal such as Weetabix or bran flakes and routinely using wholemeal bread instead of white bread. Fruit and vegetable consumption should be encouraged both at the main meal and as a between-meal snack. Vegetables can be cooked or raw

as a salad or included in a sandwich. Fresh fruit should be eaten every day and fruit should also be used for desserts, e.g. tinned fruit and custard.

THERAPEUTIC DIETS

Clients with conditions such as diabetes and hyperlipidaemia should be encouraged to manage their own diets as much as possible. In order to do this, the information they receive should be applicable to them and their lifestyle, understandable and acceptable.

Explanation of the necessary dietary modifications should be given to both the client and the key worker. The key worker has an important role in reinforcing the information given and ensuring that colleagues also understand the dietary changes necessary.

Photographs of food, packets, etc. should be used as aids, and it is helpful if the explanation is done in a kitchen or dining room where food is available and can be used as a teaching aid.

HEALTHY EATING FOR PEOPLE WITH A LEARNING DISABILITY

The recommendations for healthy eating for adults (Chapter 14) are applicable here, and all the training packs, visual aids, recipes, etc. used at social education (training) centres for adults with learning disabilities should conform to these guidelines to avoid giving conflicting messages, and ensure that clients have an understanding of the basics of a healthy diet. It has been estimated that more than 70 000 people in the UK would be using these facilities during the 1990s where they would benefit from learning the skills of independent living (CIPFA 1994). Those learning to cook or improving their cooking skills should be able to prepare and cook healthy food for themselves.

A key part of independence is to be able to choose and prepare the food that you eat, and this should be encouraged inrrespective of an individual's ability. It should always be remembered that eating meals is not just a way of providing the body with nutrients; it is a social event and a way of asserting your own identity.

Teaching programmes to help develop independent living skills need to include five basic healthy eating messages:

- Have a starchy food at each meal.
- Eat fruit and vegetables at each meal.
- Try not to eat too many fatty foods.
- Don't fry foods.
- Eating sugary foods too often is bad for your teeth.

These healthy eating messages need to be considered whenever meals are planned and food discussed. There is an enormous range of processed foods available which can be combined to make well-balanced, healthy meals, and the use of the microwave oven can make independent preparation of meals relatively easy.

Examples of easily prepared nutritious meals are:

- jacket potato with baked beans
- sliced cold meat and tinned spaghetti
- tinned spaghetti and scrambled egg
- cottage pie made from tinned meat and instant mashed potato
- sandwiches with salad and cheese, tinned fish or lean meat fillings
- baked beans on toast
- boiled pasta and sauce, e.g. tinned tuna and tinned tomatoes
- pizza and salad.

All of these meals should be served with cooked frozen vegetables or salad and are as easy to prepare as heating a meat pie and cooking oven chips. Fresh fruit, tinned fruit in natural juice, low-fat yoghurts and tinned milk puddings make convenient desserts.

The level of a client's involvement in preparing meals will vary according to their ability. Almost all will be able to carry out some tasks, e.g. taking bread out of the packet or collecting an item from the fridge. Clients who find communication difficult may find pictorial illustrations of food, either as photographs or magazine cuttings, helpful in enabling them to choose their own food.

Prader–Willi syndrome

The symptoms of Prader–Willi syndrome include short stature, hypogonadism and learning disability. There are also symptoms which are of nutritional importance. These are failure to thrive and poor weight gain in infancy and they are followed by the development of hyperphagia at the age of 2 to 4 years. If not controlled, this apparently insatiable appetite leads to the development of gross obesity. During the initial 'failure to thrive' period the infant may need tube feeding to ensure adequate nutritional intake.

The family and child need to know how to manage this eating disorder to prevent obesity from developing, as it can lead to metabolic problems such as diabetes mellitus. A multidisciplinary approach, in which the team members all provide consistent advice, support the family and use forms of behaviour modification to limit food intake, has been found to be helpful

(Wodarski et al 1988). It has been suggested that intellectual performance is improved by maintaining lower weight (Crnic et al 1980). This is seen by many families with a member with the syndrome as a very important reason for restricting energy intake. For more details on paediatric nutritional support, consult Thomas (1994).

The family's diet should be healthy, i.e. low in fat and sugar, and contain generous amounts of fruit and vegetables. The entire family needs to adopt a healthier lifestyle—encouraging regular exercise and restricting their intake of high-fat, high-sugar foods so that the child will not feel different from the rest of the family.

The child should be weighed at monthly intervals (not only to control weight gain but to ensure that carers are not over-zealous in their restriction of the child's dietary intake).

Changes in lifestyle which help the family to control their child's hyperphagia include:

- not leaving food unattended
- clearing away any food left immediately after a meal
- serving food immediately onto plates rather than putting serving dishes on the table
- having regular meal times, so that between-meal snacks are not necessary
- if necessary, locking fridges, larders, etc. to prevent stored food being taken.

Items which could be mistaken for food and are toxic, such as cleaning fluids and garden berries, should be kept safe.

It is important to maintain restrictions during adolescence. A study by Bray et al (1983) showed that some adolescents with Prader–Willi syndrome were eating more than 5000 kcal/day when their intake was unrestricted. However, the family needs to have realistic expectations of the levels of control that they can exert over their child's food intake, particularly when the child becomes adolescent and wants some independence. Although it is not usually the practice for treating or preventing obesity, some families find that calorie counting helps in the management of food intake by increasing the variety of foods available, increasing the child's independence and creating an awareness of which foods can be eaten freely and which must be kept for special treats. It also provides adolescents with a means of budgeting their energy intake. By restricting intake for a few days beforehand, they can attend a birthday party or have a treat. Whichever regime is chosen it must provide adequate minerals and vitamins.

Most children with Prader–Willi syndrome grow in height and gain weight satisfactorily on 10–11 kcal/cm actual height, the energy requirement being lower than that of a normal child. Dietary management must build on cooperation with the child, developing an understanding of the behaviour and strategies to overcome it, rather than confrontation. Many families find joining the specialist Prader–Willi syndrome support groups helpful (address at the end of the chapter).

Down's syndrome

Specific growth charts should be used to monitor the growth of infants with Down's syndrome because the rate of growth is slower than in unaffected children during the first 5 years of life (Cronk et al 1988).

Babies with Down's syndrome may have feeding difficulties in infancy and not thrive. This is due to abnormalities of bones of the skull, which can alter the positions of muscles used in chewing. It may also result in the oral cavity being small. The tongue may be of normal size, thus appearing large in a small oral cavity, or may be larger than normal. The development of teeth may also be delayed, which can result in difficulty in closing the lips, sucking and chewing. Speech therapy exercises will help to overcome these problems.

Children with Down's syndrome should be encouraged to take as much exercise as possible and to eat healthily so that they do not become obese. Hypothyroidism is associated with Down's syndrome (Dinani & Carpenter 1990) and should be excluded as the cause of obesity before a weight-reducing programme is commenced.

Phenylketonuria (PKU)

The diet required to prevent the mental retardation due to PKU is outlined in Chapter 28. It has been suggested that a protein restriction of the diet may be beneficial for those people with PKU displaying challenging behaviour who were not diagnosed in infancy and remained untreated throughout childhood.

Galactosaemia

The diet used in treatment of this condition is given in Chapter 28. It is a diet which has to be kept to for life and the long-term complications of the condition include learning disabilities. The diet has always to exclude all forms of lactose and galactose. Not only are these sugars contained in milk and foods made from milk, such as cheese and yoghurt, but they are frequently added to manufactured products such as breakfast cereals, packet soups and biscuits. In practice, the labels of all manufactured foods must be checked.

Drug/nutrient interactions

The side-effects of drugs prescribed for patients should be considered as part of the nutritional assessment. Anticonvulsants increase the need for folate and vitamin D. Dietary sources of folate are liver, fortified breakfast cereals, green vegetables and fruit. The most important source of vitamin D is exposure to the sun. Dietary sources are fortified margarine, fortified breakfast cereals and oily fish. Supplements will be required if the client is unable to get into the sunshine.

REFERENCES

Bray G A, Dahms W T, Swerdloff R S, Fiser R H, Atkinson R L, Carrel R E 1983 The Prader–Willi syndrome: a study of 40 patients and a review of the literature. Medicine 62(2): 59–79

Bryan F, Allan T, Russell 2000 The move from a long-stay learning disabilities hospital to community homes: a comparison of client's nutritional status. Journal of Human Nutrition and Dietetics 13 (4): 265–270

Chartered Institute of Public Finance and Accountancy (CIPFA) 1994 Personal social services statistics 1994–95 estimates. CIPFA, London

Cole A 1990 Teaching people how to manage their own 'special' diets: some lessons from practice. Mental Handicap 18: 156–159

Crnic K A, Sulzbacher S, Snow J, Holm V A 1980 Preventing mental retardation associated with gross obesity in the Prader Willi syndrome. Paediatrics 66: 787–789

Cronk C E et al 1988 Growth charts for children with Down syndrome: 1 month to 18 years of age. Pediatrics 81: 102

Department of Health (DoH) 1995 The health of the nation: A strategy for people with learning disabilities. Department of Health, Wetherby

Dinani S, Carpenter S 1990 Downs syndrome and thyroid disorder. Journal of Mental Deficiency Research 34: 387–392

Home Farm Trust 1993 Nutritional guidelines for people with learning disabilities. Home Farm Trust, Leamington Spa

Macdonald N J, McConnell K N, Stephen M R, Dunnigan M G 1989 Hypernatraemic dehydration in patients in a large hospital for the mentally handicapped. British Medical Journal 299: 1426–1429

Moriaty K J, Silk D A 1988 Laxative abuse. Digestive Diseases 6: 15–29

Rast J et al 1985 Dietary management of rumination: four case studies. American Journal of Clinical Nutrition 42: 95–101

Thomas B (ed.) 1994 Manual of dietetic practice, 2nd Edn. Blackwell Scientific Publications, Oxford

Wodarski L A, Bundschuh E, Forbus W R 1988 Interdisciplinary case management: a model for intervention. Journal of the American Dietetic Association 88(3): 332–335

FURTHER READING

American Dietetic Association 1997 Nutrition in comprehensive program planning for persons with developmental disabilities. Position of the American Dietetic Association. Journal of the American Dietetic Association 97: 189–193

Bender W N 1993 Learning disabilities. Butterworth Heinemann, London

Hogans 1997 A Nutritional rehabilitation program for persons with severe physical and developmental disabilities. Journal of the American Dietetic Association 97: 162

Richardson N 1993 Fit for the future. Nursing Times 89(44): 36–38

Van Dyke D C et al 1990 Problems in feeding. In: Van Dyke D C et al (eds) Clinical perspectives in the management of Down syndrome. Springer-Verlag, New York

USEFUL ADDRESSES

The Down's Association
First Floor, 12/13 Clapham Common Southside
London SW4 7AA
Tel: 020 7720 0008

Food Adviser, Home Farm Trust Ltd
Aylesford House
70–72 Clarenden Street
Leamington Spa
Warwickshire CV32 4PE
Tel: 01926 882558

Mencap
123 Golden Lane
London EC1Y 0RT
website: www.mencap.org.uk/

National Society for Phenylketonuria UK Ltd
7 Southfield Close
Willen
Milton Keynes MK15 9LL

Prader–Willi Syndrome Association (UK)
30 Follett Drive
Abbots Langley
Hertfordshire
WD5 0LP

Scottish Down's Association
158–160 Balgreen Road
Edinburgh EH11 3AU
Tel: 0131 313 4225

Therapeutic nutrition and dietetics

21

Diet in obesity

LEARNING OBJECTIVES

After studying this chapter you should be able to:

- calculate body mass index (BMI)
- define overweight and obesity
- explain the causes and consequences of overweight and obesity for both adults and children
- discuss the advantages and disadvantages of different methods of weight reduction
- provide general advice for healthy adults and children on how to achieve and maintain a healthy weight.

When energy intake from food and drink exceed an individual's immediate energy requirements, the excess energy is converted to fat and stored in the adipose tissue to be used as a source of energy at a later date. This store of energy in the adipose tissue can be beneficial. For example, the extra fat stored to meet the energy requirements of lactation confers an advantage in survival when there is a food shortage. However, in many societies there are no longer periods of food shortage and the extra energy stored is a disadvantage because of the development of obesity and its associated health risks (WHO 1990).

Distribution of body fat

Adipose tissue is not isolated in any particular areas of the body, but is spread diffusely throughout it. In women of average build, 18% of their body-weight is fat whereas in men, the percentage is lower, at 16%.

The way in which the fat is distributed falls into two categories. Fat is either deposited on hips and legs (pear-shaped—peripheral obesity) or deposited centrally around the abdomen (apple-shaped—central obesity).

Waist circumference

The distribution of fat can be assessed by calculating the waist-to-hip ratio (WHR). WHR is calculated by dividing the waist measurement by the hip measurement. The WHR should be above 1 for men and above 0.85 for women and should be considered along with the BMI in assessment of obesity. Central obesity is associated with raised plasma triglycerides and reduced plasma high-density lipoprotein (HDL) cholesterol, when compared with the plasma lipoprotein pattern of those with peripheral obesity (DoH 1994). This appears to be an important factor in the link between overweight and ill-health (Bray 1993). The apple shape is associated with a higher incidence of disease than the pear shape. It is suggested that waist circumference on its own is a good measure of intra-abdominal fat. Lean et al (1995, 1998) suggest that at a waist circumference of more than 80 cm for women and 94 cm for men no further weight should be gained, and weight loss is necessary if the waist circumference exceeds 88 cm for women and 102 cm for men.

Abdominal fat is more easily broken down than subcutaneous fat, so it is relatively easier for people with a central distribution of fat to correct this by restricting their energy intake.

MEASUREMENT OF OBESITY

A visual assessment can be a guide to whether or not a person is an appropriate weight, but it is never an adequate measure of whether the individual is over- or underweight. This is because different individuals and different cultures have different perceptions of what is an ideal weight.

A diagnosis of obesity is made from a calculation of the individual's body mass index (BMI). This method does not require sex or body build to be considered (see Appendix 8 for a body mass index chart):

$$BMI = \frac{\text{Weight in kilograms}}{(\text{Height in metres})^2}$$

The grading system for obesity in Table 21.1 removes the confusion about whether a person is overweight or obese and provides a standard way of classifying body-weight.

INCIDENCE OF OBESITY

Obesity is one of the most important preventable causes of ill-health in the UK (Kent & Bowyer 1992) and the prevalence of obesity and overweight in the population continues to increase. In the UK

Table 21.1 Grading system for obesity (Garrow & Webster 1985)

BMI	Degree of obesity	Grade
Less than 20	Underweight	
20–24.9	Desirable weight	Grade 0
25–29.9	Overweight	Grade 1
30–39.9	Obese	Grade 2
Greater than 40	Severely obese	Grade 3

17% of the population are obese (Prestcott-Clarke & Primatesta 1999).

Obesity has been identified as a risk factor for many conditions (Garrow 1988, Ravussin & Swinburn 1992), listed in Box 21.1. The role of obesity in the development of these diseases is complex and differs with different conditions. For example, in osteoarthritis the extra weight on a joint can cause mechanical damage, while in other conditions such as hypercholesterolaemia excess adipose tissue contributes to the metabolic disorder.

In some conditions the obesity does not cause the condition but aggravates it; for example conditions which cause a reduction in physical activity are frequently accompanied by an increase in BMI which aggravates the condition, so causing a 'vicious circle' of weight gain, e.g. some respiratory conditions.

It is hard to identify the mortality associated with obesity because it is associated with many diseases which are more likely to be recorded as the cause of death rather than the obesity itself (West 1994). So, although not actually recorded as the cause of death, obesity is a contributory factor.

Box 21.1 Condition for which obesity is a risk factor

- Coronary heart disease
- Stroke
- Hypertension
- Varicose veins
- Hypercholesterolaemia
- Impaired respiratory function
- Non-insulin-dependent diabetes
- Gall bladder disease
- Gout
- Impaired hepatic function
- Osteoarthritis of spine, hips and knees
- Cancer of endometrium, cervix, ovary, breast
- Menstrual irregularities
- Ovulatory failure
- Polycystic disease of the ovaries

CAUSES OF OBESITY

As already stated, a gain in weight occurs when the energy intake is greater than energy requirement. This can occur for a variety of reasons. There may have been a decrease in energy expenditure, perhaps following a change of occupation, without a corresponding decrease in food intake. Some of the weight increase which occurs in middle life may be due to the fact that activity diminishes with age, whereas established food habits tend to remain unaltered. Eventually energy intake becomes considerably in excess of expenditure.

In a society where there is an ample supply of food, a range of factors contribute to the development of obesity:

- sedentary lifestyle
- lack of information
- ill-health and physical disability
- psychological factors such as depression
- behavioural factors such as overeating
- social pressures
- genetic make-up
- endocrine disorders
- certain drug treatments
- socioeconomic status
- weight gain in childhood.

Sedentary lifestyle

The role of exercise in the treatment of obesity is discussed later in this chapter. As society changes and fewer people are involved in manual work, their energy expenditure decreases and therefore their energy requirement is also reduced. Regular exercise is important in maintenance of a desirable body-weight and preventing the development of both obesity and cardiovascular disease, and should be encouraged throughout all stages of life. See Hunt & Hillsden (1996) for information about how this can be achieved.

Lack of information

There are many misconceptions as to the energy contents of different foods and confusion about their significance.

Although packaged food is now labelled with nutritional information, there are still many people who are confused by the range of information provided, and uncertain how they should eat in order to prevent their weight from increasing. There are times when individuals are more likely to gain weight, for example during pregnancy. Pregnant women need accurate information about healthy eating during pregnancy so that they do not gain excessive weight. The establishment of good eating habits in childhood is a factor of great importance in the prevention of obesity. Teachers, school nurses, health visitors and health educators all have an important part to play (Gortmaker et al 1999).

Ill-health and disability

These can frequently cause a cyclical increase in weight. A person's physical activity can be reduced by physical incapacity, for example a back injury. However, their energy intake remains the same or increases, perhaps due to depression or boredom, thus resulting in weight gain which can further reduce mobility. People whose activity is reduced should be aware of the importance of a healthy diet at all stages of their illness or disability and encouraged to avoid weight gain and to monitor their own weight. By doing this any gradual increase in weight can be identified and the diet modified, preventing further weight gain.

Psychological factors

Many people find that eating is comforting and that they eat when they are lonely, worried or depressed. The effects of obesity on quality of life should never be underestimated. In many societies the social attitudes to obesity are such that, in addition to the physical difficulties with mobility, the obese individual is more likely to suffer from depression and low esteem (Wadden & Stunkard 1985).

Social pressures and behavioural factors

Subtle changes in behaviour, such as a change in the content of the midday meal, an increase in the number of snacks between meals, or a change of employment which leads to more eating in a social setting, can result in a slow increase in weight which will eventually cause obesity.

Genetic make-up

Two-thirds of obese patients were identified as having an obese parent in a study by Floch & McClearn (1980), but this does not demonstrate a conclusive genetic link, as children usually share the same environment as their parents so will adopt their diet and eating habits. A study of adopted children in Denmark (Stunkard et al 1986) has shown a link between BMI of adopted children and their biological parents. The identification of the obese gene and the leptin system has stimulated research into the genetic causes of and predisposition to obesity. Congenital leptin deficiency has been identified as a cause of the early development of obesity (Montague et al 1997).

Endocrine disorders

Obesity accompanies myxoedema (inactive thyroid) and Cushing's syndrome (excessive production of hormones of the adrenal cortex). These conditions can easily be identified by biochemical means and should be excluded as a cause of obesity.

The hypothalamus exerts some control over appetite and in rare conditions damage to the hypothalamus can lead to an increase in appetite and overeating.

Groups of drugs which cause obesity

The following groups of drugs can cause obesity:

- sulphonylureas
- oral contraceptives
- adrenocortical steroids
- anabolic agents
- some antidepressants—cyproheptidine.

Patients should be made aware that they may find their appetite increases and that as a consequence they may gain weight when prescribed these drugs, and they should be advised how best to avoid this happening. The best way is to change to a healthier form of diet containing fewer energy-dense, high-fat, high-sugar foods and more fruit and vegetables and starchy foods.

Socioeconomic status

In western industrialised nations obesity has a greater prevalence in lower socioeconomic groups (Stunkard 1975). The Health Survey for England 1997 showed a social class gradient in obesity for women, with those in the manual classes being almost twice as likely to be obese as those in the non-manual classes (Prestcott-Clarke & Primatesta 1999). This is due to a range of factors including financial restriction on choice of foods, lack of information, poor education, low self-esteem and lack of opportunity and facilities for exercise. The results did not show a clear pattern for men.

Weight gain in childhood

Prevention of obesity in infancy and childhood is a sensible measure, and a pattern of regular meal times, without frequent snacks between meals, should be established, as should a routine of regular exercise (Epstein et al 1990, Epstein 1995). Unfortunately, environmental and psychological factors can be difficult to resolve. For example parents who find themselves unable to give enough time and personal attention to their children may, without realising it, compensate for this by over-indulging them with sugary, fatty snacks. Children who are emotionally deprived may get comfort from eating (see Chapter 15).

Appetite control

It has been suggested that the large appetites of some obese people may be due to factors affecting their satiety mechanism, which is controlled from centres at the base of the brain in the region of the hypothalamus. These factors, however, are not fully understood.

In some cases, failure of equilibrium between energy intake and output may be the result of endocrine disturbance or genetic abnormalities, but most authorities believe this type of obesity to be relatively uncommon.

Research to see if obese people metabolise food differently from the non-obese may eventually throw more light on the problem of obesity, and work investigating the foetal origins of disease hypothesis may also contribute to this.

SOME COMPLICATIONS OF OBESITY

The incidence of overweight and obesity increases with increasing age. Of those who develop diabetes in middle life, a high proportion are overweight. In many of these middle-aged diabetics, the condition can be brought under control by weight loss. Obese people have an increased risk of developing diabetes, cardiovascular disorders, gallstones, varicose veins, abdominal hernia, flat feet and osteoarthritis of the spine, hips and knees. They are not good subjects for surgery as they present difficulties in diagnosis, surgical technique and postoperative care.

TREATMENT OF OBESITY

Most people who seek help from health care workers about weight loss have already tried unsuccessfully to lose weight.

When resources are limited, not all obese individuals can be given support in weight loss. Those categories of individuals who should be given priority in advice on how to lose weight should include:

- those with a BMI greater than 30
- those with a BMI greater than 25 who also have other cardiovascular risk factors
- those with medical conditions that are exacerbated by obesity, e.g. joint pain
- those who have an abdominal distribution of fat.

Aims of treatment of obesity

Treatment of obesity can only be considered to be truly successful if it accomplishes three things:

1. reduction of weight to within the desirable range
2. education of the obese individual into a new lifestyle which ensures that the body-weight is maintained at the new level
3. maintenance of an adequate intake of all nutrients.

However, these three goals are not always reached. It is not unusual for obese individuals to lose weight and then regain it. Repeated cycles of weight loss followed by weight gain may be associated with health risks (Jeffery et al 1992). Goldstein (1992) has produced evidence to show that there are health gains and a reduction in the incidence of weight-related disease for even a slight weight loss in those who are severely obese. A small sustained weight loss is preferable to a large weight loss followed by a return to pre-treatment weight.

Motivation to lose weight

Slow sustained weight loss is the healthiest and best way to lose weight. Unfortunately this is not the most rewarding for obese individuals who understandably want to reach their correct body-weight as quickly as possible.

People who are losing weight need encouragement and support, so that they are able to adapt to the dietary behavioural changes that they have been recommended to make and maintain them over a long period of time. It is helpful to identify for each individual the reasons why he or she wants to lose weight. It is generally the case that men are more likely to be motivated by concerns over their health, while women are motivated by a change in their physical appearance. As well as the benefits of weight loss, the benefits of increased stamina, mobility and self-confidence should be explored with the individual.

The reasons why people want to lose weight are varied and include wishing to:

- treat a specific condition
- improve their:
  — physical appearance
  — exercise tolerance

  — quality of life
  — general wellbeing.

Exercise and weight reduction

Insufficient exercise is popularly cited as the cause of weight gain or reason for unsatisfactory weight loss. It is true that for some individuals increasing activity alone will cause a reduction in body-weight, but for most individuals a combination of increased activity and decreased energy intake is the most successful.

An increase in activity may be sufficient to prevent weight gain in individuals whose weight is within the normal range and whose diet is well balanced, but who are still slowly gaining weight (Allied Dunbar et al 1992).

The actual amount of energy expended by individuals in the forms of exercise most routinely used are not very high, e.g. 420 kJ (100 kcal) is expended by walking for 1 mile. However, if incorporated into a daily routine, this can become of value. 1 mile walked every day expends the amount of energy stored in 3 kg adipose tissue over 1 year. Exercise is also beneficial for the following reasons:

- Most individuals experience an improved feeling of wellbeing during and after exercise.
- Resting metabolic rate is increased for a period after exercise.
- It is difficult to eat and exercise at the same time.

If exercise is taken after a meal, this may increase the amount of energy expended in the digestion and assimilation of the meal.

Dietary management of obesity

Whatever may be the underlying cause, the treatment of obesity necessitates either a reduction in the energy value of the diet or an increase in energy expenditure. Most successful weight loss is associated with both.

An excess weight of 10 kg (1 st 8 lb) represents an excess energy store of 336 MJ (80 000 kcal). It is obvious, therefore, that intake must be sufficiently restricted to make obese persons metabolise their own accumulated body fat in order to meet their energy requirements. The majority of moderately active people will lose weight if their daily energy intake is reduced by 2.1 to 4.2 MJ (500–1000 kcal). It is unreasonable to expect everybody to lose weight at the same rate on the same diet.

The correction of obesity in the long term requires a permanent change of eating habits and this cannot be brought about overnight. For many it may be helpful to aim for a slow weight loss based on a gradual, and it is hoped permanent, change of eating habits.

In order that satisfactory weight loss is achieved, the individual should be given dietary advice that combines the following principles:

- sound nutritional advice
- an understanding of the individual's culture and lifestyle.

Many people, particularly those with Grade 1 obesity, do not require a specific calorie-restricted diet. This imposes unnecessary restrictions on them and a far more practical approach is to encourage a change in eating habits that can be incorporated in their routine and kept to permanently. The 10 key points for change are listed in Box 21.2.

This healthy eating approach can also be successful for individuals with Grade 2 or 3 obesity, but it may also be helpful to impose a specific energy restriction to ensure a sustained weight loss.

The actual energy content of a weight-reducing diet is calculated from estimations of the individual's energy requirement derived from calculating BMR and multiplying it by the appropriate physical activity level (PAL). The daily energy intake needs to be 500 to 1000 kcal below this to achieve satisfactory weight loss (Garrow 1992). As this calculation includes body-weight, it needs to be recalculated using the new body-weight as weight is lost. This method of prescribing energy intake is more satisfactory than basing it on current estimated energy consumption calculated from a diet history, as the reported calorie intake is often an underestimate of the actual intake (Lightman et al 1992).

Box 21.2 Key points for dietary change in obesity

- Include generous portions of fruit and vegetables in meals
- Include a large portion of a starchy food at each meal
- Do not add sugar to drinks and avoid sugary soft drinks
- Do not eat large portions of meat
- Spread butter or margarine on bread very thinly or change to a low-fat spread
- Avoid between-meal snacks—if they are necessary, try to eat a piece of fruit
- Avoid fried foods
- Choose lower-fat cheeses and eat smaller portions of them
- Don't eat pastry, cakes and biscuits as part of your daily routine
- Change to a lower-fat milk (preferably skimmed milk)

The health care worker and the overweight person need to reach a realistic agreement and set goals about the weight loss hoped to be achieved, the time that this will take and how the diet will be modified.

The diet should conform, as far as possible, to the eating habits of the person concerned and should always respect the restrictions that an individual's culture or religion may impose. The modified diet must be easy to obtain and fit into established routines.

The energy content of the diet can be reduced by:

- omitting sugar and foods containing sugar
- omitting/restricting alcohol
- restricting the intake of fat and foods high in fat
- limiting intake of other foods.

It is important that adequate nutrition is maintained and a sufficient intake of protein, minerals and vitamins must always be ensured.

Excessive hunger is avoided by:

- increasing the intake of fruit (fresh or tinned in fruit juice) and vegetables
- eating wholegrain and wholemeal bread and breakfast cereals instead of the refined forms
- beginning the meal with a serving of clear soup or a glass of water; this helps for some individuals who are used to eating large quantities of food
- taking unsweetened drinks, such as tea or coffee, or a low-calorie drink, or eating raw vegetables between meals.

Examples of energy-restricted diets are given at the end of this chapter (Boxes 21.3 and 21.4).

Most people find it difficult to adhere to a strict diet and should be reassured that occasional breaking of the diet is natural although not desirable, and should not cause undue despondency. An enthusiastic attitude on the part of the dietitian or nurse is of the greatest importance in securing cooperation and achieving a BMI within the normal range.

Rapid weight loss should not be encouraged. If weight loss is rapid, not only is fat metabolised but so is the lean tissue (muscle) and the glycogen stores of the muscle and liver are depleted. The rapid weight loss which occurs on short-term, very low-energy diets is due to the metabolism of glycogen stores and the water and sodium diuresis that accompanies it. When energy intake is restored, the glycogen stores are replaced and extra weight is gained.

Eating behaviour

Changes in an individual's eating behaviour and an understanding of when or why he or she eats can be

Box 21.3 Diet suitable for the treatment of obesity

Energy value 5.0 MJ (1200 kcal) approximately
(this basic diet can easily be modified to increase/
  decrease the amount of energy provided—see Box
  21.4)

Guidelines

Daily allowances
These should all be eaten as they ensure that the diet
  provides an adequate supply of all nutrients:

250 ml semi-skimmed milk
15 g butter or margarine, or 80 g low-fat spread
Two average portions, 75 g lean meat or fish, egg or
  low-fat cheese
Six slices wholemeal bread or equivalent exchanges
Three pieces of fruit

Bread exchanges
The following foods are similar in energy value and
  may be exchanged for one another:

One medium sized portion whole grain breakfast
  cereal
One medium sized boiled or jacket potato
Three tablespoons baked beans
Two tablespoons boiled rice or pasta
One chapatti, the size of a tea plate
One small tin low-calorie soup
One piece of fruit such as an apple, orange, pear or
  small banana

Food to avoid
Sugar, glucose, syrup, honey, jam and marmalade
Sweets and chocolate
Diabetic sweets, jams, biscuits
Cakes, scones, puddings, biscuits and pastry
Soft drinks not labelled low-calorie, sugar-free or
  diet
Ice-cream, ordinary and full-cream yoghurts
Fried foods
Dried fruit and fruit tinned in syrup
Wine, beer and spirits
Full-cream milk, cream and full-cream dairy products
  including full-fat cheeses

Sample menu

Breakfast

Unsweetened grapefruit or grapefruit juice
One slice wholemeal bread with butter or margarine from
  allowance
One helping of wholegrain unsweetened breakfast cereal
  such as shredded or puffed wheat with milk from
  allowance
Tea or coffee with milk from allowance

Mid-morning

Tea or coffee with milk from allowance, or other
  low-calorie drink

Midday meal

One portion of protein food such as 75 g cooked lean
  meat, 100 g fish or portion of cooked pulses
Two slices wholemeal bread with butter or margarine from
  allowance
Large portion salad or green vegetable
One portion fresh fruit or diet yoghurt

Mid-afternoon

Tea with milk from allowance

Evening meal

One portion protein food (as midday meal)
One bread exchange as:
— medium-sized boiled potatoes (approximate weights
    6 oz or 90 g)
— large portion green vegetable
— small portion root vegetable
— piece of fruit or portion of fruit tinned in natural juice

Some suggested meals

1. Jacket potato filled with cottage cheese and chives
     with a green salad, medium-sized banana
2. Grilled tandoori chicken, boiled brown rice, sliced
     tomato and cucumber, diet yoghurt
3. Braised liver, boiled potato, green beans and carrots,
     apple
4. Portion grilled fish, jacket potato, ratatouille and
     broccoli, pear

---

very beneficial. Keeping a food diary provides a valuable insight into this; it does not have to be kept for long. It should record the type and amount of food eaten, where it was eaten, the time at which it was eaten and the individual's mood at that time (see Table 21.2).

Strategies for changing eating behaviour are outlined below.

1. Establish a routine of regular meals. This makes it easier to avoid between-meal snacks. This is not easy for people in some occupations, but most individuals can improve their current situation.

2. Try to eat when not surrounded by other distractions. This can make meals more enjoyable for some people and creates an awareness of eating. It ensures that food is eaten as part of a regular meal, rather than as habit while doing another task.

3. Serve smaller portions on smaller plates. The appearance of food is very important. Weight-reducing diets can be hard to keep to and the sight of a small

Table 21.2 Food diary—an example

Time	Food/drink	Where	Mood
7.45	2 cups coffee	Kitchen	Hungry
	Bowl cereal with milk		
9.30	Packet of crisps	In car	Bored

Box 21.4 Adjustments to the basic 5.0 MJ (1200 kcal) diet for treatment of obesity to provide the correct energy content for different individuals

Reduce to 1000 kcal (4.2 MJ)
By restricting bread exchanges to four-a-day. These should be evenly distributed throughout the day. If necessary, energy content can be further reduced by substituting low-fat spread for butter or margarine and using skimmed milk instead of semi-skimmed milk

Increase to 1400 kcal (5.8 MJ)
Daily bread allowance increased to eight exchanges
Fruit allowance increased to four pieces

Increase to 1600 kcal (6.7 MJ)
Daily bread allowance increased to nine exchanges
Both protein food portion sizes increased by 1 oz (30 g)

Daily fruit allowance increased by 2 pieces

Increase to 1800 kcal (7.5 MJ)
Fat allowance increased by 1/4 oz (7 g)
Daily bread allowance increased to 11 exchanges
Both protein food portion sizes increased by 1 oz (30 g)
Daily fruit allowance increased by 2 pieces

Increase to 2000 kcal (8.4 MJ)
Fat allowance increased by 1/2 oz (15 g)
Daily bread allowance increased to 12 exchanges
Both protein food portion sizes increased by 1 oz (30 g)
Daily fruit allowance increased by three pieces

---

meal on a large plate can reinforce the feeling of deprivation.

Other ideas which may prove useful for some people are:

- Always use cutlery to eat. This avoids 'picking' at little bits of food.
- Never go shopping for food when hungry, as you are more likely to buy foods that you had not intended to buy.

Many people are helped by meeting as part of a group where they can be given some nutrition education, helped to make their own decisions about dietary modifications, and given the opportunity to discuss mutual problems and support one another.

There are a number of commercially run slimming groups and clubs. Overweight individuals should be given the necessary information to enable them to assess whether or not the regime recommended by the organisation will be of benefit to them.

Weight maintenance

When a satisfactory weight loss has been achieved, dietary modifactions can be cautiously relaxed, so that the diet contains the appropriate energy content to maintain a healthy weight but still follows the principles of healthy eating. An ad lib low-fat, high-carbohydrate diet is more successful at maintaining weight loss than a diet with a fixed energy intake (Toubro & Astrup 1997).

Very low calorie diets (VLCDs)

For detailed information on the use of VLCDs see the COMA report (DHSS 1987). This report defines VLCDs as, 'commercially produced nutrient preparations providing less than 600 kcal per day marketed for use as a total food substitute'.

The advantages of these products to overweight individuals are that they will restrict the calorie intake and so weight is lost and, by avoiding food totally, the problems associated with trying to restrict food intake are avoided. The use of these products is not without risk. Their formulation is intended to be such that lean body mass (LBM) is preserved, but there is concern that LBM may be lost as well as stored adipose tissue. By recommending the use of these products, emphasis is placed on immediate weight loss rather than long-term dietary change leading to slow sustained weight loss.

If used, VLCDs should not be used for a period longer than 4 weeks. VLCDs should not be used by pregnant or breast-feeding women, children or elderly people and close medical supervision of people using them is essential.

The American National Task Force on the prevention and treatment of obesity (National Task Force 1993) concludes that, although the use of VLCDs is a more successful method of ensuring short-term weight loss, they are no more successful in maintaining long-term weight loss than any other dietary treatment.

Proprietary foods and sweetening agents

Foods marketed as slimming agents cannot substitute, in the long term, for re-education leading to a permanent change in eating habits. Soft drinks and confectionery intended for diabetics may be labelled as being free from sugar. They are not, however, necessarily suitable for those on reducing diets as they are often sweetened with a substitute sweetening agent, sorbitol, which has the same energy value as sugar. Other products such as low-calorie soups, diet yoghurts and drinks, and fruits tinned in juice can add variety to diets which can become monotonous. Current food labelling legislation makes it possible for individuals to decide, by looking at fat and sugar content, whether or not it is reasonable to include a manufactured food in their weight-reducing diet.

Drugs

Three types of drugs are used to help people lose weight. These are drugs which:

- reduce nutrient absorption
- increase energy expenditure
- reduce appetite.

They can be of value in selected cases. They are available only on prescription as they may give rise to uncomfortable or even serious side-effects, including in some cases possible addiction to the drug itself. It should not be forgotten that any benefit derived from drugs can only be temporary. For lasting effect a permanent change in eating habits is required.

Other methods of weight control

Surgery

Surgery has been used to treat Grade 3 (morbid) obesity, but because of the risks associated with this, all other methods of weight reduction should be tried first. It has been recommended that surgery, which is the most effective treatment for patients with morbid obesity, should be carried out more frequently (SIGN 1996). Intestinal bypass operations, in which the absorptive capacity of the small intestine is reduced by bypassing a section of it, give rise to chronic diarrhoea due to malabsorption, anaemia, vitamin deficiencies and liver damage. Gastric reduction procedures reduce the size of the stomach and so limit the amount of food that can be eaten at any one time. A recent surgical procedure that has been developed for the treatment of morbid obesity is the laparoscopic insertion of a gastric band, which resulted in weight loss that was maintained for 6 years (Belachew et al 1998).

Jaw wiring, limits the rate at which food can be consumed and its consistency. It may be successful in some situations but is not a permanent solution.

REFERENCES

Allied Dunbar, Sports Council and Health Education Authority 1992 Allied Dunbar national fitness survey. Sports Council/HEA, London

Belachew M, Legrand M, Vincent V, Lismonde M, Le Docte N, Deschamp V 1998 Laparoscopic adjustable gastric banding. World Journal of Surgery 22: 955–963

Bray G A 1993 Fat distribution and body-weight. Obesity Research 1: 203–205

Department of Health (DoH) 1994 Nutritional aspects of cardiovascular disease. Report of the Cardiovascular Review Group of the Committee on Medical Aspects of Food Policy (COMA) (Report on Health and Social Subjects 46). HMSO, London

Department of Health and Social Security (DHSS) 1987 The use of very low calorie diets in obesity. Committee on Medical Aspects of Food Policy. HMSO, London

Epstein L H 1995 Exercise in the treatment of childhood obesity. International Journal of Obesity 19 (Suppl 4): 5117–5121

Epstein L H, Valoski A, Wing R R, McCurley J 1990 Ten-year follow-up of behavioural, family-based treatment for obese children. Journal of American Medical Association 264: 2519–2523

Floch T T, McClearn G E 1980 Genetics, body-weight and obesity. In: Stunkard A J (ed) Obesity. Saunders, Philadelphia

Garrow J S 1988 Obesity and related diseases. Churchill Livingstone, Edinburgh

Garrow J S 1992 Treatment of obesity. Lancet 34: 409–413

Garrow J S, Webster J 1985 Quetelet's index (W/H) as a measure of fatness. International Journal of Obesity 9: 147–153

Goldstein J L 1992 Beneficial health effects of weight loss. International Journal of Obesity 16: 397–415

Gortmaker S L, Peterson K, Wiecha J, Sobol A M, Dixit S, Fox M K 1999 Reducing obesity via a school-based interdisciplinary intervention among youth. Planet health. Archives of Paediatric Adolescent Medicine 153: 409–418

Hunt P, Hillsdon M 1996 Changing eating and exercise behaviour. A handbook for professionals. Blackwell Science, Oxford

Jeffery R W, Wing R R, French S A 1992 Weight cycling and cardiovascular risk factors in obese men and women. American Journal of Clinical Nutrition 55: 641–644

Kent A, Bowyer C 1992 When weight gets out of control. Doctor May: 48–49

Lean M E J, Han T S, Morrison C E 1995 Waist circumference as a measure for indicating need for weight management. British Medical Journal 311: 158–161

Lean M E J, Han T S, Seidell J C 1998 Impairment of health and quality of life in people with large waist circumference. Lancet 351: 853–856

Lightman S W, Pisanska K, Bertman E R 1992 Discrepancy between self reported and actual calorie intake and exercise in obese subjects. New England Journal of Medicine 327: 1893–1898

Montague C T, Farooqi I S, Whitehead J P et al 1997 Congenital leptin deficiency is associated with severe early-onset obesity in humans. Nature 387: 903–908

National Task Force (on the prevention and treatment of obesity) 1993 Very low calorie diets. Journal of the American Medical Association 270: 967–974

Prestcott-Clarke P, Primatesta P 1999. Health Survey for England 1997. Volume 1: Findings. HMSO, London

Ravussin E, Swinburn B A 1992 Pathophysiology of obesity. Lancet 340: 404–408

Scottish Intercollegiate Guidelines Network (SIGN) 1996 Obesity in Scotland. Integrating prevention with weight management. Scottish Intercollegiate Guidelines Network, Edinburgh

Stunkard A J 1975 Obesity and the social environment. In: Howard A (ed) Recent advances in obesity research 1. Newman Publishing, London: 178–190

Stunkard A J, Sorensen T I A, Harris C et al 1986 An adoption study of human obesity. New England Journal of Medicine 314: 193–198

Toubro S, Astrup A 1997 Randomised comparison of diets for maintaining obese subjects' weight after major weight loss: ad lib, low fat, high carbohydrate diet v. fixed energy intake. British Medical Journal 314 (7073): 29–34

Wadden T A, Stunkard A J 1985 Social and psychological consequences of obesity. Annals of Internal Medicine 103: 1062–1067

West R 1994 Obesity. Office of Health Economics, London

World Health Organization (WHO) 1990 Study group on diet, nutrition and prevention of noncommunicable diseases. Diet, nutrition and the prevention of chronic diseases: report of a WHO study group (Technical Report Series 797). World Health Organization, Geneva

FURTHER READING

Anderson R E, Crespo C J, Bartlett S J, Cheskin L J, Pratt M 1998 Relationship of physical activity and television watching with body-weight and level of fatness among children. Results from the Third National Health and Nutrition Examination Survey. Journal of the American Medical Association 279: 938–942

British Nutrition Foundation 1999 Obesity. The report of the British Nutrition Foundation task force. Blackwell Science, Oxford

Centers for Disease Control 2000 Promoting health for young people through physical activity and sports. United States Department of Health and Human Services, USA

Gill T 1997 Prevention of obesity. British Medical Bulletin 53(2): 359–388

Maloney M 2000 Dietary treatments of obesity: proceedings of the Nutrition Society 59: 601–608

Pronk N P, Boucher J 1999 Systems approach to childhood and adolescent obesity prevention and treatment in a managed care organisation. International Journal of Obesity 23 (Suppl 2): S38–S42

22

Diet and cardiovascular disease

See also Chapter 3 'Fats',
Chapter 11 'Diet-related Disease',
Chapter 21 'Diet in Obesity'

LEARNING OBJECTIVES

After studying this chapter you should be able to:

- outline the different types of cardiovascular disease and describe their causes and symptoms
- discuss the effects of diet on plasma lipids
- explain the scientific basis for the dietary advice used for the prevention and treatment of cardiovascular disease.

CARDIOVASCULAR DISEASE

Cardiovascular disease is caused by a combination of atherosclerosis and thrombosis. It results in coronary heart disease, peripheral vascular disease and stroke, depending on which arteries are affected and the severity of the disease.

Atherosclerosis

Atherosclerosis is a disease of the arteries, including those which supply the heart muscle, in which fatty fibrous plaques (atheroma) develop on the inner walls of the artery. It causes a narrowing of the lumen of the artery, which results in a reduction in the amount of blood flowing through it. Atherosclerosis takes years to develop and its occurrence is linked to raised blood lipids. The narrowing of the lumen of the artery results in a reduction in the amount of oxygen and nutrients supplied to an organ by that artery. The plaque is known as atherosclerotic plaque and consists of smooth muscle cells which have migrated to the luminal side from deeper layers of the artery wall, modified lipid (usually oxidised low-density lipoproteins), fibrin and bits of thrombus. The sites of plaque formation are influenced by blood flow and usually develop in branches and bends of arteries, where the artery walls are subjected to greater stresses.

Thrombosis. This can occur when the thrombus that develops at the site of an atherosclerotic plaque is so large that it blocks the artery completely. A smaller piece of thrombus can be carried in the circulation until it reaches an artery too small for it to pass through, where it causes a blockage—an embolism.

Angina. This develops when the lumen of the coronary artery is 75% occluded, resulting in pain as the heart muscle does not receive enough oxygen. Reduced coronary artery blood flow can also result in arrhythmias. Myocardial infarction is the death of a portion of heart muscle caused by interruption of its blood supply, usually due to a coronary thrombosis.

Intermittent claudication. Atherosclerosis of the femoral arteries reduces the blood supply to leg and calf muscles leading to the pain of intermittent claudication.

FAT METABOLISM

As lipids are insoluble in water, they are incorporated into specialised proteins called lipoproteins, in the gut wall. These large triglyceride-rich lipoproteins are called chylomicrons and are secreted into the circulation. The chylomicrons are then transported to adipose tissue and skeletal muscle cells. There, the enzyme lipoprotein lipase, which is on the capillary endothelium, splits the triglycerides into:

- fatty acids and glycerol, which are used to provide energy or stored
- a chylomicron remnant.

It is the chylomicron remnant which contains cholesterol. The chylomicron remnants are assimilated by the liver.

Four other categories of lipoprotein are also found in the blood:

High-density lipoproteins (HDL). These contain cholesterol and lecithin and are produced as a byproduct of hydrolysis of chylomicrons to triglycerides and glycerol. They have an important role in transporting cholesterol back to the liver.

Very-low-density lipoproteins (VLDL). These are triglyceride-rich lipoproteins which are secreted by the liver and are carried to the tissues, where they are hydrolysed to produce fatty acids for energy production and low-density lipoproteins (LDL). The secretion of VLDL does not occur after a meal.

Intermediate-density lipoproteins (IDL). These are produced as an intermediate step before the production of LDL.

Low-density lipoprotein (LDL). These are cholesterol-rich and, like HDL, are removed from the blood by the liver, but not as quickly. It appears that the activity of the liver LDL receptors is reduced by an increased intake of saturated fat, particularly of carbon chain length 12–16 (Goldstein & Brown 1977). Studies show that the link between coronary heart disease (CHD) risk and plasma cholesterol is due to raised LDL levels.

Dietary fats

Dietary fats (lipids) are a mixture of complex fats, e.g. triglycerides, simple fats and cholesterol. In the UK, the average diet contains 70 to 100 g triglyceride and 250 to 400 mg cholesterol. Triglyceride in the diet is almost completely absorbed in all healthy individuals. The amount of cholesterol absorbed shows individual variation.

Cholesterol

Dietary cholesterol is only found in foods of animal origin. Cholesterol is essential for normal structure and function of cell membranes. It is needed by the adrenal glands, gonads and liver, as it is a precursor of steroid hormones, adrenocortical hormones and bile acids, and it is found in the fatty covering of nerves in the brain. Although plant sterols (phytosterols) have similar chemical structures to cholesterol, when eaten they inhibit intestinal cholesterol absorption, so lowering plasma total cholesterol and LDL cholesterol levels (Moghadasian & Frohlich 1999).

In humankind about one-third to one-half of the cholesterol required is manufactured by the liver, the rest being provided in the diet. Increasing the amount of cholesterol in the diet results in a decrease in production of cholesterol by the liver. It is usual for about 450 mg (12 mmol) of cholesterol to be produced by the liver each day. This means that dietary cholesterol intake is not the only factor to influence blood cholesterol levels.

Those patients whose raised total cholesterol is due to a raised HDL cholesterol are at little excess risk of CHD, in contrast to those with a raised LDL cholesterol (Neil et al 1990). As not all lipoproteins contain the same amount of cholesterol or have the same effect on CHD risk, it is important to know the levels of HDL cholesterol and LDL cholesterol, as well as total cholesterol.

Patients with a high or normal serum cholesterol concentration have been shown to benefit from cholesterol-lowering treatment by a reduction in the number of coronary events (4S Group 1994). Early studies did not show this, as they only measured total cholesterol. Variation in plasma cholesterol concentrations of populations (e.g. China 3.3 mmol/l, Japan 4.5 mmol/l, Norway 7.2 mmol/l) is mainly due to differences in LDL levels. The current treatment guidelines recommend that a treatment goal of 2.6 mmol/l for low-density lipoprotein cholesterol is set for patients with CHD (Wood et al 1998). Pignone et al (2000) have demonstrated that lipid-lowering drugs reduce CHD.

HYPERLIPIDAEMIAS

Hyperlipidaemia is the term used to described raised levels of lipids in the blood. Table 22.1 shows the normal ranges. Not all hyperlipidaemias are nutritional in origin and non-nutritional causes (see below) should be excluded before making the assumption that diet is the cause.

Table 22.1 Reference and suggested 'healthy' ranges for plasma lipids in adults under 60 years (reproduced with kind permission from Thomas 1994)

	Reference range*	Suggested range
	mmol/l	mmol/l
Total cholesterol	3.5–7.8	< 5.2
LDL cholesterol	2.3–6.1	< 4.0
HDL cholesterol	0.8–1.7	> 1.15
Triglycerides	0.7–1.8	0.7–1.7

*The reference interval is calculated from the mean of an apparently healthy population plus and minus two standard deviations. However, sex and age differences need to be considered.
Sex difference. Triglycerides are higher in men than in women. HDL levels are higher in women than in men.
Age difference. Lipids, e.g. cholesterol, may increase with age; consequently a value in the reference range of 7.0 mmol/l would be much more noteworthy in a person of 25 years than in one of 55 years.

Causes of hyperlipidaemias

Nutritional causes

- Anorexia nervosa
- Obesity
- High dietary intake of saturated fat
- High dietary intake of refined carbohydrate.

Non-nutritional causes

- Hormonal:
  — diabetes
  — hypothyroidism
  — pregnancy

- Drug treatment:
  — diuretics
  — β blockers
  — corticosteroids
- Kidney disease:
  — chronic renal failure (CRF)
  — nephrotic syndrome
- Liver disease:
  — primary biliary cirrhosis
- Genetic:
  — familial hyperlipidaemias.

It has been estimated that in a UK group practice with 10 000 patients there will be approximately 20 people with familial hypercholesterolaemia and up to 50 others with another type of hyperlipidaemia (BHA et al 1990). Many people in these categories will require and benefit from treatment with lipid-lowering drugs, as well as nutritional therapy to control their lipid levels.

Familial hypercholesterolaemia. Children are not routinely screened for cholesterol level but they should be when there is a family history of early heart disease. The aim of treatment for this group is to reduce the risk of CHD in later life by reducing blood cholesterol levels. This is done by restricting the intake of dietary fat to 30% of energy intake. It is not necessary to totally exclude all dietary sources of cholesterol, but a diet high in cholesterol should be avoided.

Dietary treatment for hyperlipidaemias

This treatment is also relevant for those patients who have cardiovascular disease, as it is likely that they will have raised lipids. Lipid-lowering diets have been shown to slow the progression of atherosclerotic plaque (Watts et al 1992).

The dietary advice given to individuals with hyperlipidaemias depends on:

- which lipids are raised
- the level to which they are raised
- the cause.

The advice should be part of a package which looks at all other cardiovascular disease (CVD) risk factors so that advice to stop smoking and increase exercise can be given at the same time.

It is usual for the primary health care team to be involved in the nutritional counselling of patients with hyperlipidaemia and there needs to be agreement to ensure that the advice given is consistent.

Weight loss should be advised for those patients with a body mass index (BMI) greater than 25. Not only is obesity a risk factor for CHD but it should also be avoided in patients with cardiovascular disorders because:

- excessive weight puts an added burden on the heart
- deposits of fat in the heart muscle itself may impair its efficiency
- large amounts of fat around the abdominal organs may interfere with respiration by impeding the movements of the diaphragm, aggravating the breathlessness of heart disease.

A weight-reducing diet should be a low-fat diet with plenty of starchy foods, fruit and vegetables and needs no further modification for treatment of hyperlipidaemias. It must be explained to the overweight person that not all diets and commercial products are suitable and will result in reduced weight and lower blood lipids—for example some weight-reducing diets have a high proportion of the energy provided by fat and are therefore inappropriate.

Dietary advice for an individual with BMI 20–25 and hyperlipidaemia

This advice should focus on the reduction of total fat consumption, change in the type of fat eaten and increased fruit and vegetable consumption as part of overall lifestyle counselling. See Table 22.2 for a summary of foods that are allowed.

The aim is to reduce total fat intake to 30% of energy intake:

- Reduce intake of saturated fat.
- Increase intake of complex carbohydrate.
- Increase intake of fruit and vegetables (at least five portions a day).
- Increase intake of oily fish (at least two portions a week).
- Increase the proportion of dietary fat intake that is provided by monounsaturates, by changing the types of fats and oils used.

Table 22.2 Summary of foods allowed on a lipid-lowering diet

	Eat freely	Eat in moderation	Try to exclude from diet
Starchy foods	Potatoes, rice, pasta, chapattis, bread, wholegrain breakfast cereals, porridge oats, crispbread	Sugar-coated breakfast cereal, roast potatoes—one per week	Chips, potato crisps, fried rice, pasta in cream sauce, croissant, pastry, biscuits
Fruit and vegetables	All fresh, dried or tinned (in water or juice) fruit and vegetables	Avocado pears—one per week	
Nuts	Walnuts	Almonds, brazils, hazelnuts, chestnuts, peanuts	Coconut
Meat/fish	Lean meat (fat and poultry skin removed before cooking), all types of white and oily fish		Shellfish, fish roe, fried fish, sausages, pâté, fatty meat
Eggs		Limit egg yolks to two per week	
Dairy products	Skimmed milk, low-fat cottage cheeses, fat-free yoghurt, fat-free fromage frais	Semi-skimmed milk, lower-fat cheeses—Edam, Camembert, low-fat Cheddar	Products containing cream, ice-cream, full-fat cheeses, full-fat yoghurt, evaporated milk
Fats/oils	Use a mono-unsaturated oil for cooking—olive/rapeseed	Low-fat spread for bread, etc.	Lard, suet, butter, vegetable oils which do not state 'high in polyunsaturates' or 'high in mono-unsaturates' on label
Confectionary and desserts	Jelly, milk puddings and custards made with skimmed milk	Boiled sweets, fruit pastilles, peppermints small portions of cakes, biscuits made with poly-unsaturated margarine	Chocolate, fudge, butterscotch, mincemeat containing suet
Miscellaneous	Tea, coffee, fruit juice	Jam, marmalade, alcohol	Mayonnaise, products which list vegetable oil or hydrogenated fat in their ingredients

Total fat, saturated fat and cholesterol intake can be reduced by making the following simple changes:

- Use a low-fat spread.
- Use a lower-fat milk such as skimmed or semi-skimmed wherever possible.
- Do not fry foods—grill, roast, bake or microwave them instead (without adding fat).
- Cut down on the foods which contain hidden fats—cakes, biscuits, pastries, etc.
- Restrict the amount of full-fat cheese you eat. Eat less cheese or substitute cottage cheese and other low-fat cheeses.
- Cut fat off meat before cooking it. Choose leaner cuts of meat and eat more fish and poultry instead of red meat.

It is foods that have a high saturated fat content that also have a high cholesterol content, so a reduction in saturated fat intake will be accompanied by a reduction in cholesterol intake. The only exception to this is egg yolk, as one egg yolk contains approximately 250 mg of cholesterol, which is why the intake of egg yolks should be restricted to two per week.

Research suggests that eating oily fish two to three times per week is associated with a reduction in mortality of men who have already suffered a heart attack (Burr et al 1989). Table 22.2 lists those foods which are low in fat and can be eaten freely, those which should be eaten in moderation and those which should be avoided by people who are trying to reduce their lipid levels.

In choosing the types of cooking oil and margarine to recommend, it must be remembered that not all vegetable oils are polyunsaturated or monounsaturated. The incorporation of margarines which contain added plant sterols or stanols into the diet reduces serum concentrations of cholesterol (Law 2000) and their use should be considered.

Raised plasma triglycerides

There is considerable individual variation in plasma triglyceride levels. The level is raised following a meal. It is also raised by increasing the amount of carbohydrate in the diet, sucrose having a greater effect than starch. This increase is transitory, usually only lasting 2 to 3 months, and is not a reason for reducing the total carbohydrate content of the diet, although it may be a reason for reducing the amount of refined carbohydrate; hence the recommendation to reduce refined carbohydrate intake in hypertriglyceridaemia. There is less evidence to support the link between raised plasma triglyceride and the risk of CHD than there is to link

raised cholesterol with CHD. A combination of raised serum triglyceride and low HDL level is predictive of CHD. A raised triglyceride level, greater than 1.7 mmol/l, can be caused by alcoholism and also occurs in many familial hyperlipidaemias.

Dietary treatment of raised triglycerides includes advice to:

- Reduce intake of alcohol.
- Reduce intake of refined carbohydrate; substitute starchy foods like bread, potatoes, rice, chapattis and fruit for cakes, biscuits and sweets.
- Increase intake of low glycaemic index carbohydrate containing foods. Jarvi et al (1999) have shown that this helps improve the lipid profile.

Cardiac rehabilitation and secondary prevention

The first step in the process of secondary prevention is to ensure that the food provided in hospitals for patients in Coronary Care Units (CCUs) should set an example of the range of appetising foods available to anyone who wants to eat healthily. This means that the process of dietary education can begin by example. All staff of the unit should be familiar with healthy eating, lipid-lowering dietary advice and be able to explain why specific foods are restricted or excluded from the diet while the increased intake of other foods is encouraged. Whether or not the patient receives formal dietary advice from a dietitian while in hospital will depend on the hospital policy and length of time the patient is in hospital. Some patients are well motivated to change at this time and benefit from advice, whereas others need time to come to terms with what has happened to them and are under too much stress to be very receptive to anything other than the simplest of explanations and briefest of lists of dietary restrictions.

It is now usual for patients from CCUs to attend group rehabilitation sessions, where they can start becoming more active and find out more about the changes in their lifestyle that they need to make. These can be very successful as the patient can attend with a relative and ask questions in a relaxed and informal atmosphere. Ideally these sessions should be run by a range of health professionals (Thompson et al 1996). Programmes do not always meet these standards. Lewin et al (1998) and the National Service Framework for Coronary Heart Disease (see Further Reading) Standard 12 for cardiac rehabilitation, address this.

Dietary topics that should be covered in the sessions are:

1. How to achieve and maintain ideal body-weight, particularly in relation to stopping smoking. Stopping smoking can lead to weight gain as smoking is an appetite suppressant. More food may be eaten, not only because it tastes better, but it is something to do. The substitution of sweets, biscuits and sugary drinks for cigarettes is not a good idea as this will lead to weight gain in the long term. Sugar-free drinks and fruit should be tried instead.

2. Understanding the different types of fat and which are limited, allowed totally or excluded from the diet.

3. Role of starchy foods, fibre, fruit and vegetables in the diet.

4. Principles of good nutrition.

5. Recipes—make healthy eating fun and restore confidence so that patients can enjoy eating. Many suitable leaflets and books are available.

Dietary treatment of hypertension

The dietary factors that influence blood pressure are obesity, sodium intake and alcohol consumption. Treatment of hypertension is an essential component of primary and secondary prevention of cardiovascular disease, particularly stroke. If patients who are hypertensive are overweight, they should be advised to lose weight and either 'healthy eating advice' or a restricted-energy diet (see Chapter 21) should be explained to them. The advice in the previous section on hyperlipidaemia is appropriate to them. Appel et al (1997) have shown that a diet rich in fruits, vegetables, low-fat dairy foods, with reduced saturated and total fat, substantially lowered blood pressure. In addition to this, they should be advised to reduce their dietary sodium intake (see p. 247 for no-added-salt diet) and to increase their dietary potassium intake by eating more fruit and vegetables.

Most of the salt in the diet comes from processed foods (see Table 22.3), so a reduction in the amount of processed foods in the diet, or the choice of lower-salt products, will significantly lower an individual's salt intake.

Table 22.3 The sodium content of portions of foods

Food	Sodium (mg)
60 g (2 oz) Cheddar cheese	370
30 g (1 slice) tinned ham	375
One packet salted potato crisps	165
3 g (thin spreading) Marmite	135

Box 22.1 Priority groups for cholesterol screening

- Those with a family history of hyperlipidaemia
- Those with a family history of premature CHD in close relatives
- Those with physical evidence of hyperlipidaemia
- Diabetics

SCREENING FOR HYPERLIPIDAEMIAS

There is considerable debate as to whether or not it is cost-effective to routinely screen everybody for raised blood lipid levels, or whether it is more appropriate to only screen those who fall into the high-CHD-risk categories (Unwin et al 1998). Different health authorities have different local policies. Box 22.1 identifies priority groups for screening.

The CHD risk depends on a number of variables which include smoking, hypertension, obesity and the amount of physical activity taken, so the additional information of a serum cholesterol value in an individual who is hypertensive, obese, smokes and takes no regular exercise may be of little value (Shaper 1988).

The Dietary and Nutritional Survey of British Adults (Gregory et al 1990) showed that:

- only 34% had a serum total cholesterol of below 5.2 mmol/l (the theoretical normal value)
- 39% had values of 5.2–6.4 mmol/l
- 20% had values of 6.5–7.7 mmol/l
- 7% had values of 7.8 mmol/l or more.

From these figures it can be extrapolated that 66% of the population have a total serum cholesterol above the ideal and that it may be more cost-effective to encourage the entire population to moderate their diet and so reduce their serum cholesterol, rather than to target a proportion of it. An individual's risk of CHD at a serum cholesterol of 6.5 mmol/l is twice that at 5.2 mmol/l, and at 7.8 mmol/l it is three times that at 5.2 mmol/l. Progress of patients on lipid-lowering diets must be monitored so that, if dietary treatment is ineffective after 3 months, they can be referred to a specialist unit.

NUTRITIONAL HYPERHOMOCYSTEINAEMIA

Homocysteine is a sulphur-containing amino acid that is derived from methionine in the diet. A raised concentration of serum homocysteine is implicated as a risk factor for vascular disease (Mohan & Stansby 1999). Circulating homocysteine is removed by conversion to an amino acid, either methionine or cysteine. Vitamin B6, vitamin B12 and folic acid are essential co-factors for these conversion processes.

Raised circulating levels of homocysteine (hyper-homocysteinaemia) are corrected by supplementation with B vitamins and folate and it may be that some individuals have a diet-induced hyperhomocyst-einaemia as a result of their low intake of B vitamins and folate.

REFERENCES

Appel L J, Moore T J, Obarzanek E, Vollmer W M, Svetkey L P, Sacks F M 1997 for the DASH collaborative research group. A clinical trial of the effects of dietary patterns on blood pressure. New England Journal of Medicine 336: 1117–1124

British Hyperlipidaemia Association (BHA), British Cardiac Society, British Hypertension Society, British Diabetic Association 2000 Joint British recommendations on prevention of coronary heart disease in clinical practice: summary. British Medical Journal 320: 705–708

Burr M L, Fehily A M, Gilbert J F et al 1989 Effects of changes in fat, fish and fibre intakes on death and myocardial reinfarction: Diet and Reinfarction Trial (DART). Lancet ii: 757–761

European Society of Cardiology (ESC) 1997 Management of stable angina pectoris. Recommendations of the task force of the European Society of Cardiology. European Heart Journal 1997; 18(3): 394–413

Goldstein J L, Brown M S 1977 The low density lipoprotein pathway and its relation to atherosclerosis. Annual Review of Biochemistry 46: 897–930

Gregory J, Foster K, Tyler H, Wiseman M 1990 The dietary and nutritional survey of British adults. HMSO, London

Jarvi A E, Karlstrom B E, Granfeldt Y E, Bjork I E, Asp N G, Vessby B O 1999 Improved glycaemic control and lipid profile and normalised fibrinolytic activity on a low glycaemic index diet in type 2 diabetic patients. Diabetes Care 22(1): 10–18

Law M 2000 Plant sterol and stanol margarines and health. British Medical Journal 320: 861–864

Lewin R J, Ingleton R, Newins A J, Thompson D R 1998 Adherence to cardiac rehabilitation guidelines: a survey of rehabilitation programmes in the United Kingdom. British Medical Journal 316: 1354–1355

Moghadasian M H, Frohlich J J 1999 Effects of dietary phytosterols on cholesterol metabolism and atherosclerosis: clinical and experimental evidence. American Journal of Medicine 107(6): 588–594

Mohan I V, Stansby G, 1999. Nutritional homocysteinaemia. British Medical Journal 318: 1569–1570

Neil H A W, Mant D, Jones L, Morgan B, Mann J I 1990 Lipid screening: is it enough to measure total cholesterol concentration? British Medical Journal 301: 584–586

Pignone M, Phillips C, Mulrow C 2000 Use of lipid lowering drugs for primary prevention of coronary heart disease: meta analysis of randomised trials. British Medical Journal 321: 983

Scandinavian Simvastatin Survival Study (4S) Group 1994 Randomised trial of cholesterol lowering in 4444 patients with coronary heart disease: the Scandinavian Survival Study. Lancet 344: 1383–1389

Shaper A G 1988 Coronary heart disease, risks and reasons. Current Medical Literature, London

Thomas B (ed) 1994 Manual of dietetic practice, 2nd Edn. Blackwell Scientific Publications, Oxford

Thompson D R, Bowman G S, Kitson A L, se Bono D P, Hopkins A 1996 Cardiac rehabilitation in the United Kingdom: guidelines and audit standards. Heart 75: 89–93

Unwin N, Thompson R, O'Byrne A M, Laker M, Armstrong H 1998 Implications of applying widely accepted cholesterol screening and management guidelines to a British adult population: cross sectional study of cardiovascular disease and risk factors. British Medical Journal 317: 1125–1130

Watts G F, Lewis B, Brunt J N H et al 1992 Effects on coronary heart disease of lipid lowering diet or diet plus cholestyramine, in the St. Thomas' Atherosclerosis Regression Study (STARS). Lancet 339: 536–569

Wood D, De Backer G, Faergeman O, Graham I, Mancia G, Pyorala K 1998 Prevention of coronary heart disease in clinical practice. Summary of recommendations of the second joint task force of European and other societies on coronary prevention. Journal of Hypertension 16: 1407–1414

FURTHER READING

British Dietetic Association 1998 Position Paper. Dietary treatment of people at high coronary risk. Journal of Human Nutrition and Dietetics 11: 273–280

Department of Health (DoH) 2000 National service framework for coronary heart disease. Website: www.doh.gov.uk/nsf/coronary.htm

Department of Health (DoH) 1994 Nutritional aspects of cardiovascular disease. Report of the Cardiovascular Review Group of the Committee on Medical Aspects of

Food Policy (COMA) (Report on Health and Social Subjects 46). HMSO, London

Ebrahim S 1998 Detection, adherence and control of hypertension for the prevention of stroke: a systematic review. Health Technology Assessment 2: 11

Irving R J, Oram S H, Boyd J, Rutledge P, McRae F, Bloomfield P, 2000 Ten year audit of secondary prevention in coronary bypass patients. British Medical Journal 321: 22–23

Lindsay G M, Gaw A 1997 Coronary Heart Disease Prevention: A handbook for the Health Care Team. Churchill Livingstone, New York

Ramsay L E, Williams B, Johnston G D et al 1999 British Hypertension Society guidelines for hypertension management 1999: summary. British Medical Journal 319: 630–635

Rosengren A 1998 Cholesterol: How low is low enough? British Medical Journal 317: 425–426

Tang J L, Armitage J M, Lancaster T, Silagy C A, Fowler G H, Neil H A W 1998 Systematic review of dietary intervention trials to lower blood total cholesterol in free-living subjects. British Medical Journal 316: 1213–1220

Truswell A S (ed) ABC of nutrition, 3rd Edn. British Medical Journal, London

Welton P K, Appel L J, Espeland M A, Applegate W B, Eltinger W H, Kostis J B 1998 for the TONE Collaborative Research Group. Sodium reduction and weight loss in the treatment of hypertension in older adults. A randomised control trial of non-pharmacological interventions in the elderly (TONE). Journal of the American Medical Association 279: 837–846

USEFUL ADDRESSES

British Heart Foundation
14 Fitzhardinge Street
London W1H 4DH
Tel: 020 7935 0185
Website: www.bhf.org.uk

Familial Hyperlipidaemia Association
PO Box 133
High Wycombe
Bucks. HP13 6LF

Family Heart Association
7 North Road
Maidenhead
Berks SL6 1PE
Tel: 01628 628638
Website: www.familyheart.org

23

Hospital-related malnutrition and nutritional support

LEARNING OBJECTIVES

After studying this chapter you should be able to:

- discuss the causes, consequences and prevention of hospital-related malnutrition
- explain the processes of nutritional screening and assessment and use them to identify patients who are at risk of becoming malnourished and so are likely to need nutritional support
- describe the different types of nutritional support and explain their advantages and disadvantages.

Hospital-related malnutrition is an acknowledged cause of medical and surgical complications for hospital patients. It has been estimated that up to 50% of hospital patients are malnourished (Bistrian et al 1977, Hill et al 1977). Subsequent reports show that it remains a problem (Twomey & Patchings 1985, Jendteg et al 1987, Allison 1999, Elia 2000) which results in increased patient morbidity, increase in length of hospital stay and increased need for convalescent care. These consequences are significant for both the patient and health care provider.

This delay in recovery has both social and economic consequences for the patient caused by:

- loss of income and employment
- loss of social contact with family, friends and colleagues.

There is an economic cost for the health care provider caused by:

- increased length of treatment
- need for additional and sometimes more expensive treatment
- reduction in the number of patients who can be treated.

The complications of malnutrition in hospital include:

- loss of muscle power
  — cardiac (Heymsfield et al 1978)
  — respiratory (Arora & Rochester 1982)
- reduced mobility (Barstow et al 1983)
- predisposition to thromboembolism and bedsores (Holmes et al 1987)
- impaired immune response (Bistrian et al 1977)
- depression, apathy and loss of concentration (Keys et al 1950).

These effects have been demonstrated in all areas of medicine and surgery (Barstow et al 1983, Reilly et al 1987, Sullivan et al 1990).

The study by McWhirter & Pennington (1994), which was designed to determine the incidence of malnutrition among patients admitted to hospital and to monitor any changes in nutritional status occurring during the stay in hospital, concluded that:

- On admission to hospital 40% of patients were already malnourished.
- Two-thirds of hospital patients lost weight during their hospital stay.
- Hospital staff lacked awareness of the importance of nutrition.

In addition to the clinical evidence for the need to improve hospital nutrition, the experience of the patients is now also well documented. The poor quality of hospital food and the difficulties encountered by patients at meal times were identified in a report published by the Patients Association in 1993 and followed by the Influential Association of Community Health Councils Report, *Hungry in Hospital* (Burke 1997). These reports, along with the Kings Fund Report, *A Positive Approach to Nutrition as Treatment* (Lennard-Jones 1992) and the BAPEN report *Hospital Food as Treatment* (Allison 1999), have ensured that good nutrition is now seen as an essential component of good hospital care, and that in order to achieve this, the organisation of the catering services and attitudes of all hospital staff towards the provision of food in hospital needs changing.

Allison (1999) investigated the existing inadequacies in the provision of food for patients in hospital and identified ways in which the situation could be improved. Box 23.1 lists the factors identified in this report that were preventing patients from eating in hospital.

In the UK, hospitals have tried a range of new initiatives to reduce the incidence of hospital-related malnutrition, which have included reviewing the hospital menu, changing meal times and the appointment of diet assistants and ward hostesses. In 2001 a new

---

Box 23.1 Factors that prevent people from eating in hospital (Allison 1999)

- Problems in ordering food. For instance, some people may need help in ordering their meals due to language or literacy difficulties or disability. There are also inefficient ordering systems.
- The menu choice available does not take into account the results of patient surveys of preferences, cultural differences or special needs.
- The general appearance and presentation of food is often poor and the preparation, transportation and serving methods do not always ensure the preservation of nutrient content and palatability.
- Meal times are disrupted for some patients due to ward rounds, investigations and procedures. The consequence of this is that some patients miss meals.
- Patients who require special help are not identified on wards and busy nurses do not have the time to help patients eat.
- Other factors in the ward environment—for example other patients' medical conditions—can often put patients off eating.
- There is break-down in communication between nursing, catering and dietetic staff on the ward.
- Health managers have failed to design protocols or set standards and policies.
- Surveys have shown that there is a low nutritional knowledge among medical and nursing staff.

National Health Service Menu was introduced which aimed to ensure that the food provided in hospitals was of a uniform high standard nationally. As well as providing standard recipes for dishes, this menu also stipulated the types of snack meal that should be available for patients who had missed a main meal. Another UK initiative to improve hospital nutrition has been the introduction of Benchmark Standards for Food and Nutrition (DoH 2001). These standards identify best practice for enabling patients and clients to eat enough food so that their nutritional needs are met and are listed in Box 23.2

These changes to the ways in which food is provided in hospitals will help to ensure that many patients/clients achieve an adequate nutritional intake. However, there will always be a large group of patients who, because of the nature of their condition, their high nutritional requirements or their frailty, will require nutritional support.

NUTRITIONAL SUPPORT

Nutritional support is:

'The provision of an adequate nutritional intake by means other than the eating of normal meals. The extent of support

---

Box 23.2   Benchmark standards for food and nutrition (from DoH 2001, with permission)

- Routine nutritional screening is in place and progresses to further nutritional assessment for all patients/clients who have been identified as at risk of malnutrition.
- Care plans that are based on ongoing nutritional assessment are devised, implemented and evaluated.
- The meal-time ward environment has acceptable sights, sounds and smells, so making it conducive to eating.
- Patients/clients receive the care and assistance they require with eating and drinking.
- Patients/clients/carers, whatever their communication needs, have sufficient information to enable them to obtain their food.

- Food that is provided by the service meets the needs of individual patients/clients.
- Patients/clients have set meal-times and are offered a replacement meal if a meal is missed, and can access snacks at any time.
- Food is presented to patients/clients in a way that takes into account what appeals to them as individuals.
- The amount of food a patient actually eats is monitored and recorded and leads to action when there is cause for concern.
- All opportunities are used to encourage the patient/client to eat to promote their own health.

---

can vary from supplementing an inadequate diet to providing the sole source of nutrition.'

(Sizer 1996)

Nutritional support can be divided into three categories:

1. oral supplementation
2. enteral feeding
3. parenteral feeding.

The types of patient who may require nutritional support are listed in Box 23.3

The type of nutritional support that is necessary for an individual patient is decided upon following nutritional screening and assessment. There are two components to a nutritional assessment: anthropometric measurements and a diet history. In some situations biochemical measurements will also be undertaken.

Box 23.3   Patients who may require nutritional support

Preoperative patients

These patients are malnourished prior to surgery either as a consequence of their condition, for example those requiring surgery for disorders of the gastrointestinal tract, or because of their age, other medical conditions or social circumstances.

Postoperative patients

These patients may require nutritional support because they have a poor appetite following surgery or because of the consequences of the surgery, for example surgery to the head and neck, or because their nutritional requirements are increased due to complications such as postoperative infection.

Patients with diseases of the gastrointestinal tract

The symptoms of nausea, vomiting, diarrhoea, anorexia and abdominal pain can all reduce the oral intake of the patient and nutritional requirements are increased by the losses through vomiting, diarrhoea and fistulae.

Patients with high nutritional requirements

Trauma patients, burns patients and patients with sepsis all have increased nutritional requirements which cannot be met by a normal diet.

Patients with dysphagia

Enteral nutrition is necessary for all patients who are unable to swallow or for those whose swallowing is unsafe, for example stroke patients, and those with neurological conditions that effect their ability to swallow.

Patients with cancer

Intake may be reduced as a side-effect of radiotherapy and chemotherapy treatment, and requirements may be increased by cachexia.

Patients with chronic illnesses and or chronic intractable pain

For example, shortness of breath for those with chronic chest conditions makes eating very difficult and chronic pain may be accompanied by depression, lethargy and loss of appetite.

Patients who are unconscious

These patients are unable to eat and will require enteral or parenteral nutrition.

ANTHROPOMETRIC MEASUREMENTS

On admission to hospital the patient should be weighed. This weight is used to calculate body mass index (BMI) and also as a reference point to assess past and future changes in weight. The published standards should be used for children (Tanner et al 1966). Regular weighing is necessary to ensure that slow gradual weight loss is identified promptly and treated with the appropriate intervention. This also enables the calculation of percentage weight loss for an individual:

$$\% \text{ weight loss} = \frac{\text{usual weight–actual weight}}{\text{usual weight}} \times 100$$

An unintentional weight loss of greater than 10% in the preceding 3 to 6 months suggests the probable development of undernutrition and is usually an indication that nutritional support is necessary.

Patients with a BMI of greater than 25% while classified as overweight or obese are still at risk of undernutrition and it is very important that any unintentional weight loss in this group is identified. This group of patients appears well nourished; this masks the physical effects of starvation and can mean that malnutrition develops without being recognised.

The body-weight of an individual is an unreliable indicator of nutritional state for patients with oedema, for example those with renal or liver disease, and for those patients with muscle wasting either due to immobility or neurological conditions and during pregnancy.

Other anthropometric measures that are sometimes used are:

Triceps skinfold thickness (TSF). This measures endogenous fat stores (Gurney & Jelliffe 1973) and is measured using specially designed callipers, and the result obtained is compared with standard tables (Bishop et al 1981). Accuracy of measurement is improved by measuring the patient's non-dominant arm, with the same person routinely conducting the patient measurements (Heymsfield & Caspar 1987).

Mid-arm circumference (MAC). This measures skeletal muscle mass. A tape measure is used to measure the patient's mid upper-arm circumference. Error is reduced by marking the site of measurement and ensuring that the same person routinely performs the patient measurement (Bishop et al 1981).

Mid-arm muscle circumference (MAMC) is calculated from the TSF and MAC.

$$\text{MAMC} = \text{MAC (cm)} - \text{TSF (mm)} \times 0.314$$

Dynamometry. The measurement of muscle grip-strength using a hand dynamometer is sometimes used as a measure of muscle function, however results are difficult to interpret because grip-strength decreases with age and debility and increases with training.

Dietary history. An evaluation of the patient's usual and current dietary intake is an important part of nutritional assessment. Its accuracy and usefulness depend on the memory and cooperation of the patient and the skill of the interviewer in obtaining dietary information and assessing its significance. It can be very valuable in giving indications of specific nutrients which the patient is likely to be deficient in. For example, a patient who seldom eats fruit or vegetables is likely to have a low vitamin C intake. Dietary history is also useful for identifying specific problems that an individual may have in the preparation and consumption of food.

CLINICAL ASSESSMENT

This detects the physical signs and symptoms associated with malnutrition which include:

- hair—dull and dry
- skin—loses its natural colour and elasticity and appears dry and flakey and bruises easily
- muscles—appear wasted, patient may comment on muscular weakness
- cardiovascular—increased heart rate (above 100).

In addition to clinical assessment, anthropometric assessment and dietary history, laboratory biochemical tests may be used to identify sub-clinical deficiencies of specific micronutrients.

Nutritional screening tools

It is good practice to ensure that all patients are routinely screened on admission to hospital, in order to identify those who are malnourished and those who are at risk of becoming malnourished. Many hospitals have developed their own screening tool which has been developed to meet their specific needs and those of their patients. The Malnutrition Advisory Group (MAG) of BAPEN has designed, validated and produced a nutrition screening tool which can be used for adults in the UK to identify both patients who are malnourished and those who are at risk of developing protein–energy malnutrition. The screening tool is available from MAG (see useful addresses). This tool is suitable for use with both hospital inpatients and outpatients, as well as in primary care situations. This tool divides nutritional screening into three steps:

Step 1—gathering nutritional measurements

- Calculation of BMI
- Calculation of recent weight loss as a percentage of BMI
- Identification of factors which suggest recent weight loss such as loose-fitting clothes and jewellery, difficulty eating, poor appetite.

Step 2—categorising the risk of malnutrition

The nutritional measurements gathered in step 1 are used to categorise the individual as at high, medium or low risk of malnutrition. The categories are summarised in Table 23.1.

Step 3—set an appropriate care plan

An individual's care plan will depend on their risk category and may include nutritional support either as extra food, nutritional supplements and enteral or parenteral feeding. An essential component of the care plan is continued monitoring of the patient's nutritional status, including weight, to assess the effect of the nutritional support and review its provision.

AIMS OF NUTRITIONAL SUPPORT

Nutritional support aims to:

1. ensure an adequate energy intake—this prevents weight loss and metabolism of lean tissue to provide energy
2. prevent negative nitrogen balance—negative nitrogen balance is associated with loss of lean body mass, reduced immune response and impaired liver function
3. provide adequate amounts of all micronutrients and trace elements—this will prevent the development of deficiency symptoms and aid recovery and repair of tissues
4. maintain fluid balance—this is essential for the normal functioning of the renal, cardiovascular and respiratory systems.

The choice of type of nutritional support used depends on the nutritional requirements of the individual and his or her ability to meet them by consuming normal food. Some individuals will need all their nutrient needs to be met by nutritional support, while others will just require a small amount.

Nutritional requirements and nutritional support

Energy. An individual's energy requirement in health depends on their basal metabolic rate, physiological status and physical activity (DoH 1991). In ill-health, energy requirement is increased by injury, surgery, sepsis, burns and infection (Scrimshaw 1991). Activity and injury factors have been identified which, when multiplied together with the basal metabolic rate (BMR) can be used to estimate an individual's energy requirements.

Protein. Protein is lost from the body in the faeces and from the exudates of fistulae and burns (where the loss can exceed 4 g protein/100 ml (Molnar et al 1983) lost tissue), blood-loss and as urea in the urine. When the individual's diet does not contain sufficient protein, negative nitrogen balance develops. Positive nitrogen balance is essential for tissue repair following major trauma (Larsson et al 1990).

Nitrogen balance can be estimated by comparing the amount of urea excreted in the urine with the actual protein intake. For an individual who is receiving all their nutrition by enteral or parenteral nutrition the actual intake may be calculated accurately.

$$\text{g protein lost in 24 h} = \frac{\text{mmol urinary nitrogen excreted in 24 h}}{5}$$

If positive nitrogen balance is being achieved, the dietary protein intake will exceed the amount of protein that is being lost.

Water. For patients who are receiving all their nutrition from enteral or parenteral nutritional support, careful monitoring of fluid balance is essential to ensure that the patient becomes neither fluid overloaded nor dehydrated. The fluid allowance for such patients with normal renal function is usually calculated as:

Table 23.1 Categories of nutritional risk

	BMI and weight loss	Action
High-risk	less than 18.5 18.5 to 20 + recent weight loss	need nutritional support
Medium-risk	18.5 to 20 + weight loss of less than 5%	observe, may need nutritional support
Low-risk	> 20 + weight loss less than 5%	no action required unless clinical deterioration expected

Fluid = urine + 500 ml + Abnormal
input output (for insensible losses (diarrhoea,
 losses via skin vomiting, fistula,
 and respiration) pyrexia exudate)

In pyrexia an additional 500–750 ml water and 30 mmol sodium should be given for each 1°C above 37°C (Elwyn 1980).

Adequate intakes of sodium and potassium are necessary for the maintenance of fluid balance. The actual requirements depend on renal function and any abnormal losses (i.e. from fistulae, vomiting, diarrhoea). Serum electrolytes should be reviewed regularly to ensure that the nutritional intake is appropriate to the patient's specific needs.

ORAL SUPPLEMENTATION

In addition to supplementing the diet with fortified foods and oral dietary supplements, the oral intake of normal food should be maximised by ensuring that:

- food is of a suitable texture and attractively presented in small portions
- help is provided to ensure that the patient is comfortably seated
- help is provided for those who are unable to feed themselves
- the meal time environment is pleasant and stress-free.

Fortified foods

The nutrient content of many commonly consumed foods can be increased by changing the type of ingredient used or the cooking method. An advantage of this method of nutritional support is that a normal meal pattern with familiar foods can be maintained. Examples of ways in which foods can be fortified are listed in Box 23.4.

A range of commercially available prepared fortified soups and puddings are also available which may be used as part of a meal.

Sip-feeds. A wide range of sip-feeds are available. These are milk- or juice-based drinks, which are normally presented as a 200 or 250 ml tetrapak with straw

---

Box 23.4 Ways in which foods can be fortified to increase their nutrient content

- Adding powdered dried milk to liquid milk and routinely using this instead of milk for cooking and drinks.
- Adding cream or evaporated milk to soups and milk puddings and deserts.
- Adding cream, butter or margarine to vegetables and potatoes.
- Adding energy supplements such as glucose polymers, protein powders and liquid fat emulsions to drinks, soups and desserts.

---

or as a can, and are available in a range of sweet and savoury flavours. Typically they contain 10 g of protein and provide 200–300 kcal. Some examples of sip-feeds are listed in Table 23.2.

Specialised supplements

It is possible to add protein, fat or carbohydrate separately to food to meet an individual patient's specific needs. These supplements may come in powder or liquid form, vary in palatability and some of the products are often low in electrolytes, so they are very useful in ensuring adequate nutrient intake for patients with renal and liver diseases.

These supplements include:

- glucose polymers (carbohydrate)
  — powder form: approximately 400 kcal/100 g
  — liquid: approximately 200 kcal/100 ml
- liquid fat emulsions—usually 50% with water supplying approximately 225 kcal/100 ml
- protein powders—containing 80–90 g protein/100 g, some of which also contain carbohydrate and fat.

Examples are given in Table 23.3.

PRE- AND POSTOPERATIVE NUTRITION

Preoperative nutrition

Preoperative nutrition is about planning for surgery and ensuring that the patient is not malnourished

---

Table 23.2 Sip-feeds

Sip-feed	Manufacturer	Protein content per carton (g)	Energy content per carton (kcal)
Provide Xtra	Fresenius Kabi Ltd	7.5	250
Ensure	Abbot Nutrition	10	250
Entera	Fresenius Kabi Ltd	11.2	300
Fortisip	Nutricia Clinical Care	12.0	300

Table 23.3 Examples of specialised supplements used in nutritional support

Manufacturer	Carbohydrates	Fat	Protein
Scientific Hospital Supplies		Calogen (LCT emulsion)	
Scientific Hospital Supplies	Duocal Supersoluble (fat and glucose polymer)		
Scientific Hospital Supplies	Liquigen (glucose polymer, low in electrolytes)		
Scientific Hospital Supplies		MCT oil	
Nutricia Clinical Care	Polycal liquid and powder (glucose polymer)		
H J Heinz & Co Ltd			Casilan 90
Unigreg			Forceval (protein powder)
Abbott Nutrition	Promod (protein powder also contains fat and carbohydrate)		
Nutricia Clinical Care	Protifor (protein powder also contains fat and carbohydrate)		

prior to surgery. This is of course only possible with elective surgery, but it is important, particularly for elderly patients and those with a BMI below 20. If assessment has indicated poor nutritional status, measures should be taken to improve intake, possibly with the use of supplements.

If patients are obese, because obesity is a major risk factor for surgery, measures should be taken to reduce their weight by sensible eating prior to surgery. Rapid weight loss is not appropriate because it is accompanied by loss of lean body tissue and can result in reduced stores of some vitamins and minerals. Such diets will reduce the body protein and glycogen stores and compromise vitamin and mineral status. (See Chapter 21).

Postoperative nutrition

Postoperatively, malnutrition may occur if the patient is not allowed, or is unable, to eat sufficient for more than 5 to 7 days following surgery. If the patient was malnourished prior to surgery, this situation will become even worse. Protein–energy malnutrition has been shown to occur in 40–50% of UK and US surgical patients 1 week after surgery (Hill et al 1977). In the event of malnutrition being undetected and/or untreated, wound healing is delayed (Moghissi et al 1977). It has been shown that the incidence of wound infections can be reduced by nutritional support (Williams et al 1977).

It has been normal practice following surgery to support a patient with dextrose or dextrose saline to meet fluid and electrolyte requirements. One litre of 5% dextrose supplies approximately 48 kJ (200 kcal).

An average calorie requirement for an adult female is approximately 48 MJ (2000 kcal) per 24 hours, so even if she were given 3 litres of dextrose, neither her nitrogen nor energy requirements would be met; consequently she would become malnourished.

After surgery involving the gut, feeding is not normally commenced until gastric emptying and bowel sounds recur. Sips of water, 15–30 ml, are given hourly, gradually increasing in volume as tolerated.

In surgery not involving the gut, most patients are able to eat within 1 day of surgery. However, it has been documented that following major surgery such as cardiopulmonary bypass, protein and energy intakes are very low (Walesby et al 1979).

ENTERAL NUTRITION

Systems and methods

In the past, tube feeds were usually administered by giving a measured bolus of feed at intervals throughout the day. It is now usual to give the same total volume of feed steadily over a 12- to 24-hour period via a continuous-gravity drip system or preferably through a feeding pump (see Box 23.5). The advantages of the continuous system are in Box 23.6.

It is thought desirable by some authorities to have a rest period of at least 4 hours, usually during the night, to allow the gastric pH to recover as this seems to reduce the incidence of pneumonia.

Box 23.5 Advantages of using feeding pumps for enteral feeding

- They are safe and simple to use after appropriate training
- Their accuracy is ± 10% of expected volume
- There is a reduction in nursing time
- Most pumps are alarmed, warning if the flow of feed has become reduced or obstructed

> **Box 23.6** Enteral feeding: advantages of continuous feeding over bolus method
>
> - Reduces risk of nausea and vomiting; less distension of stomach
> - Makes starter regimes unnecessary
> - Allows use of fine-bore tubes
> - Enables use of more viscous feeds
> - Enables better utilisation of nutrients by the body

In the continuous-flow system, a fine-bore (1 mm internal diameter) tube is used, which is much simpler to manage and more pleasant for the patient. Most tubes are made of polyvinyl chloride (PVC) or polyurethane. Plasticisers from PVC tubes leach out after about 10 days causing the tube to harden, which can damage the gastric and intestinal mucosa. Polyurethane tubes are resistant to acid-hardening and can remain in place for up to 6 months. Both types of tube may have a guide-wire to help positioning. It is possible to aspirate through these tubes to check gastric pH and absorption of feed.

The nasogastric tube is passed into the stomach through the nose. Its position can be checked by:

- auscultating over the stomach as a bolus of air is injected and listening for bubbling through the gastric juice
- aspirating gastric juice and testing its pH with litmus paper
- making an abdominal radiograph—all nasogastric tubes are radio-opaque (see Fig. 23.1).

Percutaneous endoscopic gastrostomy (PEG)

A percutaneous endoscopic gastrostomy (PEG) makes it possible to feed a patient enterally without using a nasogastric tube.

The use of a *gastrostomy button* in feeding adults and children is increasing. However, the disadvantages of this system are that a delay of 3 months is necessary after the formation of the gastrostomy before the button can replace the catheter, and that leakage can occur around the button site.

Gastrojejunal, duodenostomy and jejunostomy feeding can also be achieved.

Jejunostomy feeding, when used after major upper gastrointestinal resections, has had better results in terms of nitrogen balance and nutrient retention than parenteral feeding (Hoover et al 1980). Jejunostomy feeding is contraindicated in Crohn's disease, radiation enteritis and malabsorption. All these methods of feeding carry a risk of aspiration of the stomach con-

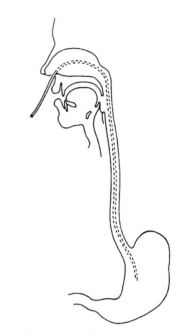

Figure 23.1 Positioning of nasogastric tube.

tents into the lungs. The higher up the site of entry to the alimentary tract, the greater is the risk of aspiration (see Fig. 23.2).

Delivering the feed

Whichever method of access to the gut has been chosen, the tube or catheter is attached, using aseptic technique via a giving set, to a reservoir of feed. This is usually the feed bottle or a bag set. Ideally the giving set will be routed through a feeding pump (see Box 23.6) and the delivery (flow) rate of the feed set. If no pump is available, the flow rate will have to be checked regularly.

There are many feeding pumps available, either for fixed use, i.e. over the patient's bed, or portable to enable the patient's full mobility. The pump manufacturers also make giving sets and nasogastric tubes and may also produce enteral feeds.

Hospitals should ideally use one system throughout their unit, as it means that staff will be familiar with the system used on whichever ward they work.

The choice of feed is normally made by the dietitian or medical staff, who, after calculating the patient's nutrient requirements, will prescribe a specific feed, volume and flow rate. This information should be entered on a chart kept by the patient's bed. The flow rate is usually built up over 2 to 3 days to ensure that the patient is able to tolerate the feed,

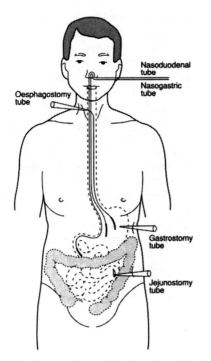

Figure 23.2 Routes of enteral feeding (reproduced with kind permission from Thomas 1994).

but this depends on the period of time that the patient was not eating prior to feeding being commenced. Maximum volume per hour is approximately 250 ml.

Many giving sets have a 'medicine port', which allows medicines to be given directly into the tube without disconnecting the feed. However, some medicines such as iron supplements and acidic solutions are incompatible with enteral feeds and so cannot be added to the feed. Once opened the chosen feed must be attached to a sterile giving set, poured into a sterile enteral feed bag (if a large volume of feed or a mixture of feeds is to be used) or discarded. The giving set should be changed after a maximum of 24 hours.

Feeds should not normally be diluted, so extra water, if required, can be given at the end of the feeding time, either via a bag, sterile bottle or as a syringe bolus. Water can normally be delivered at a faster rate than the feed. If the patient is immunocompromised sterile water should be used.

It is important to remember that the feed is part of the patient's treatment and it is essential that the patient receives the actual volume prescribed. If the patient requires procedures that need the feed to be disconnected, care should be taken to start it again as soon as possible and to ensure, where possible, that the full volume is given, even if this means extending the feeding time.

Complications of enteral feeding

The complications most usually associated with enteral feeding are diarrhoea, constipation and vomiting.

Diarrhoea

If an enterally fed patient develops diarrhoea or fails to absorb all of the feed, the flow rate of the feed should be reduced. It is not necessary to stop the feed in the first instance.

Common causes of diarrhoea include:

- antibiotic therapy—antibiotics particularly likely to cause diarrhoea are those of the penicillin and tetracyclin groups
- too fast a flow rate, particularly if the patient was nil by mouth for a long period of time prior to the commencement of feeding
- poor hygiene in setting up feed—giving sets should be changed every 24 hours; although the feeds are initially sterile they can easily become contaminated
- malabsorption of the feed—consider changing to an elemental or peptide feed

All possible causes of diarrhoea should be eliminated before the feed is stopped. Some patients may require:

- feed with added fibre
- a milk-free feed, e.g. a soya-based feed
- an elemental or peptide feed.

Constipation

Common causes of constipation include:

- dehydration—check fluid balance chart and ensure patient is receiving sufficient fluid
- immobility—this may be a consequence of drugs being prescribed which reduce gut motility or lack of non-starch polysaccharides (NSP) in the diet reducing gut motility. Changing to a fibre-containing feed is often beneficial.

Nausea and vomiting

Common causes of nausea and vomiting include:

- poor gastric emptying—ensure the patient's head and shoulders are raised 30° and consider the use of drugs which increase the rate of gastric emptying

- rapid infusion of feed—use a slower infusion rate, but increase the duration of the feeding time to ensure adequate nutritional intake.

There are many proprietary feeds available, the majority being milk-based. The composition of these feeds varies to accommodate the altering nutritional requirements of individuals and the requirements of different conditions, for example:

- feeds with additional fibre, either soluble or insoluble—for constipation and diarrhoea
- low-carbohydrate feeds—for respiratorily compromised patients
- higher-protein feeds—for patients with increased protein needs, e.g. burns
- low-sodium feeds—for liver, renal and cardiovascular diseases
- paediatric feeds—for children over 1 year
- peptide feeds
- elemental feeds.

Monitoring of enteral feeding

Patients receiving enteral feeding must be regularly monitored. Weekly weighing is ideal, but if impossible the nursing staff must be especially alert to the patient's physical appearance, changes of bulk, skin condition and muscle tone. Anthropometric measurements such as skinfold thickness and mid-arm circumference are important in the unconscious patient, as is routine biochemical monitoring.

Choice of feed

Most feeds contain 1 kcal/ml but some have 1.5 kcal/ml. It is usual to use commercially prepared feeds rather than feeds prepared at the hospital because:

- they come in a convenient form for immediate use
- they are nutritionally complete
- they can be stored without refrigeration
- they are manufactured under sterile conditions
- they remain sterile until opened, thus considerably reducing the risk of gastrointestinal infections
- their composition is accurately controlled
- they have a known osmolarity and feeds of lower osmolarity can be chosen if necessary.

Two categories of enteral feed are available. These are the whole-protein feeds and the elemental/peptide feeds.

Whole-protein feeds are also known as polymeric feeds. These feeds are available in a wide range of formulations to meet specific dietetic needs. An intact and functioning gastrointestinal system is essential for them to be digested and absorbed.

Protein is provided as milk protein, hydrolysed casein or soya protein. Carbohydrate is provided as maltodextrins, corn syrup solids, glucose and sucrose. Fat is provided usually as a vegetable oil derivative.

Elemental/peptide feeds. The major difference between this category of feeds and the whole-protein category is that protein is provided as peptides and amino acids which do not need to be digested. This type of feed is used when digestion and absorption are impaired. As with protein feeds, a range of formulations are available, some of which provide fat as medium-chain triglycerides.

All of these products can be used as an enteral feed for total nutrition or as an oral supplement. Some are flavoured. However, the elemental diets are generally unpalatable, but flavourings are available to improve their palatability.

Some patients, unable to eat sufficient food during the day, are tube-fed overnight, e.g. some patients with cystic fibrosis.

Enteral feeding and diabetes

Diabetes is not a contraindication to enteral feeding, but additional care needs to be exercised. There are no specially formulated diabetic tube feeds, so a standard formulation (1 kcal/ml) is usually given. Those feeds with a higher energy content (1.5 kcal/ml) are not usually suitable for patients with diabetes. The patient's total calorie requirements are given at a fairly slow infusion rate of 80 to 100 ml/hour. A feeding pump should be used to prevent an uneven delivery rate. If the feeding regime has a rest period, this should occur at night. Blood glucose levels should be monitored regularly, 2- to 4-hourly initially. If glucose levels rise, small amounts of soluble insulin can be given.

Babies

Babies under 1 year normally receive an infant formula milk. Baby milks are not fed continuously as they block the feeding tube (due to the fat composition). Instead, they are given as 1-, 2-, 3- or 4-hourly boluses by syringe. After the age of 1 year it is usual to use an enteral feed specifically formulated for paediatric use.

Home enteral feeding

Many patients, both adults and children, are successfully fed in their own home. The patient and/or carers are trained in use of the feeding system and are supported via the hospital and their district nursing service. Portable feeding pumps are available and are usually carried in a waistband or rucksack and are invaluable for patients who are mobile, enabling them to return to their normal activities and occupations.

In 1997 it was estimated that 10 000 patients were receiving home enteral nutrition. This is obviously advantageous for the patient who can be cared for in familiar surroundings and regain their independence. However the British Artifical Nutrition Survey (Elia 1997) showed that many patients and carers were receiving unsatisfactory support.

PARENTERAL NUTRITION

Parenteral nutrition should only be initiated if it is not possible to feed the patient by the enteral route. Total parenteral nutrition (TPN) is only effective if it is to be used for more than 3 to 5 days. This is probably due to the need for the liver to establish its enzyme systems to deal with intravenous nutrients. The use of TPN for longer than 6 weeks can lead to gut atrophy in up to 50% of patients (Williamson 1984). Current research shows adding glutamine to TPN mixtures may be protective for the gut, and solutions are already available. Their use is being evaluated.

Once it has been decided to feed a patient parenterally, a peripheral or central venous line is inserted under aseptic conditions, preferably in the operating theatre.

Peripheral feeding is normally chosen if:

- it is intended to feed the patient for less than 7 days
- nutrient requirements are not high
- the volume required is more than 2000 to 2500 ml/24 hours.

Central feeding is normally chosen if:

- it is intended to feed the patient for more than 7 days
- nutrient requirements are high
- the volume of fluid is likely to be or needs to be restricted

The central vein that is usually used is the subclavian vein. Here the rapid blood flow quickly dilutes the infused hypertonic nutrient solution, reducing the risk of thrombophlebitis.

Parenteral solutions

Nitrogen source

Protein is given in the form of pure amino acid solutions. All essential amino acids must be present. A range of non-essential amino acids are also present. It is thought that some conditions require greater amounts of specific amino acids. Glutamine is thought to be necessary to protect gut integrity.

A sufficient amount of energy must be present simultaneously with the amino acids, otherwise the amino acids will be used as an energy source and not for protein synthesis.

Energy sources

Energy is provided both as carbohydrate and fat.

Hypertonic glucose. This is a suitable source of carbohydrate (glucose providing 4 kcal/g to the central vein) and can be supplied in concentrations of up to 70%. In stress situations, notably after surgical operations, severe burns and hypothermia, endogenous insulin secretion for this carbohydrate load may be insufficient. If the patient becomes hyperglycaemic additional insulin may be needed.

Any extra energy given that exceeds the patient's energy requirements will be converted to fat and stored in adipose tissue.

Fat (lipid) emulsions. These have a high energy content relative to volume, therefore they are invaluable in TPN, not only as they provide energy but also essential fatty acids.

Electrolytes, trace elements and vitamins

In TPN lasting longer than a few days, provision of electrolytes, trace elements and vitamins must be comprehensive and complete. Some solutions used may already contain electrolytes, but additions can be made as necessary depending on the clinical condition of the patient. Sodium and potassium are particularly important where there are large gastrointestinal losses, for example as a result of vomiting, diarrhoea or substantial gastric aspiration. Sweating is another route for large losses of sodium.

The trace elements, including cobalt, copper, fluorine, iodine, selenium, magnesium, manganese and zinc, are all important for human metabolism and can be added to intravenous nutrients satisfactorily. Mineral and trace-element solutions are available, giving the daily requirements of minerals such as calcium and trace elements. Patients receiving intravenous feeding may require increased amounts of some vitamins; water-soluble vitamins are rapidly excreted from the body and a proportion may be destroyed in the TPN feeding solution. A source of both water-soluble and fat-soluble vitamins needs to be administered.

Patient monitoring

It is necessary to monitor the patient continuously while TPN is introduced, to ensure any changes in biochemistry are detected early. Accurate estimation of daily fluid balance is essential in the early stages of TPN and all fluid input needs to be considered, not just that from TPN. A careful watch must be kept for early signs of sepsis. As TPN becomes well established, the frequency of monitoring can decrease.

Complications of parenteral feeding

There are three main types of complications—technical, metabolic and infective:

1. Technical resulting from catheter placement. For example pneumothorax
2. Metabolic. This type is the most commonly occurring. For example hyperglycaemia and hypophosphataemia
3. Infective. For example sepsis resulting from poor catheter care. Sepsis occurs in 2–7% of all patients receiving TPN (Sitzmann & Pitt 1989).

Before TPN is stopped, the patient should be being nourished via the enteral route, whether by tube or by encouraging the patient to eat. It is often necessary to run an enteral regime concurrently with TPN for a few days.

Home parenteral feeding

Although not as common as home enteral feeding, it is possible for patients to receive TPN at home.

NUTRITIONAL SUPPORT AND CANCER CARE

Nutritional assessment is an essential part of the care of the patient who is being treated for cancer. Many patients will require and benefit from nutritional support at some stage of their illness (Celeya Perez & Valero Zanuy 1999). Nutritional support will prevent or reduce the severity of malnutrition, improve tolerance of treatment and resistance to infection and increase the feeling of wellbeing. Malnutrition in cancer patients is associated with a poor prognosis (Ingaki et al 1974, O'Gorman et al 1999).

The causes of malnutrition are biochemical, physical and psychological. Some are due to the condition itself while others are due to side-effects of the treatment that is being undergone. Weight loss is usually more severe in the people who have cancer of the upper gastrointestinal tract or lung than in those who have other types of cancer.

Both chemotherapy and radiotherapy can cause unpleasant side-effects which lead to poor nutritional status. The type of symptom and its severity will depend on the individual and their actual treatment.

Possible adverse effects of chemotherapy

- Anorexia, nausea and vomiting
- Constipation
- Diarrhoea and malabsorption
- Change in taste acuity and sensation
- Anaemia
- Fatigue.

Possible adverse effects of radiotherapy

Adverse effects depend on the site of the tumour and the field of treatment:

- Sore mouth, dry mouth
- Change in taste acuity and sensation
- Anorexia, nausea and vomiting
- Diarrhoea, malabsorption
- Intestinal obstruction
- Colitis.

Those patients with cancer of the head and neck or gastrointestinal tract are also likely to have had a reduced oral intake before treatment was commenced. This is due to the symptoms associated with the cancer such as nausea, vomiting, malabsorption, anorexia and difficulties in eating and swallowing.

The anxiety that accompanies the diagnosis of cancer and its treatment can also lead to loss of appetite and enjoyment of food, which results in a reduced dietary intake.

Sympathetic dietary counselling and the use of dietary supplements are important parts of the patient's treatment.

Cancer cachexia

Cachexia is the term used to describe the syndrome that includes anorexia, nausea, lipolysis, loss of both muscle and visceral protein and weight loss and it develops in most patients who have advanced cancer. The consequences of cachexia are decreased survival, increased complications of surgery, radiotherapy and chemotherapy, weakness, anorexia, chronic nausea and psychological distress to the patient and family (Bruera 1998).

Cancer cachexia used to be thought to be due to an increase in metabolic requirements, which was due to the presence of the tumour, associated with a reduced dietary intake, in turn caused by factors released by the tumour that caused anorexia. Current understanding is that the cachexia syndrome develops as a result of major metabolic disorders caused by disturbances in the functioning of the cytokine system. The metabolic changes that occur in cancer cachexia are reviewed by Inui (1999). It is the changes in the cytokine system which cause the negative nitrogen balance, lipolysis and anorexia (Bruera 1998).

Intensive support, as enteral feeding or total parenteral nutrition, is not appropriate for all cases of cancer cachexia. However, it is important for those cachexia patients who are recovering from surgery or waiting for chemotherapy as it will improve their healing and tolerance of the treatment. For those patients for whom intensive nutritional support is not considered suitable, nutritional support should still be given. This will optimise oral intake, by encouraging the use of sip-feeds, and give carers information about the type of diet that is suitable and best-tolerated by the individual to overcome some of the side-effects of the treatment, such as alterations in taste perception and a sore mouth (see Chapter 29).

Some people with cancer try alternative diets to treat their disease. If this is the case, nutritional status should be monitored regularly and the individual's actual nutritional requirements and intake explained. While it is the patient's decision whether or not to follow a particular dietary regime, it is the health care worker's role to ensure that the patient is able to make an informed decision. The disadvantage of some alternative diets is that, because they tend to exclude refined and processed food products and encourage the consumption of very large amounts of fruit and vegetables, they are likely to be bulky and have a low energy content.

REFERENCES

Allison S P 1999 Hospital food as treatment, A report by a working party of the British Association for Parenteral and Enteral Nutrition. The British Association for Parenteral and Enteral Nutrition, Maidenhead

Arora N S, Rochester D F 1982 Respiratory muscle strength and maximal voluntary ventilation in undernourished patients. American Review of Respiratory Diseases 126: 5–8

Barstow M D, Rawlings J, Allison S P 1983 Benefits of supplementary tube feeding after fractured neck of femur: a randomised controlled trial. British Medical Journal 287: 1589–1592

Bishop C W, Bowen P E, Ritchey S J 1981 Norms for nutritional assessment of American adults by upper arm anthropometry. American Journal of Clinical Nutrition 34: 2530–2539

Bistrian B R, Sherman M, Blackburn G L et al 1977 Cellular immunity in adult marasmus. Archives of Internal Medicine 137: 1408–1411

Bruera E 1998 Anorexia, cachexia, and nutrition. In: Falon M, O, Neill B (eds) ABC of palliative care. BMJ Books, London

Burke 1997 Hungry in hospital. The Association of Community Health Councils, London

Celeya Perez S, Valero Zanuy M A 1999 Nutritional management of oncologic patients. Nutrition in Hospital 4 (Suppl 2): 435–525

Department of Health (DoH) 1991 Dietary reference values for food energy and nutrients for the United Kingdom. Report of the Panel on Dietary Reference Values of the Committee on Medical Aspects of Food Policy (COMA) (Report on Health and Social Subjects 41). HMSO, London

Department of Health (DoH) 2001 The essence of care patient to use benchmarking for health care practitioners. HMSO, London

Elia M 1997 The 1997 Annual report of the British Artificial Nutrition Survey. British Association for Parenteral and Enteral Nutrition. BAPEN, Maidenhead

Elia M (ed) 2000 Guidelines for detection and management of malnutrition: Malnutrition Advisory Group, British Association for Parenteral and Enteral Nutrition. BAPEN, Maidenhead

Elwyn D H 1980 Nutritional requirements of adult surgical patients. Clinical Care Medicine 8: 9–20

Gurney J M, Jelliffe D B 1973 Arm anthropometry in nutritional assessment. American Journal of Clinical Nutrition 26: 912–915

Heymsfield S B, Casper K 1987 Anthropometric assessment of the adult hospitalised patient. Journal of Parenteral and Enteral Nutrition 11(S): 36S–41S

Heymsfield S B, Bethel R A, Anstey J B, Gibbs D M, Felner J M, Nutter D O 1978 Cardiac abnormalities in cachectic patients before and during nutritional repletion. American Heart Journal 95: 584–594

Hill G L, Blackett R L, Pickford L et al 1977 Malnutrition in surgical patients—an unrecognised problem. Lancet 1: 689–692

Holmes R, Macmhiano K, Jhangiani S S, Agarwal N R, Savino J A 1987 Combating pressure sores—nutritionally. American Journal of Nursing 1301–1303

Hoover H C Jr, Ryan J A, Anderson E J, Fischer J E 1980 Nutritional benefits of immediate postoperative jejunal feeding of an elemental diet. American Journal of Surgery 139: 153–159

Ingaki J, Rodriguez V, Bodey G P 1974 Causes of death in cancer patients. Cancer 35(2): 568–573

Inui A 1999 Cancer anorexia-cachexia syndrome: are neuropeptides the key? Cancer Research 59(18): 4493–4501

Jendteg S, Larsson J, Lindgren B 1987 Clinical and economic aspects of nutritional supply. Clinical Nutrition 6: 185–190

Keys A, Brozek J, Henschel A, Michelsen D, Taylor H L 1950 In: Keys A, Brozek J, Henschel A (eds) The biology of human starvation. University of Minnesota Press, Minneapolis (vol I: 703–748, vol II: 819–918)

Larsson J, Lennmarken C, Martensson J, Sandstear S, Vinnars E 1990 Nitrogen requirements in severely injured patients. British Journal of Surgery 77: 413–416

Lennard-Jones J 1992 A positive approach to nutrition and treatment. King's Fund Centre, London

McWhirter J P, Pennington C R 1994 The incidence and recognition of malnutrition in hospitals. British Medical Journal 308: 945–948

Moghissi K, Hornshaw S, Teasdale P R, Dawes E A 1977 Parenteral nutrition in carcinoma of the oesophagus treated by surgery: nitrogen balance and clinical studies. British Journal of Surgery 64: 125–128

Molnar J A, Wolfe R R, Burke J F 1983 Burns. Metabolism and nutritional therapy in thermal injury. In: Schneider H A, Anderson C E, Cousin D B (eds) Nutritional support of medical practice, 2nd Edn. Harper & Row, Philadelphia: 260–281

O'Gorman P, McMillan D C, McArdle C S 1998 Impact of weight loss, appetite and the inflammatory response on quality of life in gastrointestinal cancer patients. Nutrition and Cancer 32(2): 76–80

Reilly J J, Hull S F, Albert N, Waller A, Bringardener S 1987 Economic impact of malnutrition: a model system for hospitalised patients. Journal of Parenteral and Enteral Nutrition 12: 372–376

Scrimshaw N S 1991 Effect of infection on nutrient requirements. Journal of Parenteral and Enteral Nutrition 15(6): 589–600

Sitzmann J V, Pitt H A, Patient Care Committee of the American Gastroenterological Association 1989 Statement on guidelines for total parenteral nutrition. Digest of Disease and Science 34(4): 489–496

Sizer T 1996 Standards and guidelines for nutritional support of patients in hospitals. BAPEN, Maidenhead

Sullivan D H, Paleh G A, Walls R C, Lipschitz D A 1990 Impact of nutrition status on morbidity and mortality in a select population of geriatric rehabilitation patients. American Journal of Clinical Nutrition 51: 749–758

Tanner J M, Whitehouse R H, Takaishi M 1966 Standards from birth to maturity for height, weight, height velocity and weight velocity for British children in 1965. Archives of Disease in Childhood 41: 454–471

Thomas B (ed) 1994 Manual of dietetic practice, 2nd Edn. Blackwell Science, Oxford

Twomey P L, Patchings S C 1985 Cost-effectiveness of nutritional support. Journal of Parenteral and Enteral Nutrition 9: 3–10

Walesby R K, Goode A W, Spinks T J, Herring A, Ranicar A S, Bentall H H 1979 Nutritional status of patients requiring cardiac surgery. Journal of Thoracic and Cardiovascular Surgery 77: 570–576

Williams R H P, Heatley R V, Lewis M H, Hughes L E 1977 In: Baxter D H, Jackson G M (eds) Clinical parenteral nutrition. Geistlich Education, Chester: 52

Williamson R C N 1984 Disuse atrophy of the intestinal tract. Clinical Nutrition 34: 393–399

FURTHER READING

Allison S P 1996 The management of malnutrition in hospital. Proceedings of the Nutrition Society 55 (3): 855–862

Anderton A, Howard J P, Scott D W 1986 Microbiological control in enteral feeding: a guidance document. British Dietetic Association, Birmingham

Anderton A 1995 Reducing bacterial contamination in enteral tube feeds. British Journal of Nursing 4: 368–376

British Dietetic Association 1996 Malnutrition in hospital. Position Paper. British Dietetic Association, London

Carr C S, Ling K D E, Boulos P, Singer M 1996 Randomised trial of safety and efficacy of immediate postoperative enteral feeding in patients undergoing gastrointestinal resection. British Medical Journal 312: 869–871

Cologiovanni L 1997 Parenteral nutrition. Nursing Standard 12:9 34–45

Elia M 1990 Artificial nutritional support. Medicine International 82: 3392–3396

Griffith C D M, Clark R G 1984 A comparison of the 'Sheffield' prognostic index with forearm muscle dynamometry in patients from Sheffield undergoing major abdominal and urological surgery. Clinical Nutrition 3: 147–157

Hamaoui E, Leftowitz E, Olender L et al 1990 Enteral nutrition in the early postoperative period: A new semi-elemental formula versus total parenteral nutrition. Journal of Parenteral and Enteral Nutrition 14: 501–507

Jeejeebhoy K N 1990 Assessment of nutritional assessment. Journal of Parenteral and Enteral Nutrition 14(5): 193S–196S

Kennedy J F 1997 Enteral feeding for the critically ill patient. Nursing Standard 11:33 39–43

King's Fund 1992 A positive approach to nutritional treatment. King's Fund, London

Lennard-Jones J 1998 Ethical and legal aspects of clinical hydralin and nutritional support. BAPEN, Maidenhead

Maes J, Fry J 1988 Gastrostomy tube feeding: a review. Nutritional Support Services 8: 29–31

Moran B, Taylor M 1989 Percutaneous endoscopic gastrostomy. Clinical Nutrition Update 2(7): 4

Norton B, Homer-Ward M, Donnelly M T, Long R G, Holmes G K T 1996 A randomised prospective comparison of percutaneous endoscopic gastrostomy and nasogastric tube feeding after acute dysphagic stroke. British Medical Journal 312: 13–16

Payne-James J J, Silk D B A 1988 Enteral nutrition: background indications and management. Bailliere's Clinical Gastroenterology 2: 107–143

Potter J, Langhorne P, Roberts M 1998 Routine protein energy supplementation in adults: a systematic review. British Medical Journal 317: 495–501

Richards D M, Deeks J J, Sheldon T A, Shaffer J L 1997 Home parenteral nutrition: a systematic review. Health Technology Assessment 1(1)

Taylor S, Goodinson-McLaren S 1992 Nutritional support: a team approach. Wolfe Publishing, London

USEFUL ADDRESS

Malnutrition Advisory Group
10th Floor
10 Cabot Square
Canary Wharf
London E14 4QB

24

Diet in disorders of the gastrointestinal tract

LEARNING OBJECTIVES

After studying this chapter you should be able to:

- describe the scientific basis for the dietary treatments used for treatment of the range of commonly encountered disorders of the gastrointestinal tract
- explain how the diet can be modified to meet the specific needs of these different conditions.

Improved understanding of the physiology of the gastrointestinal tract, new and improved treatments for alimentary disorders and a critical appraisal of the effectiveness of the previously prescribed diets, have led to changes in the dietetic treatment of disorders of the gastrointestinal tract.

The conditions which require specific dietary modifications are outlined in this chapter. Most patients with a gastrointestinal disorder expect to be given dietary advice. To them, it seems obvious that the food they eat will affect their condition. The best advice for patients where there is no evidence for the benefit of a specific therapeutic diet is:

- eat a varied diet
- avoid the foods that upset you, but only if you are certain that they do.

Even if this seems unnecessary, this advice should be given because, without it, patients may exclude a large number of foods, leading to the development of malnutrition and unnecessary restrictions on the individual's life. If a large number of foods are excluded from the diet the patient should be referred to a dietitian to ensure that the diet is nutritionally adequate.

DYSPEPSIA

This is the term used to describe a range of gastrointestinal symptoms, the occurrence of which is associated with the ingestion of food. These symptoms include nausea, heartburn, discomfort and epigastric pain and they have many different causes. In a proportion of sufferers no actual disease of the gastrointestinal tract is identified.

Causes of dyspepsia

- Food intolerance
- Psychological factors
- General disease such as cardiac failure and chronic nephritis
- Ulceration or inflammation of the gut mucosa as in peptic ulcers.

Peptic ulcers

Peptic ulcers may be either in the stomach (gastric) or the duodenum (duodenal). The isolation of *Helicobacter pylori* in the stomachs of patients with peptic ulcer and gastritis by Marshall & Warren (1984) led to a revolution in the treatment of this condition. Peptic ulcer is due to one of two causes:

- *Helicobacter pylori* infection (Blaser 1998)
- intake of non-steroidal anti-inflammatory drugs.

Gastric ulcers. These are less common than duodenal ulcers and can be acute or chronic. The pain that they cause usually occurs shortly after eating.

Duodenal ulcers. In this condition it is usual for the pain and dyspeptic symptoms to occur when the stomach is empty, i.e. before meals and during the night. Treatment is no longer based on a bland diet and antacids. Instead, it is usual for treatment to consist of a course of antibiotics with a gastric-acid suppressant. For those patients in whom peptic ulcer is associated with the intake of non-steroidal anti-inflammatory drugs (e.g. aspirin and ibuprofen), alternatives to these drugs need to found. This group of drugs is used for self-medication, as a painkiller for arthritic pain and to prevent cardiovascular disease.

Stress and irregular meal frequency may contribute to the development of duodenal ulcers. Some people find their symptoms relieved by regular small meals.

Acute oesophagitis, gastritis and duodenitis

These are inflammation of the mucosa of the oesophagus, stomach and duodenum, which can occur without mucosal ulceration and produce similar symptoms to those accompanying peptic ulceration. Common causes of gastritis are the ingestion of gastric irritants such as alcohol and the excessive use of anti-inflammatory and analgesic drugs.

Principles of dietary treatment for dyspepsia

These are summarised in Box 24.1. The dietary modifications should incorporate the minimum of restrictions and interfere as little as possible with the eating habits of the patient. This treatment has been included as it may still be used for those people for whom drug therapy is inappropriate.

Box 24.1 Summary of dietary treatment for dyspepsia

- Take a snack at bedtime and between meals. Food in the stomach buffers the acid gastric juice and stimulates the production of bicarbonate-rich pancreatic secretion, which neutralises acid in the duodenum.
- Patients usually feel more comfortable if they eat small, frequent meals.
- Avoid foods that upset you. Foods which may upset individuals include onions, cucumber, raw vegetables and coffee.
- Alcohol, nicotine, aspirin and highly spiced foods are gastric irritants and should be avoided.

THE DUMPING SYNDROME

In some cases gastric surgery is necessary, as a response to severe ulceration, malignant disease or trauma to the upper gastrointestinal tract.

A small proportion of patients who have had gastric surgery develop a range of symptoms shortly after eating food. These symptoms are known as dumping syndrome and may include faintness, muscular weakness, epigastric discomfort, giddiness and sweating. In the majority of cases, the symptoms gradually disappear or lessen in severity, but in a few they persist. In some instances, symptoms are alleviated if the patient lies down for half an hour after taking food.

There are two types of dumping syndrome, known as early dumping syndrome and late dumping syndrome. They are caused by different mechanisms. The physiological responses to the rapid emptying of the hypertonic stomach contents into the small bowel is, however, the common cause of symptoms in both types of dumping syndrome.

Early dumping

Early dumping occurs within 30 minutes of eating a meal. The rapid passage of the hypertonic meal draws large amounts of fluid into the intestine. This causes a decrease in the circulating plasma volume, and it is this that produces the early symptoms of faintness, weakness, distension and discomfort.

Dietary advice for early dumping

- Eat small, frequent, dry meals.
- Take drinks between, not with, meals.
- Avoid any foods which you know worsen your symptoms.

Late dumping

Late dumping occurs 1 1/2 to 2 hours after a meal. A rapid rise in blood glucose follows the rapid gastric emptying. This stimulates an overproduction of insulin, which causes a rapid drop in blood glucose and the symptoms of hypoglycaemia.

Dietary advice for late dumping

- Avoid sugar and sugar-containing foods.
- Eat carbohydrate as starch instead of sugar.
- Avoid any foods which you know worsen your symptoms.

Long-term complications of gastric surgery

Following gastric surgery, reduced absorption of some essential nutrients may occur. These nutrients include iron, folic acid, vitamins B_{12}, D and K, and calcium, and can present as nutritional deficiencies once the body's stores of them have been depleted. The condition should be treated by providing dietary supplements. The necessity for supplements depends on the severity of the surgery and the patient's habitual diet. The vitamin B_{12} supplement will need to be given by injection as the intrinsic factor produced for its absorption is only produced by the stomach.

ATROPHIC GASTRITIS

Atrophic gastritis does not produce abdominal symptoms, but causes a macrocytic anaemia due to vitamin B_{12} malabsorption. This is of nutritional importance because, along with the acid- and pepsin-secreting cells of the stomach, the cells which produce the intrin-

sic factor necessary for vitamin B_{12} absorption atrophy. These patients are likely to develop a deficiency of this vitamin and require B_{12} injections to prevent this. Oral supplements of B_{12} are of no use as they cannot be absorbed.

CONSTIPATION

Delay and difficulty in evacuation of faeces is known as constipation. In most cases, constipation is not related to any organic disease but is due to long-established habits and a diet that is deficient in dietary non-starch polysaccharides (NSP). It frequently develops as a result of physical inactivity and prolonged bed-rest.

Constipation is a rare condition in areas where there is a high intake of dietary NSP. It is the cause of considerable discomfort, leading to abdominal distension, headache, nausea, loss of appetite and, in extreme conditions, vomiting. Chronic constipation can lead to haemorrhoids. Dietary treatment must include education so that the condition is not allowed to develop again.

When the diet lacks NSP, the faeces are not bulky enough to be passed effectively by normal peristalsis. This results in an increase in the activity of the muscles of the colon, colonic spasm and chronic constipation. The use of laxative and aperient drugs can be avoided in many cases of constipation by increasing the intake of all types of dietary NSP from cereals, vegetables and fruit and accompanying this with an increase in the fluid intake. Table 24.1 shows the NSP content of some commonly eatern food portions. Different people require different amounts of NSP in their diet. An adequate amount of NSP is the amount required to allow the patient to pass a soft stool without effort.

Figure 24.1 shows the mechanisms by which unabsorbed carbohydrates, including NSP, increase stool bulk and prevent constipation.

Table 24.1 Non-starch polysaccharide (NSP) content of food portions

Food	NSP content (g)
One slice white bread	0.5
One slice wholemeal bread	1.9
Average portion of corn flakes	0.3
Average portion of All Bran	7.4
Two Weetabix	3.4
One orange	2.0
Average portion of baked beans	4.2

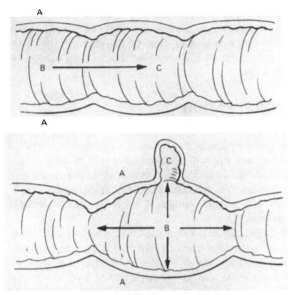

Figure 24.1 Normal colonic movement. *Upper:* Contraction of the colonic segment at A propels colonic contents from B to C. *Lower:* If the colonic contents are small and hard, this cannot occur. Instead, pressures build up in B, resulting in herniation of the colonic wall and the formation of a diverticulum at C.

High-NSP (fibre) diet

The NSP content of the diet can be increased by making the simple dietary changes that are listed in Box 24.2.

When this type of diet is used it is important that caterers understand the need to increase dietary NSP from fruit and vegetables and that a palatable diet is provided, rather than the substitution of wholemeal flour for refined flour and incorporation of bran into all dishes, which can make the diet unpalatable and unappetising. Table 24.2 shows a comparison of the NSP contents of two different days' food intakes.

Box 24.2 Advice for increasing the NSP content of the diet

- Eat a wholegrain or bran-enriched breakfast cereal, for example Weetabix, puffed wheat, Shredded Wheat, or All Bran.
- Eat wholemeal bread instead of white bread, and eat more of it.
- Eat more fruit and vegetables, fresh, frozen or tinned.
- Avoid refined cereal products, for example cakes, biscuits, polished rice and pasta. Use wholegrain products and brown rice instead.
- Increase fluid intake—dietary NSP in the gut makes the stool bulkier and softer by absorbing water.

DIVERTICULAR DISEASE AND DIVERTICULITIS

A colonic diverticulum is formed when the colonic mucosa is pushed through the colonic muscle wall to form a blind sac. These diverticula are frequently found in people who have a low-NSP diet, which results in the formation of small hard stools that require increased colonic muscular activity for their passage (Painter & Burkitt 1971). The presence of asymptomatic diverticula, known as diverticular disease, increases with age. These diverticula are usually multiple.

The mechanism of formation of a diverticulum is illustrated schematically in Figure 24.1.

The symptomatic form of diverticular disease is called acute diverticulitis and is due to acute inflammation of an obstructed diverticulum. After treatment of the acute inflammation, treatment is usually based on increasing the amount of NSP in the diet. The dietary recommendations are the use of a high-NSP diet as for the treatment of constipation, discussed above. In some cases, it may be necessary to increase the cereal NSP content of the diet while reducing the fruit and vegetable content, as fruit and vegetables can cause mucosal irritation and diarrhoea.

DIARRHOEA

Diarrhoeal diseases are a major public health problem in developing countries. They are caused by inadequate water supplies, poor quality of water, poor sanitation and malnutrition, and result in the death of children and adults, the young, the old and the unwell being particularly vulnerable. The prevention and treatment of diarrhoeal diseases in developing countries is not addressed in this chapter. An overview of the prevention and treatment of diarrhoeal disease in an emergency situation can be found in *Refugee Health—an Approach to Emergency Situations* (Medecins Sans Frontieres 1997).

Acute diarrhoea has many causes, the commonest being dietary indiscretion and bacterial food poisoning. It is usually mild and does not require dietary treatment, though generous fluids and a simple light diet (i.e. one that does not include fried foods and strongly flavoured or highly spiced foods) probably speed recovery. Chronic diarrhoea is a less common symptom than constipation but can be equally troublesome and have a profound effect on an individual's quality of life. Diarrhoea means the passage, often frequently, of loose unformed stools (usually more than 200 ml/day).

Chronic diarrhoea can be caused by:

Table 24.2   Ways of increasing the non-starch polysaccharide (NSP) content of a typical diet

Typical diet (low in NSP)	NSP content* (g)	Suggested diet (high in NSP)	NSP content* (g)
Cornflakes and milk	0.3	Weetabix and milk	3.4
Two slices white toast, butter and honey	1.0	Two slices wholemeal toast, butter and chunky marmalade	3.8
Cheese sandwiches (four slices white bread)	2.0	Cheese sandwiches (four slices wholemeal bread)	7.6
Fruit scone	1.0	Tomato	2.5
Fruit yoghurt		Wholemeal fruit scone	1.0
		one orange	2.0
Lamb chop		Lamb chop	
Boiled potatoes	1.8	Potato baked in jacket	5.4
Carrots	1.8	Carrots	1.8
		Peas	3.3
Fruit pie (made with white flour)	1.6	Tinned plums	1.1
Custard		Custard	
Daily total	9.5	Daily total	31.9

*Figures for NSP content taken from McCance and Widdowson's Composition of Foods, 5th Edition (Holland et al 1991), NSP analysed by Englyst method (Englyst & Cummings 1988).

- diseases of the gastrointestinal tract, such as ulcerative colitis, Crohn's disease, diverticulitis and intestinal neoplasm
- malabsorption syndrome
- food allergy
- excessive alcohol consumption
- uraemia
- antibiotic treatment.

Antibiotics, particularly of the penicillin and tetracyclin groups, alter the gastrointestinal bacterial flora resulting in diarrhoea. This usually stops once the antibiotic treatment is finished.

The symptoms may be severe enough to require fluid and electrolyte replacement. Management involves diagnosis and treatment of the underlying disorder, and administration of dietary supplements to correct nutritional deficiencies that have developed as a consequence of the diarrhoea. In some cases of intractable diarrhoea, a low-residue diet may be used, but other individuals may find that an increase in the cereal NSP content of the diet is beneficial.

Diarrhoea that occurs after a gastrointestinal infection may be due to a temporary lactose intolerance. This should be treated with a milk-free diet (see Chapter 28).

Foods to avoid on a low-residue diet

- Bread and biscuits made from brown or wholemeal flours
- Breakfast cereals which contain the whole grain or are fortified with bran

- Seeds and skins of fruit
- Fruit which has a specific laxative effect, e.g. prunes, rhubarb
- Pulses and fibrous vegetables.

THE IRRITABLE BOWEL SYNDROME

The irritable bowel syndrome (IBS) is a functional bowel disorder which affects about 20% of adults in the industrialised world. Most people with the condition (60–75%) do not consult a doctor (Farthing 1995). It is thought to occur when colonic motor responses to a range of stimuli including food, stress and colonic distention, are increased. The actual causes of these increased responses are poorly understood. The range of symptoms associated with this syndrome are listed below.

Symptoms of IBS

- Abdominal discomfort and pain
- Diarrhoea
- Constipation
- Abdominal bloating
- Passing of mucus
- Flatulence
- Nausea and occasional vomiting.

Different combinations of these symptoms occur in different IBS sufferers and different combinations will occur at different times for the same individual. So an IBS sufferer can have constipation at one time and diarrhoea at another.

IBS is a common cause of referral to gastroenterology clinics and was thought to account for 50% of the referrals in a study by Harvey et al (1983).

Dietary treatment

There is no specific dietary treatment—some patients' symptoms are relieved by a high-NSP diet, others by a low-NSP diet. Although modifying the NSP content of the diet is a popular treatment, there is no consensus of opinion as to its value (Rees et al 1994). There has been considerable interest in the idea that IBS is a symptom of a food-intolerance and sufferers have been treated by excluding specific foods such as dairy products, wheat or citrus fruits. A high incidence of food-intolerance with IBS was found by Hunter (1985). This method of treatment is successful for some patients, but as exclusion diets are potentially very harmful, this approach should only be pursued under medical and dietetic supervision.

Some patients are particularly sensitive to sorbitol and caffeine (Farthing 1995). These patients find the exclusion of foods which are sweetened with sorbitol such as some soft drinks, preserves and sweets and the exclusion of caffeine-containing drinks (coffee, tea and cola) beneficial. Dietary advice for most people with IBS is that they should:

- try to eat a diet that is as varied as possible
- avoid the foods that they know aggravate their condition
- increase their intake of cereal NSP.

A review of the dietary treatment of IBS (Burden 2001) highlights the need for the diet of the individual with IBS to be assessed, so that dietary treatment can be targeted to the symptom profile of the individual.

MALABSORPTION SYNDROMES

Malabsorption of nutrients results from a wide range of diseases and disorders of the gastrointestinal tract. If the disorder results in damage to the intestinal mucosa, it can generally be assumed that there will be a reduction in intestinal enzyme secretion and damage to the sites of nutrient absorption. This will reduce the ability of the intestine to digest and absorb foods, resulting in malabsorption.

Protein, fat, carbohydrate, vitamins and minerals can all be malabsorbed. The type of nutrient and amount malabsorbed depends on the area and length of gastrointestinal tract affected (see Fig. 24.2).

The causes of malabsorption

The causes of malabsorption are divided into groups:

1. *Impaired gastric function*. This can develop after gastric surgery (see 'Dumping Syndrome' above) and sometimes in atrophic gastritis.
2. *Diarrhoea*. Diarrhoea due to either intestinal hurry or bacterial colonisation of the small intestine, as in blind loop syndrome, can cause malabsorption.
3. *Impaired digestion within the intestine*. In pancreatitis and cystic fibrosis, the pancreatic secretion, which contains lipase and is necessary for the emulsification of fat, is reduced, causing malabsoption of fat. In biliary disease the reduced production of bile salts will prevent fat from being emulsified, so it cannot be absorbed.
4. *Impaired digestion and absorption by small intestine brush border cells*. The final stages of protein and carbohydrate digestion take place on the surface of the cells lining the small intestine. If the surface area has been reduced by damage to the intestinal villi, then the amount of nutrients absorbed will be reduced. This reduction may be due to:
   a. surgical resection
   b. mucosal damage by infection
   c. radiation
   d. drugs
   e. gluten-sensitive enteropathy—see page 240.

Symptoms of malabsorption

The symptoms of malabsorption include:

- diarrhoea
- steatorrhoea
- abdominal distension
- weight loss
- development of nutritional deficiency diseases, e.g. iron deficiency anaemia, osteomalacia.

Steatorrhoea is an excessive loss of fat in the stools. They normally contain 5 to 6 g/day when dietary intake is 70 to 100 g fat/day. When fat malabsorption occurs, they can contain as much as 50 to 60 g/day and are greasy, pale in colour, unformed and smell offensive.

Dietary treatment of malabsorption

The principles of dietary treatment for malabsorption are:

1. Restore fluid and electrolyte balance immediately.
2. Maintain optimal nutrition by the provision of a diet or dietary supplements which contain nutrients in a form that are not malabsorbed.

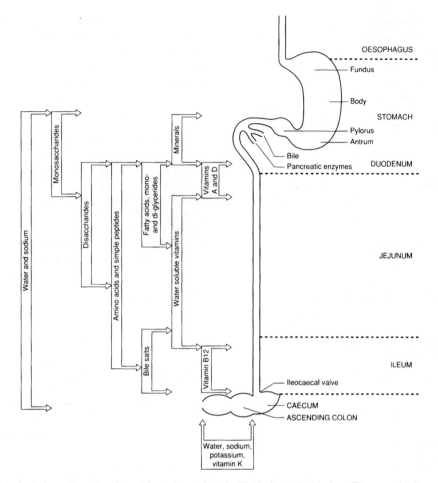

Figure 24.2 Principal absorption sites for nutrients (reproduced with kind permission from Thomas 1994).

3. Exclude or reduce the intake of foods that contain the nutrient that is malabsorbed or causes malabsorption and replace with suitable alternatives.

Hypolactasia

Congenital alactasia, that is, absence of the enzyme lactase, is very rare and is discussed in Chapter 28. However, 70 to 80% of the non-Caucasian population develop low lactase levels after childhood (acquired primary hypolactasia). Most of these individuals are free from the symptoms of malabsorption, are unaware they have a low lactase level and are not on a strict lactose-free diet. Most of these adults can tolerate 12 g/day of lactose (the amount contained in about 250 ml milk). However, if they take large amounts of lactose, such as in large quantities of milk, malabsorp-tion does occur, usually resulting in symptoms. This point should be considered when providing nutritional support (see Chapter 23), as many preparations contain milk or milk products and may not be suitable for individuals who habitually have a low lactose intake, since their consumption would cause abdominal discomfort and diarrhoea.

Chronic pancreatic exocrine insufficiency

This disorder occurs in adults as a result of chronic pancreatitis and is related particularly to alcohol-induced pancreatic damage. Not only is the exocrine function of the pancreas damaged, but its endocrine function is often impaired too. This means that diabetes mellitus may be an added complication and further dietary modification will be needed to maintain normoglycaemia. The nutritional treatment of chronic pancreatic exocrine insufficiency is a reduced-fat diet (see Box 24.3) with pancreatic enzyme supplements. It is not usually practical to restrict the dietary fat intake to below 40 g/day and this should not be continued if the severity of symptoms does not improve. If diabetes is also present, then the type and amount of carbohydrate in the diet will need to be regulated (see Chapter 27). The amount of fat restriction and enzyme supplementation depends on the residual activity of the pancreas. Only when pancreatic exocrine output is reduced to less than 10% of normal is malabsorption a problem and enzyme supplementation necessary.

Box 24.3 Reduced-fat diet

Reduced fat: approximately 45 g, 4.3 MJ (1800 kcal)
Suitable for malabsorption steatorrhoea

Guidelines
Avoid:
Whole milk and whole-milk products such as cheese, cream, full-cream yoghurts
All cooking oils and fats
Fried foods, visible fat on meat, sausages
Pastries
Cakes and biscuits, unless home-made without fat
Ice-cream, chocolate, cream sauces and cream soup

Include:
Semi-skimmed milk, low-fat spread
Lean meat, fish, poultry (cooked without fat), pulses
Bread, breakfast cereals, rice, pasta
Potatoes, fruit and vegetables (fresh, tinned and frozen)
Jam, honey, marmalade, sugar

Sample menu
500 ml semi-skimmed milk
30 g low-fat spread

Breakfast
Cereal, semi-skimmed milk and sugar
Grapefruit and sugar
Toast, low-fat spread and marmalade

Lunch
Four slices of bread
Lean ham/tomato
Fat-free yoghurt
Banana

Evening meal
Lean roast lamb (gravy made with stock cube, vegetable-water and cornflour)
Boiled potatoes
Carrots/peas
Milk pudding and tinned fruit

Later
Currant bun

It is always important to remember that a reduction in fat intake results in a reduction in energy intake and steps must be taken to prevent this either by including medium-chain triglycerides (MCT) in the diet and/or including high-energy supplements.

Medium-chain triglycerides (MCT) oil

Most of our dietary fats are mixtures of long-chain triglycerides (LCT). These require bile and pancreatic lipase for their digestion and subsequent absorption. MCT are of value when fat digestion is impaired, because even when pancreatic lipase and bile-salt activity is absent some absorption still occurs. This is because a proportion of the MCT enters the mucosal cells as triglyceride. MCT oil is prepared commercially from coconut oil and does not contain all the essential fatty acids, so a dietary source of LCT, particularly essential fatty acids, is necessary if MCT is used as the major dietary fat source.

Elemental and semi-elemental products

These products contain nutrients in forms that require the minimum of digestion before being absorbed. They are used for patients with severe disorders of digestive or absorptive function and come in a range of formulations. Some contain very little fat, while others contain fat as MCT. Their use reduces malabsorption and stool bulk and may enable some degree of bowel rest to be achieved. These products are unpalatable and are used with greatest success when the patient is very well motivated, or it may be necessary to feed them via a nasogastric tube (see Chapter 23).

Inflammatory bowel disease

The two major forms of inflammatory bowel disease are Crohn's disease and ulcerative colitis. They both cause similar symptoms—abdominal pain, diarrhoea, weight loss and anaemia, depending on the severity of the disease and the site of the gastrointestinal tract that is affected. If the small bowel is affected, steatorrhoea will also occur, and if the large bowel is affected, the stools will contain blood and mucus. Crohn's disease can occur anywhere along the entire length of the gastrointestinal tract, while ulcerative colitis occurs predominantly in the large bowel.

Both conditions show periods of remission and relapse and vary in severity. The causes of the conditions are unknown. They are thought to include genetic, immunological and infective mechanisms. There is no conclusive evidence that diet has a role in their development. Drug therapy is an important part of the treatment and maintenance of remission in both Crohn's disease and ulcerative colitis. Drugs used include corticosteroids and immunosuppressants.

Crohn's disease

The incidence of Crohn's disease has increased. It now affects 1 in 1500 people (Rampton 1999).

In an acute relapse, total parenteral nutrition (TPN) or enteral feeding using an elemental diet has been shown to induce remission. The length of time taken for this to happen varies (Teahon et al 1990).

In those patients for whom TPN or an elemental diet induces a remission, a return to a normal diet is slow and food intolerances must be identified. Then the diet which is followed during remission should be nutritionally adequate and exclude those foods of which the patient is known to be intolerant. Nutritional support may be necessary if weight was lost during the acute stage of the illness and if oral intake is poor. In those patients who have had a gut resection resulting in short bowel syndrome, dietary modification will be necessary to prevent malabsorption.

Ulcerative colitis

There is no evidence to show that TPN or elemental diets induce remission in ulcerative colitis, nor is there any evidence to suggest the involvement of food-intolerances. The diet should provide adequate protein, energy, vitamins and minerals and no specific foods need excluding. Nutritional support will also be of value during the recovery stage if weight has been lost.

ILEOSTOMY

An ileostomy is fashioned when the colon has been totally removed. If the ileum is normal, it is able to adapt to increase absorption of fluid and electrolytes, thus compensating for the removal of the colon. Following surgery, a period of adjustment occurs in which the ileum adapts. This period of adjustment takes up to 6 weeks. Once the ileostomy has settled down, a daily ileostomy output of 400 to 800 ml should be expected. Care should always be taken to ensure that dietary fluid intake is adequate; at least 8 cups of fluid a day should be encouraged. It is not usual to supplement the patient with extra sodium to cover that which is lost in the ileostomy fluid, because the normal dietary intake exceeds the normal require-

ment. However extra sodium may be needed in the immediate period postoperatively or during periods of very hot weather.

Most people with an ileostomy are able to enjoy a diet that is far more varied than that which they were able to eat before their surgery (Andrews 1993).

Following surgery, the range of foods in the diet should be slowly increased to be as varied as possible, with fruit and vegetables reintroduced gradually. There is considerable individual variation as to which foods upset people and the level of symptoms that they are prepared to tolerate. Increased stoma output, flatulence, liquid motions and odour of ileostomy effluent can all be caused by particular foods in susceptible individuals (see Box 24.4).

Gazzard et al (1978) recommend that food items which cause symptoms should be tested on at least three occasions before being totally excluded from the diet.

Dietary advice

1. Encourage a liberal fluid intake. This is important to prevent water depletion.
2. Avoid foods that you are certain cause symptoms. If it is necessary to exclude a wide range of foods, dietetic advice should be sought to ensure that the diet is nutritionally adequate.
3. Reintroduce fruit and vegetables into the diet in small portions. Mix high-NSP foods with lower-NSP ones in a meal.
4. Chew food well.

If necessary, the ileostomy output at night can be minimised by eating more food in the first half of the day than during the late afternoon and evening.

Box 24.4 Foods which may cause discomfort for individuals with an ileostomy

- Peas, onions, beans, cabbage, cauliflower, fizzy drinks and beer may cause flatulence.
- Prunes increase ileostomy output.
- Strongly coloured foods will colour output, e.g. beetroot.
- Alcohol may make ileostomy output more watery.
- Raw vegetables, dried fruit and sweetcorn may cause colic.
- A high intake of dietary NSP, particularly cellulose, can cause discomfort at the stoma site as it may be difficult for the stoma to pass the semi-solid mass. Nuts, apples and celery in particular may cause this sensation.

COELIAC DISEASE (GLUTEN-SENSITIVE ENTEROPATHY)

Coeliac disease is diagnosed as the cause of malabsorption in infants, children and adults and the incidence of diagnosis is rising among adults, although there are still thought to be many adults with undiagnosed coeliac disease. It has been suggested that the condition may affect 1 in 200 of the general population (Feighery 1999). The incidence of diagnosis among children is declining and this may be due to changes in weaning practice with the later introduction of gluten-containing foods (Stevens et al 1987).

The condition, which affects the upper small intestine, is due to the effect on certain susceptible individuals of the protein gluten, which occurs in both wheat and rye flours. Gluten is a mixture of two proteins, glutenin and gliadin. Gliadin is the fraction which gives rise to coeliac disease. The mechanism of action of gliadin in bringing about its harmful effect is not yet fully understood but it may be that it causes an abnormal immunological response.

Structural changes occur in the mucosa of the small bowel. This includes villus atrophy which is identified by jejunal biopsy. Following the introduction of a gluten-free diet, the structural appearance of the mucosa returns to normal slowly. Most patients show a rapid improvement in clinical symptoms but it can take years for histological improvement to be complete.

Symptoms of the disease include loss of appetite, muscle wasting, flatulence, abdominal distension and nutritional deficiencies. Malabsorption of fat gives rise to steatorrhoea, which can lead to deficiencies of fat-soluble vitamins and calcium. It has been recommended that all patients with osteoporosis should be screened for coeliac disease (Lindh et al 1992). Anaemia due to reduced absorption of iron and folic acid is usually present. The severity of the symptoms varies between individuals.

Dietary treatment of coeliac disease

The treatment consists of ensuring that the diet is completely free of gluten, wheat, barley and rye. Traditionally oats were also excluded from the diet. The studies of Janatuinen et al (1995) and Srinivasan et al (1996) provided evidence that the ingestion of oats did not damage the intestinal mucosa of patients with coeliac disease. It is now accepted that moderate amounts of oats can be included in the diets of most people with coeliac disease.

This is a diet that needs to be adhered to throughout life and its impact on the choices that individuals are able to make, and the impact on their families, should not be underestimated. A study of coeliacs by Twist & Hackett (1992) showed that 24% of the group surveyed thought that it was impossible for coeliacs to have a normal social life.

Coeliacs are at greater risk than non-coeliacs of developing cancer. Holmes (1989) has shown that adherence to a strict gluten-free diet reduces this risk. In Box 24.5 are listed some foods which may, and some which may not, be included in a gluten-free diet. In some cases, foods generally regarded as being unsuitable are available in a gluten-free form.

Gluten-free wheat starch, rice flour, cornflour, soya flour and potato flour are used as substitutes. Gluten-free products are available on prescription for people with coeliac disease and those with dermatitis herpetiformis, but not for other conditions requiring a gluten-free diet.

As soon as coeliac disease is diagnosed, a gluten-free but otherwise normal diet is started. Vitamin and iron supplements may be necessary, particularly if the condition has been undiagnosed into adulthood when the adult may initially present with malnutrition, e.g. osteomalacia and anaemia, or if a child has presented as failing to thrive.

At diagnosis, the child may be unhappy and have a poor appetite. If this is the case, the nurse, dietitian and child's family must be prepared to spend a lot of time encouraging the child to eat and try the special gluten-free products. Initially children usually find the gluten-free biscuits more palatable than the gluten-free bread. Once a gluten-free diet has been started, improvement is rapid and this helps to convince and motivate children and their families to continue the diet. Time needs to be spent discussing the diet, and how it can be incorporated into their routine, with the children and their carers. It is important that children feel confident about managing their diet as this will help them to enjoy a normal social life and not to feel too different from their peers.

In some children, damage to the intestinal mucosa may be such that digestion of disaccharides is impaired—notably digestion of lactose. In this event, the diet should be free from milk as well as free from gluten. Occasionally a multiple malabsorption state is encountered involving the disaccharides, protein and fat, and this will need to be treated with an elemental product suitable for children.

Prognosis

If a gluten-free dietary regimen is consistently maintained, normal health and development can be expected.

Box 24.5   Classification of foods for a diet free from wheat or rye gluten

Foods not allowed
- Bread, biscuits, cakes or puddings which contain ordinary flour
- Proprietary cake and pudding mixes
- Bought baking powders
- All pasta and semolina
- Shredded Wheat, Weetabix, puffed wheat, mixed-grain breakfast cereals
- Ryvita, Bemax, some infant cereal foods
- Vegetables canned in sauce, unless labelled 'gluten-free'
- Canned and packed soups, unless labelled 'gluten-free'
- Canned meats, canned fish in sauce, fish coated with batter or crumbs, fish and meat pastes, sausages, prepared gravy mixtures
- Some cheese spreads
- Malted milk drinks
- Salad creams, bottled sauces, pickles in sauce, commercial chutneys (unless labelled 'gluten-free')
- Sweets, chocolates and ice-cream
- Commercially prepared lemon curd

It may not be necessary to exclude all of these foods. For example, some companies do produce gluten-free sausages. The packaging of a product states if it is gluten free.

Foods allowed
- Bread, biscuits, cakes, etc. made from gluten-free flour substitute; yeast, or a gluten-free chemical raising agent, may be used for leavening
- Rice, ground rice, sago, tapioca, oatmeal, pure cornflour, custard powders prepared from cornflour
- Cornflakes and Rice Krispies
- All fresh, frozen or dried vegetables, and vegetables canned in brine
- All fruits—fresh, frozen, canned or dried
- Home-made soups, which may be thickened with lentils, split peas, gluten-free flour, or a suitable cereal such as rice
- All freshly cooked meat and fish; gravy may be thickened with cornflour; Bovril or Marmite may be added if desired
- Milk, eggs, cheese, butter, margarine, cooking oils
- Cocoa, Ovaltine, coffee, tea, soft drinks, fruit juices
- Vinegar, salt, flavouring essences and herbs, pickles in clear vinegar, pepper and spices
- Jam, marmalade, sugar, glucose, treacle, syrup, clear boiled sweets, jellies

---

Everyone must understand that occasional lapses, although apparently trivial, will impair the beneficial effects of the diet. It is generally accepted that for optimum benefit a gluten-free diet must be maintained for life.

The Coeliac Society (address at end of chapter) produces lists of manufactured foods which are gluten free. Care must be taken to ensure that the most recently produced list is consulted because the recipes used for products are often changed. The organisation runs a telephone hotline which has a monthly recorded message of any changes to the list. The Coeliac Society also publishes a wide range of literature of interest to coeliacs and a video entitled 'The Coeliac Condition'. It has local branches which provide helpful support and local information such as local suppliers of gluten-free bread.

Dermatitis herpetiformis

In this condition, which responds to the exclusion of gluten from the diet, there is a skin rash and small intestinal enteropathy.

REFERENCES

Andrews C 1993 Mixed meals. Nursing Times 89(43): 56–58
Blaser M J 1998 Helicobacter pylori and gastric diseases. British Medical Journal 316: 1507–1510
Burden S 2001 Dietary treatment of irritable bowel syndrome: current evidence and guidelines for future practice. Journal of Human Nutrition and Dietetics 14: 231–241
Englyst H N, Cummings J H 1988 An improved method for the measurement of dietary fiber as non-starch polysaccharides in plant foods. Journal of the Association of Analytical Chemistry 71: 808–814
Farthing M J G 1995 Fortnightly review: irritable bowel, irritable body or irritable brain? British Medical Journal 310: 171–175
Feighery C 1999 Coeliac disease. British Medical Journal 319: 236–239

Gazzard B G, Saunders B, Dawson A M 1978 Diet and stoma function. British Journal of Surgery 68: 642–644
Harvey R F, Salih S Y, Read A E 1983 Organic and functional disorders in 2000 gastroenterology out-patients. Lancet 1: 632–634
Holland B, Welch A A, Unwin I D, Buss D H, Paul A A, Southgate D A T 1991 McCance and Widdowson's composition of foods, 5th Edn. Royal Society of Chemistry, Cambridge
Holmes G K T 1989 Malignancy in coeliac disease—effects of gluten free diet. Gut 30: 333–338
Hunter J O 1985 The dietary management of Crohn's disease. In: Hunter J O, Alun Jones V (eds) Food and the gut. Baillière Tindall, Eastbourne

Janatuinen E K, Pikkarainen P H, Kemppainen T A et al 1995 A comparison of diets with and without oats in adults with coeliac disease. New England Journal of Medicine 333: 1033–1037

Lindh E, Ljunghall S, Larsson K, Lavob 1992 Screening for antibodies against gliadin in patients with osteoporosis. Journal of Intestinal Medicine 234: 403–406

Marshall B J, Warren J R, 1984 Unidentified curved bacilli in the stomach of patients with gastritis and peptic ulceration. Lancet 1: 1311–1315

Medecins sans Frontières 1997 Refugee health: An approach to emergency situations. Macmillan Education, London

Painter N S, Burkitt D P 1971 Diverticular disease of the colon: a deficiency disease of western civilization. British Medical Journal 2: 450–454

Rampton D S 1999 Management of Crohns disease. British Medical Journal 319: 1480–1485

Rees G A, Trevan M, Davies G J 1994 Dietary fibre modification and the symptoms of irritable bowel syndrome—a review. Journal of Human Nutrition and Dietetics 7(3): 179–189

Srinivasan U, Leonard N, Jones E et al 1996 Absence of oats toxicity in adult coeliac disease. British Medical Journal 313: 1300–1301

Stevens F M et al 1987 Decreasing incidence of coeliac disease. Archives of Disease in Childhood 62: 465–468

Teahon K, Bjarnason I, Pearson M, Levi A J 1990 Ten years' experience with an elemental diet in the management of Crohn's disease. Gut 31: 1133–1137

Thomas B (ed.) 1994 Manual of dietetic practice, 2nd Edn. Blackwell Scientific, Oxford

Twist S R, Hackett A F 1992 An investigation of some implications of coeliac disease. Journal of Human Nutrition and Dietetics 5: 343–350

FURTHER READING

Akehurst R, Kaltenthaler E 2001 Treatment of irritable bowel syndrome: a review of randomised controlled trials. Gut 48: 272–282

Bingham S, Cummings J H, McNeil N I 1982 Diet and health of people with an ileostomy. British Journal of Nutrition 47: 399–406

British Nutrition Foundation 1990 Clinical implications of complex carbohydrates for irritable bowel syndrome and constipation. In: complex carbohydrates in foods. The report of the British Nutrition Foundation's task force. Chapman & Hall, London: 94–98

Delaney B, Wilson S, Moayyedi P, Oakes R et al 2000. The management of dyspepsia: a systematic review. Health Technology Assessment 4: 39

Guthrie E and Creed F 1994 The difficult patient treating the mind and the gut. European Journal of Gastroenterology and Hepatology 6: 489–494

Royle J A, Walsh M (eds) 1992 The person with disorders of motility, secretion and absorption in the intestines. In: Watson's medical–surgical nursing and related physiology, 4th Edn. Baillière Tindall, London: 478–502

Solomon M J, Schritzler M 1998 Cancer and inflammatory bowel disease: bias, epidemiology, surveillance and treatment. World Journal of Surgery 22: 352–358

Woolner J T, Kirby G A 2000 Clinical audit of the effects of low-fibre diet on irritable bowel syndrome. Journal of Human Nutrition and Dietetics 13(4): 249–254

USEFUL ADDRESSES

British Colostomy Association
15 Station Road
Reading
Berks RG1 1LG
Tel: 0118 939 1537
Website: www.bcass.org.uk

Digestive Disorders Foundation
3 St Andrew's Place
Regents Park
London NW1 4LB
Tel: 020 7486 0341
website: www.digestivedisorders.org.uk

Coeliac Society of the UK
P O Box 220
High Wycombe
HP11 2HY
Tel: 01494 437278 (Hotline: 01494 473510)
website: www.coeliac.co.uk

Illeostomy and Internal Pouch Support Group
PO Box 132
DN15 9YW
Tel: 0800 0184724
website: www.lleostomyPouch.Demon.co.uk

National Association of Colitis and Crohn's Disease
4 Beaumont House
Sutton Road
St Albans
Herts. AL1 5HH
Tel: 01727 844296

Oesophageal Patient Association
16 Whitfields Cresent
Solihull
West Midlands B91 3NU
Tel: 0121 704 9860

25

Diet in disorders of the liver and biliary system

LEARNING OBJECTIVES

After studying this chapter you should be able to:

- outline the roles of the liver in protein and carbohydrate metabolism
- explain the scientific basis for the dietary treatment of diseases of the liver and biliary system
- explain how the required changes in dietary intake can be achieved.

FUNCTIONS OF THE LIVER

The liver is the largest internal organ of the body. The hepatic portal vein carries blood from the spleen, stomach and intestine to the liver. This blood contains the products of digestion and absorption. The liver is still able to function adequately when over 75% of its cells have been damaged or destroyed. Liver cells have a remarkable ability to regenerate and recover from injury. The liver is a vital organ, with many complex functions. These include:

Protein metabolism

Products of protein digestion are carried to the liver where some amino acids are used for protein synthesis to form blood proteins, enzymes and structural proteins. Other amino acids are deaminated. In this process urea is produced, which is excreted via the kidneys, and the remainder of the amino acid is used for glucogenesis with the eventual production of energy.

Fat metabolism

Cholesterol, phospholipids, lecithin and lipoproteins are all produced by the liver.

Carbohydrate metabolism

Glucose is converted to glycogen and stored in the liver. This is then mobilised to provide an energy source in response to hypoglycaemia. Any glucose in excess of that amount which can be stored by the liver as glycogen is converted to fat by the liver and stored in adipose tissues throughout the body.

Detoxification of harmful substances

The liver destroys hormones produced by the body, so preventing circulating levels from becoming too high. It also detoxifies some drugs such as barbiturates.

Production of bile

The normal liver secretes 500 to 1000 ml of bile per day, of which 90 to 97% is water. However, this water content is reduced when the bile is concentrated by and stored in the gall-bladder, which has an average capacity of 40 to 50 ml.

Bile is a strongly alkaline fluid containing bicarbonate ions and chloride ions: it also contains bile pigments, salts of the bile acids, cholic and chenodeoxycholic acids, sodium and calcium salts, cholesterol, phospholipids and lecithin.

Bile pigments

There are two bile pigments, bilirubin (red) and biliverdin (green). They are produced by the breakdown by the liver of red blood cells and some of the products of digestion. Bilirubin occurs in greater concentration in humans, whereas biliverdin predominates in species with a mainly vegetable diet (Royle & Walsh 1992). Once bile has been secreted into the intestine, intestinal bacteria act on the bile pigments to produce urobilinogen, which is excreted in the faeces giving them their usual brown coloration. Some urobilinogen is reabsorbed and is reconverted into bile pigments by the liver.

Bile salts

Bile salts have a role in the emulsification of fats prior to their digestion and in the absorption of fats, fat-soluble vitamins and calcium. They are sodium and potassium salts of certain amino acids and are reabsorbed from the intestine and carried to the liver in the portal circulation, where they stimulate the liver to secrete bile and are again secreted into the bile.

Storage

The liver has an important role in maintaining an individual's nutritional status. The liver stores the fat-soluble vitamins A, D and K and is the site where vitamin D is hydroxylated to the active form. It also stores vitamin B_{12} and iron, which are essential for healthy red blood cell production. Energy is stored as glycogen which can be rapidly mobilised as an energy source. Small amounts of protein and fat are also stored.

CAUSES OF LIVER DAMAGE

Liver damage is caused by:

- The action of *infective agents*, such as the virus of acute infective hepatitis.
- *Toxic substances*, such as carbon tetrachloride, chloroform, some drugs and some plant alkaloids (nitrogen-containing substances which may be contained in some plants and some herbal remedies). As the blood from the gastrointestinal tract reaches the liver before any other organ, the liver receives any absorbed toxins in high concentrations. The liver protects other organs by detoxifying these substances, but is often damaged in the process.
- *Malnutrition*. A diet which contains sufficient energy but an inadequate amount of protein can lead to the deposition of fat droplets in the liver cells. This condition is known as fatty liver and may be found in kwashiorkor, inadequate parenteral nutrition and alcoholism. The condition is reversible if the dietary imbalance is detected early and corrected, but may progress to further permanent liver damage.

JAUNDICE

The yellow pigmentation of the skin and mucous membranes is a common feature of liver and biliary disease. It is caused by an increased concentration of the bile pigment bilirubin in the blood. An excessive amount accumulates in the blood if:

- too much bile is produced by the liver (haemolytic jaundice)—this is associated with some forms of anaemia, e.g. sickle cell anaemia
- the liver is unable to dispose of the bilirubin because the function of the liver cells has been impaired, e.g. in infective hepatitis
- the bile ducts are obstructed so that the bilirubin does not enter the intestine, e.g. in biliary cirrhosis and carcinoma of the head of the pancreas.

Dietary treatment of jaundice

Jaundice is a symptom of a disease, not a specific disease, so there is no specific dietary treatment for it. The dietary treatment used depends on the cause of the jaundice.

DIETARY TREATMENT OF LIVER DISEASE

The dietary treatment of a patient with liver disease depends on:

- nutritional status when the condition is diagnosed
- existing level of liver function
- symptoms of the individual.

Malnutrition, ascites, encephalopathy, steatorrhoea, oesophageal varices and anorexia are all symptoms of liver disease and all require dietary modification.

The severity of liver injury varies greatly. In some instances it is so mild that no symptoms are apparent or there are only minor symptoms which are followed by complete recovery. On the other hand, the patient may be seriously ill with the condition progressing to acute or chronic liver failure. The most usual causes of acute liver failure are toxins such as drugs, e.g. paracetamol or alcohol, and viral infections, particularly viral hepatitis. In all types of liver disease it is essential to monitor nutritional status and adjust the diet accordingly.

Hepatic cirrhosis

Hepatic cirrhosis is a chronic condition which can result from various forms of liver damage, including damage caused by a high alcohol intake or infective hepatitis. It is thought that an inadequate food intake may contribute to the development of the cirrhosis, which frequently occurs in association with alcoholism. In many cases, the cause of the disease remains unknown. The liver glycogen stores are reduced in hepatic cirrhosis, so it is necessary to provide frequent small meals and a late-night snack of food containing complex carbohydrate (Verboeket-van de Venne 1995). These frequent meals will help to prevent the metabolism of body fat and protein stores and also prevent hypoglycaemia. Both the protein and energy requirements are increased in cirrhosis. The diet should provide 75 kJ/kg and 1 g protein/kg (Plauth et al 1997).

General diet

For those individuals whose liver damage is not so severe as to cause ascites or encephalopathy, a balanced diet, adequate in all nutrients, should be given. It is important to prevent malnutrition from developing in these patients, who often have a poor appetite. Care should be taken to monitor dietary intake and nutritional status regularly. An adequate intake can be encouraged by ensuring that in the choice of food for these patients:

- portions are small, well presented and appetising
- between-meal snacks such as milk drinks and biscuits are available to maintain nutrient intake
- likes and dislikes are considered
- nutritional supplements are provided for those patients who require them.

If dietary intake is poor, dietary supplements should be used (see Chapter 23). Sip-feed products may be suitable, providing both protein and energy, or it may be more appropriate to use a supplement which only provides carbohydrate e.g. Polycal (Nutricia Clinical Care), Maxijul (Scientific Hospital Supplies) and Caloreen (Nestle Clinical Nutrition), depending on individual patients and their actual dietary intake. The use of glucose polymers and sip-feeds will help to maintain adequate nutritional intake. A protein intake of 1 g/kg body-weight is sufficient and this is easily provided by a normal diet. An excessive intake of protein-rich foods should be discouraged as in certain instances higher protein intakes can precipitate encephalopathy.

Vitamin supplementation in liver disease

It should be assumed that all individuals with liver disease will be deficient in most vitamins. The factors which lead to these deficiencies are:

- inadequate dietary intake
- abnormal metabolism of damaged liver leading to increased vitamin requirements
- increased vitamin losses.

Specific vitamin deficiencies which have been observed include:

- vitamin A deficiency occurring in chronic alcoholic liver disease and cholestasis
- vitamin D deficiency developing when cholestasis jaundice reduces skin photolysis
- vitamin K deficiency occurring when chronic or acute liver disease reduces absorption of vitamin K
- vitamin B_1 and B_2 and vitamin C deficiencies are common in patients with alcoholic liver disease and are caused by poor dietary intake
- folate is deficient in most individuals with liver disease.

Iron deficiency is common in alcoholic liver disease and is caused by both poor dietary intake and increased iron losses from gastrointestinal bleeding. It can also develop in patients with oesophageal varices because of the blood-loss.

DIETARY TREATMENT OF SPECIFIC FEATURES OF LIVER DISEASE

Ascites

Ascites is the retention of a protein-rich fluid in the abdominal cavity. Its cause is unclear but contributory factors are:

- inability of the damaged liver to synthesise an adequate amount of albumin; this leads to a lowering of the plasma osmotic pressure
- portal hypertension arising from restriction of the outflow of blood via the portal vein due to liver damage, causing fluid to enter the peritoneal cavity.

The accumulation of fluid results in the retention of sodium and water by the kidneys. This is to compensate for the reduction in effective body fluids, and oedema usually develops. The aim of dietary treatment is to reduce sodium and water reabsorption by the renal tubules and so reduce fluid retention and prevent electrolyte imbalances from developing.

The presence of ascites makes the estimation of nutritional status by body-weight and body mass index (BMI) very inaccurate. It has been proposed that severe ascites can add an extra 14 kg to an individual's weight (James 1989).

Sodium restriction

If the dietary sodium intake is restricted, there will be less available to be retained by the kidneys. It is important to ensure that if the sodium content of the diet is restricted, this is not accompanied by a reduction in protein content—unless this has been specifically prescribed, for example when encephalopathy is also present. A reduction in protein intake can occur because the high-protein foods—meat, fish, milk and eggs—also have a relatively high sodium content. The level of sodium restriction prescribed depends on:

- local policy
- the resistance of the ascites to treatment
- the patient's appetite
- the patient's social circumstances
- the level of cooperation of the patient
- whether or not the patient is an inpatient or outpatient.

Too severe a restriction can result in an inadequate intake of energy and protein. A diet that is very low in sodium (22 mmol a day, see Box 25.1), is unpalatable and very restrictive and can result in a low energy intake, particularly if the patient is anorexic. Although this lower sodium intake may resolve the ascites more quickly, it may be preferable to restrict the sodium intake to a slightly more generous 40 mmol to ensure that the patient maintains optimal nutritional status. This more generous diet is similar to the diet containing 22 mmol, except it also includes three slices of ordinary bread. Salt-free bread is found unpalatable by many.

The no-added-salt diet (see Box 25.2) may be suitable when the ascites is less severe.

Fluid restriction is sometimes imposed and can be as low as 500 ml a day, particularly if the patient is hyponatraemic.

Anorexia is a symptom of ascites, as the physical effect of fluid in the peritoneal cavity results in early satiety and also causes abdominal discomfort. Small frequent meals are necessary. This can result in a poor

---

Box 25.1 Sample menu for a low-sodium, high-protein diet

Sodium: 500 mg (22 mmol)

Breakfast
Fruit or fruit juice
Low-sodium cereal such as unsalted porridge, Puffed Wheat or Sugar Puffs (Quaker Oats Ltd) or Shredded Wheat (Nabisco Foods)
Unsalted bread, with unsalted butter or margarine
Marmalade or honey
Tea or coffee with milk from allowance

Mid-morning
Low-sodium, high-protein milk drink

Midday meal
Fruit juice
Average helping unsalted meat or fish
Unsalted vegetable as desired
Low-sodium sweet such as fruit or jelly with cream, or pastry or sponge pudding prepared from low-sodium ingredients
Tea or coffee with milk from allowance

Tea
Unsalted bread, toasted or made into sandwiches
Tea with milk from allowance

Evening meal
Average helping unsalted meat, fish or egg dish
Unsalted vegetables
Unsalted bread, with unsalted butter or margarine
Sweet as at midday
Tea or coffee with milk from allowance

Bedtime
Remainder of milk allowance: 250 ml daily

oral intake. The energy intake can be increased by use of dietary supplements if enteral feeding is necessary. It may be necessary to use an enteral feed specifically designed for the treatment of liver disease such as Generaid (Scientific Hospital Supplies) or Heptamine (Scientific Hospital Supplies).

It may be necessary to use a low-sodium milk, salt-free bread and unsalted butter, in order to achieve a low sodium intake while maintaining an adequate protein and energy intake.

If a less strict sodium restriction is required then a no-added-salt diet (see Box 25.2) is suitable.

Choice of foods

Chapter 26 should be consulted regarding choice of foods, and also suggested seasonings, for sodium-restricted diets. Box 25.1 gives a sample menu for a low-sodium, high-protein diet, and there are guidelines for a no-added-salt diet in Box 25.2.

Oesophageal varices

These are sub-mucosal veins in the lower oesophagus and fundus of the stomach which, because of the increased venous pressure, become grossly enlarged.
  Rupture of varices is due to:

- ulceration of the mucosa caused by gastric acid secretion
- increased intra-abdominal pressure—this can be caused by vomiting and coughing.

Bleeding varices cause anaemia, contribute to hypoalbuminaemia and can precipitate encephalopathy.

Soft diets, although beneficial immediately after sclerotherapy for treatment of varices, do not prevent rupture of the varices.

Oesophageal varices are in some circumstances a contraindication for nasogastric feeding and gastrostomy feeding may be considered.

Hepatic encephalopathy

Some patients suffering from liver disease develop signs of impaired function of the nervous system which are so severe that they result in coma. This is known as hepatic encephalopathy.

The physical symptoms of encephalopathy are caused by the production of false neurotransmitters from protein in the gut. In liver diseases encephalopathy is precipitated by:

- constipation—lactulose is used to reduce transit time and so reduce constipation
- fluid and electrolyte imbalances
- diarrhoea and vomiting
- excess alcohol
- high protein intake, tolerance to different types of dietary protein varies. Encephalopathic patients are more tolerant of dairy protein and vegetable protein than meat protein.

The ESPEN consensus group (Plauth et al 1997) recommends that restricting the protein intake of patients with established encephalopathy should be avoided wherever possible. If it is necessary to restrict the protein intake, additional dietary nitrogen should be provided as an amino acid supplement. It is important during this period that the diet should still provide enough energy, because if the energy supply is inadequate, breakdown of tissue protein to provide an energy source will occur.

Use of branched-chain amino acids in treatment of encephalopathy

During encephalopathy the ratio of the branched-chain amino acids (BCAAs)—valine, leucine and isoleucine—to aromatic amino acids changes. This results in a relative deficiency of BCAAs. There are specialised products available which have a high BCAA content. These are used in specialist units in situations where patients who are encephalopathic have a high nitrogen requirement, for example following trauma or surgery. Their use is currently being reviewed.

ALCOHOLIC LIVER DISEASE

Alcohol now provides a significant proportion of the total energy intake of many people. Their actual intake is always difficult to establish (Watson et al 1984). It is absorbed quickly from the stomach and transported by the hepatic portal vein to the liver, where it is metabolised. Alcohol damages the liver tissue of both normal and alcoholic individuals and can cause liver disease. It is excluded from the diets of all patients with liver disease.

It should be assumed that patients admitted to hospital with alcoholic liver disease (ALD) are malnourished, but it is usually difficult to perform an accurate nutritional assessment. This is because oedema and ascites increase body-weight and mid-arm muscle circumference measurements, and an accurate dietary history including the amount of alcohol is difficult to obtain.

There are two types of liver damage occurring in alcoholic liver disease:

- alcoholic hepatitis—acute and potentially reversible
- alcoholic cirrhosis—chronic and progressive.

Alcohol has a range of metabolic effects on the liver:

- it acts as a toxin
- it impairs glucose synthesis
- it accentuates glycogen breakdown leading to rapid depletion of muscle glycogen
- it increases sensitivity to some drugs.

Alcohol contributes to the development of malnutrition by:

- providing empty calories, i.e. energy without vitamins, minerals or protein
- suppressing appetite
- causing pancreatic damage leading to pancreatic insufficiency and consequent malabsorption of that food which is eaten
- causing gastritis which leads to anorexia and nausea.

Following a nutritional assessment of the patient, dietary treatment should aim to restore and maintain nutritional status and treat the symptoms which will respond to dietary modification (see Nutritional Care Plan 25.1). As ascites and encephalopathy resolve, the anorexia and nausea will also improve.

The nutrients commonly found to be deficient are iron, zinc, folate, nicotinic acid, pyridoxine, thiamin and vitamin C. These deficiencies develop because of a reduced dietary intake of nutrients. Alcoholic drinks are an energy source but contain negligible amounts of vitamins and minerals. An increased requirement for vitamins of the B group is caused by the high carbohydrate content of the diet. Ethanol is poisonous and causes gastrointestinal bleeding, the blood-loss leading to iron deficiency. Pancreatic damage caused by alcohol reduces the amounts of pancreatic enzymes produced, which gives rise to maldigestion and malabsorption of fats.

Dietary treatment should correct malnutrition by providing an adequate supply of all nutrients, treating

Nutritional Care Plan 25.1	For patient with liver disease		
Patient problem	Goal	Nutritional intervention	Outcome
Anorexia and poor appetite due to abdominal distension caused by presence of ascites	Achieve negative fluid balance until ascites no longer present	Weigh daily Record fluid intake and output Nutritional assessment Increase energy intake by using high-energy supplements Restrict sodium intake Restrict fluid intake	Weight returns to pre-ascites level Ascites no longer present Patient's energy is assessed as meeting his energy requirements Negative fluid balance achieved
Patient malnourished due to poor diet prior to hospital admission	Patient no longer malnourished BMI within range 20–25	Record dietary history Vitamin and mineral supplements to correct malnutrition Prevent further malnutrition by nutrition education	Nutritional assessment shows patient well nourished Patient understands roles of different nutrients in the diet and is able to obtain a nutritionally adequate diet

clinical symptoms and protecting the liver from further damage. A well balanced normal diet may be sufficient for some patients, whereas other patients will require sodium restriction to treat their ascites. The provision of these diets has already been discussed in this chapter.

DISORDERS OF THE BILIARY SYSTEM

Bile is secreted by the liver cells into a system of canaliculi and ductules, which join to form the common bile duct. This duct drains into the gall-bladder, where the bile is concentrated and stored. Bile has an important role in the digestion of fat. The bile salts and lecithin emulsify the fat in the duodenum so that it can be hydrolysed by pancreatic lipase. The release of bile into the duodenum via the common bile duct occurs in response to the presence of food in the stomach and duodenum. This is under both nervous and hormonal control.

Cholecystitis

Cholecystitis, or inflammation of the gall bladder, is usually associated with gallstones. The most commonly occurring type of gallstone to be found in industrialised nations is rich in cholesterol. It is composed of cholesterol, bile pigment and calcium salts. These stones can only be formed when the bile stored in the gall bladder is supersaturated with cholesterol. Gallstones are frequently accompanied by obesity—being found in 20% of autopsies (Garrow & James 1993)—and are more common among women than men. Many studies have shown an increased level of cholesterol saturation of bile in obese people, and that a decrease in this level accompanies weight loss. The increased incidence of gallstones in industrialised societies is thought to be linked to the low-fibre, high-fat diet, but this has not been proved.

There is no evidence to show that increasing fibre intake prevents the recurrence of gallstones (Bouchier 1990).

Acute cholecystitis

Acute cholecystitis is usually due to infection or is associated with obstruction of the cystic duct or neck of the gall bladder.

During an acute attack, which is not sufficiently severe to require surgical intervention, the dietary treatment is similar to that employed in the treatment of other acute febrile conditions. The patient should drink plenty of fluid and optimum nutrition should be maintained. If appetite is poor, dietary supplements should be used (see Chapter 23).

As the presence of fat in the duodenum stimulates gall bladder contraction, a low-fat diet may be helpful so that the contraction is reduced to a minimum during the period of acute inflammation. However, this is not invariably the case. While many patients find that they are intolerant of fatty foods, others find that such foods do not influence the pain.

Chronic cholecystitis

In the case of patients for whom surgery is not advised, a suitable long-term regime is required.

Entry of fat into the duodenum is necessary for contraction of the gall bladder and excretion of bile. In the case of patients with chronic cholecystitis, therefore, a normal fat intake helps to counteract atony of the gall bladder, promotes the drainage of the biliary system and helps to prevent the formation of further gallstones, so a diet that is very low in fat is not indicated.

Persons with chronic gall bladder disease frequently suffer from flatulence and epigastric discomfort following meals, and it should be noted that the fats in milk and eggs are usually tolerated in moderate quantities, and that lard, dripping and fried foods are best avoided. Other foods best avoided are onions and cucumbers, as these frequently cause dyspepsia.

A diet suitable for weight reduction, such as that outlined in Chapter 21, is suitable if there is associated obesity. However, rapid weight loss should be discouraged as it is linked with increased incidence of gall stones (Liddle et al 1989).

Obstructive jaundice

Obstruction to the flow of bile along the biliary tract may give rise to jaundice, in this case termed obstructive jaundice. Two causes of obstructive jaundice are the presence of gallstones in the common bile duct and carcinoma of the head of the pancreas. Where possible, surgical measures are employed for the relief of the obstruction, but where surgery is not practicable, an important aspect of treatment is the provision of a suitable diet.

Since bile is a factor of importance in the digestion of fat, obstructive jaundice is associated with failure of fat digestion and absorption and the excretion of an excessive amount of fat in the faeces (steatorrhoea). Diarrhoea may also be present. A low-fat diet is required (see Box 25.3), which may need to include nutritional supplements to ensure an adequate energy intake. Fat intake may be subsequently increased in accordance with the ability of the patient to tolerate fat. It is usually necessary to give the fat-soluble vitamins by intramuscular injection. The patient's weight should be closely monitored because restricting fat intake can result in a reduced energy intake.

Box 25.3 Low-fat diet

Fat: 20 g (approximately)

Guidelines

Foods to avoid

- Whole milk, ice-cream, butter, eggs, cheese, except cottage cheese
- Margarine, lard, and all fats and oils
- Visible fat on meat and fatty meats such as bacon, tongue and sausages
- Most canned meats, e.g. luncheon meat, chopped ham and pork and corned beef
- Fatty fish such as herring and salmon
- Soups, unless known to be low in fat content
- Pastry, cakes and most biscuits
- Chocolate, toffee, fudge, nuts, marzipan and lemon curd

Increase of the fat content
The fat intake may be increased to 40 g daily by the inclusion of 500 ml semi-skimmed milk and 30 g low-fat spread.

Sample menu
Breakfast
Fruit or fruit juice with added sugar, glucose or glucose polymer
Cereal
Bread, toast or a roll, with marmalade or honey, but without butter
Tea or coffee with skimmed milk and sugar

Mid-morning
Drink made with skimmed milk

Midday
Fruit, fruit juice or tomato juice
Average helping of lean meat or fish, e.g. stewed beef, liver, kidney, poultry, ham or white fish
Potato and other vegetables
Low-fat sweet such as jelly and fruit, or a pudding made with skimmed milk
Tea or coffee with skimmed milk and sugar

Mid-afternoon
Low-fat sandwiches, e.g. banana, preserves *or*
Water biscuits or Ryvita Crispbread with honey or preserves

Evening meal
Lean meat or fish as at midday *or*
A low-fat savoury dish such as baked beans or spaghetti in tomato sauce *or*
Salad vegetables with cottage cheese and pineapple
Toast or a roll without butter
Tea or coffee with skimmed milk and sugar

Bedtime
Skimmed milk drink as at mid-morning

Diets low in fat are correspondingly low in energy value. Provided the patient is not overweight, glucose, sugar and glucose polymers should be added to fruit and fruit drinks.
Boiled sweets are unrestricted

REFERENCES

Bouchier I A D 1990 Gallstones. British Medical Journal 300: 592–597

Garrow J, James P 1993 Davidson's human nutrition and dietetics, 9th Edn. Churchill Livingstone, Edinburgh

James R 1989 Nutritional support in alcoholic liver disease. Journal of Human Nutrition and Dietetics 2: 315–323

Liddle R A, Goldstein R B, Saxton J 1989 Gall stone formation during weight reduction dieting. Archives of Internal Medicine 149: 1750–1753

Plaugh M, Merli M, Kondrup J, Weimann A, Ferenci P, Muller M J 1997 ESPEN guidelines for nutrition in liver disease and transplantation. Clinical Nutrition 16: 43–55

Royle J A, Walsh M (eds) 1992 Caring for the patient with disorders of the liver, biliary tract and exocrine pancreas. In: Watson's medical–surgical nursing and related physiology, 4th Edn. Baillière Tindall, London: 515–544

Verboeket-van de Venne W P H G, Westerherp K R, Van Hoek B, Swart G R 1995 Energy expenditure and substrate metabolism in patients with cirrhosis of the liver: effect of the pattern of food intake. Gut 36: 110–116

Watson C G, Tilleslejor B, Hoodecheck-Schaw B, Pikel J, Jacobs L 1984 Do alcoholics give valid self reports? Journal of Studies in Alcohol 45: 344–348

FURTHER READING

Bateson M 1999 Gall bladder disease. British Medical Journal 318: 1745–1748

Gauthier A, Levy V G, Quinton A et al 1986 Salt or no salt in the treatment of cirrhotic ascites?—a randomised study. Gut 27: 705–709

Kalman D R, Saltzman J R 1996 Nutrition status predicts survival in cirrhosis. Nutrition Reviews 54: 217–219

Runyon B 1994 Care of patients with ascites. New England Journal of Medicine 330: 337

Sherlock S 1989 Diseases of the liver and biliary system, 8th Edn. Blackwell Scientific Publications, Oxford

Thomas B (ed) 2001 Manual of dietetic practice, 3rd edn. Blackwell Science, Oxford

26

Diet in disorders of the kidneys

LEARNING OBJECTIVES

After studying this chapter you should be able to:

- outline the roles of the kidney in maintaining homeostasis
- explain the scientific basis for the dietary treatments used in the treatment of kidney disease
- describe the range of dietary modifications that are used for the treatment of kidney disease and the conditions that they are used to treat.

By excreting a urine of variable composition and volume, the kidneys play a major part in maintaining the constant volume and composition of the body fluids. Metabolic waste products are excreted in the urine, while materials necessary for body function are retained. Renal disease is associated with metabolic disturbances due to impairment of the kidney's regulatory activities. In the management of renal failure, dietary modifications are required either as the only treatment or, more commonly, to play a supporting role in conjunction with some form of renal replacement therapy such as haemodialysis, intermittent peritoneal dialysis, continuous ambulatory peritoneal dialysis or renal transplantation.

In all of these situations the dietary advice should aim to fulfil four objectives (see Box 26.1).

Box 26.1   Aims of dietary treatment for renal disease

1. Maintain optimal nutritional status.
2. Reduce production of waste products.
3. Promote a satisfactory quality of life. This is particularly difficult if the diet is very restrictive.
4. Slow the rate of renal deterioration.

CHRONIC RENAL FAILURE

Chronic renal failure (CRF) is a progressive and irreversible condition in which the nephrons of both kidneys are damaged. It has a variety of causes, of which the most frequently occurring are:

- glomerulonephritis
- renal vascular disease
- diabetic nephropathy
- polycystic kidney disease.

This condition is progressive and passes through three stages:

Stage 1: Diminished renal reserve. This stage is asymptomatic and can last for many years, depending on the cause of the condition, and may be first noticed when albuminuria is detected in a routine medical examination.

Stage 2: Renal insufficiency. The glomerular filtration rate is reduced to about 25% of normal at this stage and levels of blood urea and serum creatinine become raised.

Stage 3: End-stage renal failure. This develops when the kidneys are no longer able to compensate for the effects of the damaged nephrons and the glomerular filtration rate is reduced to less than 10% of normal. This results in an accumulation of metabolic waste products, causing the blood urea and serum creatinine levels to rise.

Dietary modification is essential for the conservative management of CRF and it will require frequent reviewing as the patient's condition progresses. The dietary prescription is adjusted so that water and electrolyte balance are maintained and the amount of nitrogenous waste retained is reduced to a minimum.

As this diet will be kept to long-term, it is important that the patient and carers understand it fully and that their needs, preferences and meal-pattern routines are included in its formulation. For some patients it will be the only form of treatment they receive. It must be remembered that a raised blood urea affects the ability to concentrate and an individual's cognitive abilities, so teaching sessions should be short with facts clearly presented. Patients should be provided with written information that can be reviewed by them and discussed again.

Key points for dietary treatment of chronic renal failure

Regular nutritional assessment to prevent or detect and treat protein–energy malnutrition is essential, as protein–energy malnutrition is associated with increased morbidity and mortality from chronic renal failure and the success of renal replacement therapy is affected by the nutritional status of the patient (Walker 1997). Both Bergstrom (1995) and Ikrizler & Hakim (1996) have correlated the poor outcome of renal replacement therapy with reduced muscle mass, low serum albumin concentration and low transferrin concentration at the start of renal replacement therapy.

Energy

An adequate energy intake is essential to ensure that the limited amount of protein provided by the diet and the individual's existing body protein (muscle) are not catabolised to produce energy. If this happens, there is an increased amount of nitrogenous waste produced, which the kidneys have to excrete.

Weight loss is a symptom of this condition and should be prevented by ensuring that the energy content of the diet is assessed for the individual and is sufficient to maintain the individual's ideal body-weight. The diet should provide 35 kcal/kg body-weight (146 kJ/kg body-weight). This is approximately 10 460 kJ (2500 kcal) for a 70-kg man and most of this energy will be provided by carbohydrate and fat, as it may be necessary to restrict protein intake.

Special low-protein products, such as low-protein biscuits, flour, pasta and bread are used to increase the energy content and variety of a low-protein diet. These products are important, because a restriction in the amount of protein in the diet means that the protein content of cereals and cereal products needs to be considered. They will be restricted so that the protein included in the diet is provided from high biological value sources which include milk and eggs. Patients need to be encouraged to try these special low-protein products and to include them in their diet, otherwise it is very difficult to ensure an adequate energy intake. They also increase the variety of foods available, so making the diet less monotonous. These products can be incorporated in puddings, sauces and biscuits; recipes and instructions as to how best to use them will be supplied by the dietitian. Hadfield (1992) has shown that the optimum energy intake of patients with CRF can only be achieved on a protein-restricted diet if these foods and glucose polymers are included in the diet. It is likely that there will still be an energy deficit which should be met with energy supplements such as glucose polymers.

Use of glucose polymers

Anorexia and nausea are frequently associated with raised blood urea and many patients need a lot of encouragement to maintain an adequate energy intake. They need to get into the routine of adding extra energy to the food they eat, for example glucose polymers to drinks, sugar to breakfast cereals and fruit jam onto bread.

Products that are available include:

- Caloreen (Nestle Clinical Nutrition)
- Maxijul (Scientific Hospital Supplies)
- Polycal (Nutricia Clinical Care)
- Polycose (Abbot Nutrition)
- Vitajoule (Vitaflow).

Protein

The kidneys have an important role in protein metabolism and the excretion of nitrogenous waste. A reduction in protein intake is necessary when their ability to excrete the nitrogenous material has been reduced.

The aim of the protein restriction is to reduce the symptoms of uraemia, which include nausea, vomiting, anorexia, pruritus and fatigue. It has also been proposed by workers that reducing the protein intake also slows down the rate of renal deterioration. A study by Oldrizzo et al (1989) showed that a protein intake of 0.6 g/kg body-weight has no detrimental nutritional effect and reduces the rate of progression of kidney function deterioration.

For patients with CRF, 0.6 g protein/kg body-weight is occasionally recommended, which is in practice 40 g protein for a 70-kg man (see Box 26.2). If protein intake is restricted, at least 70% of the daily protein allowance should be as protein with a high biological value (see Chapter 4), such as egg, meat or milk. However, this diet is difficult to keep to, unpalatable and may result in a low energy intake, leading to malnutrition. It is usual for a system of protein exchanges to be used to plan the type of diet. These protein exchanges are listed in Table 26.1.

The high biological value (HBV) protein is allocated in portions distributed throughout the day and the allowance should not be saved up and eaten all at one meal. Some hospitals allow four portions containing 6 g HBV protein a day, while others allow three portions containing 7 g protein a day. The remaining protein allowance is spread throughout the day as 2 g protein exchanges of foods which have a lower protein content, such as potatoes and cereal products. It must be remembered that bread, biscuits, breakfast cereals, certain fruit and vegetables all contain some protein which needs to be restricted if the total protein intake is to be controlled.

Sodium

The sodium content of the diet can be either increased or decreased. This depends on the site and severity of the kidney damage and how it affects the ability of the kidneys to excrete sodium, and the symptoms produced. An increase in the sodium content of blood causes a rise in blood pressure and fluid retention. The aim of the sodium restriction is to keep the patient normotensive and prevent oedema. There are three levels of sodium-restricted diet, progressing from the least restrictive no-added-salt diet to the most restrictive salt-free diet. The amount of sodium these diets contain and the foods which are restricted are compared in Table 26.2.

The most frequently used form of sodium restriction in chronic renal failure is the no-added-salt diet. Most people find this easy to adhere to if they have had the reason for the restriction clearly explained to them.

Salt substitutes. It is generally inappropriate to use a salt substitute for patients with CRF because of their high potassium content. However, the dietitian's advice should be sought if patients find their diet unpalatable. Alternative flavouring such as herbs, spices, vinegar and olive oil may make the food more palatable. Some patients require supplementary sodium. This is provided either as sodium chloride or sodium bicarbonate supplements. A negative sodium balance will lead to dehydration, and so must be prevented.

Potassium

Some patients retain potassium and, for these, a potassium restriction is necessary to prevent hyperkalaemia, the severity of the dietary restriction depending on the level of potassium retention. Foods with a very high potassium content are excluded from the diet. These include coffee, dried fruit and fruit juices.

Like the daily protein allowance, the daily potassium allowance should be spread throughout the day and is usually allocated as portions of fruit or vegetable which contain 4 mmol potassium, so are known as 4 mmol potassium exchanges (see Table 26.3) (Bower 1989).

Box 26.2 Restricted-protein diet

Approximately 40 g protein.
This diet only contains approximately 1600 kcal.

Guidelines
Extra energy will need to be included in the form of glucose polymers.

Daily allowances
200 ml (1/3 pt) milk
Three of 7-g protein exchanges, six of 2 g protein exchanges

The following are unrestricted:

- Sugar, preserves and confectionery
- Tea and coffee (some instant coffees have a high potassium content)
- Vegetables, fruit and fruit juices, providing the diet is not restricted in potassium
- Butter or salt-free margarine may be necessary
- Polyunsaturated and monounsaturated cooking oils
- Boiled sweets and fruit pastilles
- Fruit squashes and cordials.

To help ensure adequate energy intake:

- Use full-cream milk, not skimmed or semi-skimmed
- Add sugar to foods, for example to drinks and stewed fruit
- Take butter and preserves with bread
- Use frying as a method of cooking, where practicable
- Include energy supplements as recommended by dietitian.

The following foods are not allowed:

- Extra milk, meat, egg, fish or cheese
- Pulses unless exchanged for meat, fish or eggs
- Yoghurt or ice-cream unless exchanged under the guidance of a dietitian
- Products made from milk
- Tinned and packet soups and sauces.

Protein-free products

- Low-protein flour, semolina, pasta, crispbread and biscuits are produced by Ultrapharm Ltd, PO Box 18 Henley-on-Thames, Oxon RG9 2AW, and SHS International Ltd, 100 Wavertree Boulevard, Wavertree Technology Park, Liverpool L7 9PT.
- Low-protein biscuits and pastry may be prepared at home using any of the special flours already mentioned, along with fat and sugar.

Sample menu
Breakfast
One egg, two large thin slices bread with margarine or butter and jam, honey or marmalade
Drink with milk from allowance

Mid-morning
Drink using milk from allowance
Three low-protein biscuits

Lunch
1 oz cooked lean meat (28 g)
4 oz boiled potatoes (122 g)
3 oz portion green vegetables (84 g)
Tinned fruit or fruit pie made with low-protein pastry served with double cream

Mid-afternoon
Tea with milk from allowance
Three low-protein biscuits or low-protein bread with butter or jam

Evening meal
1 1/2 oz cooked lean meat (42 g)
One slice white bread
1 oz sponge cake (28 g)
Tinned fruit

Bedtime
Drink using remaining milk allowance
Low-protein biscuits

Phosphorus

It may be necessary to impose an extra phosphorus restriction on patients with chronic renal failure if their protein intake is not restricted It is these protein-containing foods which have a high phosphorus content. A 40 g protein diet usually contains 600 to 700 mg of phosphorus. Phosphate binders containing calcium carbonate or calcium acetate may also be prescribed to bind the phosphate and regulate its absorption from the small intestine. These should be taken with protein/phosphorus-containing meals.

Fluid s

If the patient is oliguric, then fluid intake will need to be restricted to 400 to 700 ml a day, plus an amount equal to any urine passed the previous day. If there is vomiting, extra fluid should be allowed to compensate for this loss. The allocation of this fluid throughout the day depends on the individual's personal preferences.

Fat

Although fat is a valuable source of energy, an increased intake of fat, particularly saturated fat, should not be encouraged because of its effects on blood lipid levels. Many patients with chronic renal failure also have hyperlipidaemia. Restriction of animal protein will automatically reduce saturated fat and cholesterol intake, as animal fats present in milk, dairy products such as cheese, and meat are rich sources of saturated fat.

Table 26.1 Protein-exchange lists

Food	Portion containing 7 g protein	Portion containing 6 g protein
Milk	1/3 pt	180 ml
Cheddar cheese	1 oz	25 g
Cottage cheese	2 oz	45 g
Yoghurt	5 oz	120 g
Hen's egg	1 large	1 small
Lean cooked meat	1 oz	25 g
Cooked poultry	1 oz	25 g
Liver	1 oz	25 g
White fish	1 oz	40 g
Fish fingers	2	2
Peanuts, unsalted	$1\frac{1}{2}$ oz	25 g
Baked beans	5 oz	125 g
Haricot beans, raw	1 oz	25 g
Mung beans, raw	1 oz	25 g
Peas, fresh or frozen	4 oz	100 g
	Portions containing 2 g protein	
Bread, one large thin slice	1 oz	25 g
Cornflakes	1 oz	25 g
Rice crispies	1 oz	25 g
Shredded Wheat	1 ($\frac{1}{2}$ oz)	1 (15 g)
Wheat flour	$\frac{1}{2}$ oz	15 g
Pasta, raw	$\frac{1}{2}$ oz	15 g
Rice, raw	1 oz	25 g
Rice, boiled	$3\frac{1}{2}$ oz	100 g
Biscuits, semi-sweet	4 small	4 small
Cream crackers	3	3
Sponge cake	1 oz	25 g
Chapatti	1 small	1 small
Cream, double	2 oz	50 g
Green vegetables (average portion)	3 oz	75 g
Sweetcorn	2 oz	50 g
Potatoes	4 oz	125 g
Crisps	1 small pkt	25 g

Table 26.2 Sodium-restricted diets

Type of restriction	Sodium content	Dietary restriction
No-added-salt	80–100 mmol	Small amount of salt can be used in cooking No salt added at table No salty foods such as cheese, bacon, ready salted potato crisps and nuts, preserved meat and fish allowed
Low-salt	50–60 mmol	No salt in cooking No salt added at table No salty foods
Salt-free	22 mmol	No salt in cooking No salt added at table No salty foods Salt-free bread and butter must be used instead of ordinary bread and butter, which contain salt

The progress of a patient on a restricted diet for chronic renal failure should be monitored carefully. When a dietary protein restriction is introduced, the patient's urea:creatinine ratio should drop. A subsequent increase in this ratio can be a sign that the protein restriction is not being kept to, as can an elevation of the blood phosphorus level.

Falling levels of serum albumin, protein and transferrin can be due to an inadequate energy intake and/or inadequate protein intake. Some patients further restrict their protein intake in the mistaken belief that their health will benefit. This sort of complicated dietary regime will only be successful if the patient, relatives and carers all understand the restrictions it

Table 26.3 Food portions which contain 4 mmol potassium (approximately)

Food	Portion
Beetroot, boiled	40 g
Brussels sprouts, boiled	60 g
Cabbage, boiled	130 g
Carrots, old, boiled	180 g
Cauliflower, boiled	100 g
Celery, raw	60 g
Cucumber	110 g
French beans, boiled	150 g
Lettuce	80 g
Mushrooms, fried	30 g
Onion, fried	60 g
Onion, spring, raw	70 g
Potato, boiled	50 g
Tomato, raw	50 g
Apples, raw, weighed with skin and core	180 g
Apricots, canned, fruit and syrup, weighed	60 g
Banana, weighed with skin	80 g
Grapes	60 g
Orange, weighed without peel	80 g
Peaches, fresh, weighed with stones	70 g
Peaches, canned, fruit and syrup, weighed	100 g
Pears, weighed with skin and core	170 g
Plums, victoria dessert, weighed with stones	90 g
Raspberries	70 g
Strawberries	100 g

Vegetables should be cooked in as large a pan of water as possible and this cooking water should be discarded, not used for gravy or soup as it will contain the potassium that has been leached out of the vegetables.

imposes and the reasons why these restrictions are necessary.

It is difficult to use weight as an assessment tool for the adequacy of energy intake because the development of oedema masks weight loss.

The dietary modifications that are used in the treatment of chronic renal failure are summarised in Box 26.3.

When conservative treatment for CRF is no longer able to control the fluid and electrolyte balances and concentrations of waste products in the blood, some form of renal replacement therapy is necessary. The

---

Box 26.3 Summary of dietary modifications used in CRF

- Encourage adequate energy intake.
- Reduce protein intake if it is high
- Modify sodium/potassium/phosphorus intake—depends on blood level.
- Modify fluid intake—depends on urine output.
- Check fat type.

---

introduction of renal replacement therapy is accompanied by a change in dietary restrictions.

Diet during long-term haemodialysis

During dialysis blood is pumped from the body through the dialyser and then returned into the patient. The dialyser contains a semi-permeable membrane. Urea, creatinine, phosphorus and potassium diffuse across this membrane and are removed in the dialysis fluid. Fluid is also removed from the blood by ultrafiltration through the semi-permeable membrane. Regulation of the ions in the dialysis fluid means that normal levels of calcium, magnesium, sodium and chloride can be maintained. Dietary restrictions are necessary for patients on haemodialysis to ensure that too high a concentration of metabolites such as protein, urea, creatinine, phosphorus and potassium do not accumulate between dialyses, and that the individual does not become fluid overloaded. Dialysis is a catabolic process and it is important that the patient's dietary intake meets this increased demand. Because of the risk of malnutrition the nutritional status of the patient undergoing long-term haemodialysis must be reviewed regularly.

Protein. The diet should contain 60 to 80 g protein a day. This is the average UK daily protein intake, so there is no need for any formal restrictions other than the advice to eat 'sensible-sized' portions and explanation as to what constitutes a 'sensible-sized' portion, i.e. 3 to 4 oz (90–120 g) of meat at a meal. For some patients whose diet normally contained large portions of meat there will be an actual reduction in their protein intake.

Some patients who have previously been treated by diet for CRF find it difficult to adjust to their increased protein allowance. It is necessary for them to increase their protein intake to maintain an adequate nitrogen status and compensate for protein loss during dialysis. Malnutrition can occur among patients with CRF undergoing long-term haemodialysis (Allman 1990).

Fat. Patients should be encouraged to reduce their intake of saturated fat to reduce the risk of cardiovascular disease, which is the major cause of death in people with end-stage renal failure.

Sodium. A no-added-salt diet is usually advised because fluid intake is still restricted and salty foods tend to make people thirsty, so making adherence to a fluid restriction more difficult. The sodium restriction is modified for changes in blood pressure and fluid weight gain. If blood pressure and weight gain occur, the sodium intake will be further restricted.

Nutritional Care Plan 26.1	For patient with chronic renal failure		
Patient problem	Goal	Nutritional intervention	Outcome
Increased circulating fluid volume due to inability to excrete water	Patient achieves fluid balance	Fluid intake and output recorded Fluid intake restricted	Fluid intake and output are balanced Weight remains stable
Raised blood lipids	Serum cholesterol drops	Reduce intake of saturated fat	Serum cholesterol within acceptable range
Raised serum levels of sodium and potassium due to inability of kidneys to excrete sodium and potassium	Serum potassium and sodium within normal range	Restrict dietary sodium intake Restrict dietary potassium intake	Serum electrolyte concentrations within normal ranges
Poor nutrient intake causing loss of lean body mass	No loss of lean body mass	Increase energy content of diet Ensure high-energy supplements included in diet	Serum creatinine and blood urea levels are within acceptable ranges for patient Rate of rise in serum creatinine and blood urea slowed
Anorexia and confusion due to effects of uraemia	Serum creatinine and blood urea within acceptable range	Assess current nutritional intake Increase dietary energy Restrict dietary protein content	Serum creatinine and blood urea within acceptable range for patient
Anxiety about how diet will be managed at home due to lack of knowledge	Patient and relatives understand diet	Explain dietary restrictions to patient and relatives Provide written information Provide follow-up appointment	Patient and relatives can identify dietary sources of protein, energy, sodium, phosphate and potassium, understand limits and are confident in planning meals

Potassium. This is usually restricted to 70 mmol a day, allocated as 17 of 4-mmol exchanges (see Table 26.3), which need to be spread throughout the day rather than being kept for one meal. The daily allowance is adjusted by increase or reduction in the number of exchanges allowed, to maintain serum levels within the normal range.

Phosphorus. This is usually restricted to 1 g a day by avoiding large amounts of protein and processed foods such as biscuits, cakes and fizzy drinks, all of which have a high phosphorus content. Phosphate binders may also be prescribed as in CRF.

Fluid. 500 ml a day is allowed to cover insensible fluid loss, plus an amount equivalent to the previous day's urine output.

Dietary supplements. It is usual for patients on long-term haemodialysis to be routinely prescribed supplements of water-soluble vitamins and iron because these are lost during dialysis.

It is normal for dietary restrictions to be relaxed during the dialysis period. They should be reimposed 3 hours before the end of the dialysis session.

Diet following transplantation

Those patients who have a successful kidney transplant are able to have a relatively unrestricted diet. They should be given healthy eating advice, as this will help to prevent the development of obesity and hyperlipidaemia, which are both associated with steroid therapy.

CONTINUOUS AMBULATORY PERITONEAL DIALYSIS (CAPD)

This method of dialysis provides continuous dialysis, requires very little equipment, can be adjusted to fit in with individuals' normal routines and need not restrict patient mobility. There are three stages to CAPD:

1. Dialysate containing glucose and small amounts of electrolytes flows into the peritoneal cavity through a permanent access tube.
2. The empty dialysate bag remains attached, is rolled up and strapped to the waist or leg for the next 4 to 8 hours, usually 6 hours.
3. The empty bag is lowered and the dialysate drains out.

The dialysate solution commonly used contains glucose. Dialysate is available in 1-, 2- and 3-litre bags. It is usual for four 2-litre bags to be used in 24 hours. The glucose absorbed from the dialysate is a source of energy and can contribute to the development of obesity and hypertriglyceridaemia. To compensate for this extra energy the individual's energy requirement from the diet is only 25 kcal/kg body-weight (110 kJ/kg body-weight) (the diet of a 70-kg man would only need to provide 1750 kcal).

Energy. Initially the extra energy gained from the dialysate is beneficial, as it helps the patient regain weight. Many patients are underweight prior to dialysis. Once they have returned to their ideal body-weight, further weight gain should be prevented by ensuring that patients are aware of foods that have a high energy content and by limiting the intake of sugar and sugary foods and high-fat foods.

Protein. This is not usually restricted. 1.2 to 1.5 g/kg body-weight should be aimed for (84–135 g/day for a 70-kg man). This intake is needed to compensate for the amino acids and proteins lost in the dialysate effluent. It has been shown that up to 3 g a day of amino acids and 5 to 15 g of protein can be lost in this way. During peritonitis these losses are increased further. If the protein intake is not high enough to compensate for these losses, hypoalbuminaemia will develop (Bennett et al 1990).

Patients with a poor appetite and some vegetarians may find it difficult to eat enough protein. In this situation a protein supplement or sip-feed might be used. This is particularly important during peritonitis, when regular monitoring of the albumin level should be carried out to ensure that hypoalbuminaemia is not developing. Protein foods, such as meat and fish, which have a low phosphorus content, should be encouraged, and no more than one egg per day, rather than milk, cheese and shellfish which have a higher phosphate content.

Sodium. A no-added-salt diet is usually recommended to prevent excessive thirst and hypertension from developing.

Potassium. This is not usually restricted, although patients should be weighed daily to check fluid balance.

Phosphorus. High-phosphate foods should be discouraged.

Fluid. 700 ml per day plus the amount of the previous day's urine output is the usual allowance.

Non-starch polysaccharides (NSP). Patients who have CAPD frequently become constipated. A high NSP intake including wholemeal bread and high-fibre cereal should be encouraged to prevent this, as constipation can affect the drainage of the dialysate.

Water-soluble vitamins. Supplements are needed to replace those lost in the dialysis effluent.

Meal times. The absorption of glucose from the infused fluid and the pressure of fluid against the stomach may make the patient feel full and not hungry. If meal times can coincide with drainage times when the individual is most likely to feel hungry, this may help.

Many patients who receive CAPD are elderly, so the considerations applied to the dietary treatment of older people (Chapter 17) should be applied. For example: are their teeth functioning properly; have they other disabilities; or is their taste impaired? This is important to ensure that their diet is varied, nutritionally adequate and will contribute to enhancing their quality of life.

ACUTE RENAL FAILURE (ARF)

Acute renal failure (ARF) describes the syndrome which develops when the kidneys are no longer able to excrete the waste products of metabolism.

There are many causes of acute renal failure including:

- reduced circulating blood volume resulting from surgery, trauma or gastrointestinal bleeding
- reduced blood supply to the kidneys, for example following renal artery thrombosis
- obstruction, as in cancer of the bladder or cervix
- damage to the kidney by certain poisons (nephrotoxins), such as mercury and carbon tetrachloride
- infections such as acute nephritis and pyelonephritis
- septicaemia.

The type of dietary treatment that ARF patients receive will depend on their metabolic state and whether or not they are receiving any renal replacement therapy.

Where possible, the immediate cause of the condition is dealt with, e.g. by restoration of blood volume in circulatory failure or removal or obstructions. Modifications of the diet are directed to reducing, as far as possible, the accumulation of metabolic end-products requiring excretion by the kidneys, and ensuring adequate nutrition. The high mortality and morbidity rates that have occurred in patients with ARF were in part due to malnutrition, one of the causes of which was an over-restrictive protein allowance.

Lee (1980) has divided patients with acute renal failure into three categories (Table 26.4).

Table 26.4 Categories of acute renal failure (Lee 1980)

Category	Catabolic state	Cause of ARF
1	Normocatabolic	Obstructive uropathy or drug reaction
2	Catabolic	Post-surgery
3	Hypercatabolic	Multiple trauma, burns, road traffic accidents

Patients in the first category are managed in a similar way to the conservative treatment for CRF. However, the protein intake should not be restricted below 0.6 g/kg ideal body-weight as this leads to a negative nitrogen balance. Anorexic patients may benefit from the use of high-energy supplements. If the patient does not respond to this treatment and renal replacement therapy is used, the diet will need to be reviewed, as the protein requirements for all types of replacement therapy are higher than 0.6 g/kg.

Dietary treatment of ARF for catabolic and hypercatabolic patients

Most patients who are catabolic or hypercatabolic will need some sort of nutritional support in the form of either enteral or parenteral feeding, to ensure that their nutritional requirements are met.

A high protein and high energy intake are needed because of the catabolism caused by the underlying disease. The sodium, potassium, phosphate and fluid intake all depend on the type of replacement therapy used and the clinical state of the patient.

Patients with ARF either have a decreased urine flow or are anuric—in 98% of cases the urine flow drops below 400 ml/day (Thomas 2001), so fluid intake is restricted.

Dietary treatment of ARF for normocatabolic patients

The treatment follows the same principles as for CRF. However, as these patients are normally nauseated and anorexic, an adequate energy intake must be ensured by the use of high-energy supplements. It is important to remember that if the high-energy supplements used contain fluid, that their fluid content is included in the daily allowance. The allocation of the daily allowance should be discussed and agreed with the patient in order to make the diet as acceptable as possible. For example, some patients find a meal served without gravy both unpalatable and unattractive, while others are quite happy to have their meals without sauce or gravy.

During recovery from ARF, a period of diuresis usually occurs as kidney function returns to normal. During this time it is necessary to replace losses of water, sodium and potassium. Salts of these minerals are given by mouth and part of the fluid intake may be given in the form of fruit juices which have a high potassium content.

THE NEPHROTIC SYNDROME

The dietary treatment of all individuals with renal disease depends on their biochemistry and clinical status. Nephrotic syndrome is the term used to describe a syndrome in which the characteristic symptoms are:

- oedema
- proteinuria
- hypoalbuminuraemia
- hypercholesterolaemia.

The disease runs a protracted course and is caused by a wide variety of glomerular disorders. It occurs when the permeability of the glomeruli to plasma proteins is increased, leading to loss of protein in the urine. It is now usual to prescribe nephrotic patients a normal-protein, low-salt diet (Mason & Pusey 1994).

Protein. The traditional treatment for the nephrotic syndrome was to increase the protein intake to at least 100 g/day. The aim of this increase was to compensate for urinary loss and prevent the depletion of body tissues. Recent research has shown that the progress of the disease can be slowed by a reduction in the protein and phosphorus intake.

Sodium. A restriction of the sodium intake to 40 mmol or a no-added-salt diet may be necessary to help counteract the oedema which follows the fall in the plasma albumin level. The actual restriction will depend on clinical symptoms and sodium levels.

Fat. Because one of the features of the disease is hyperlipidaemia, most patients develop raised triglyceride and total serum cholesterol levels. Patients should be advised to reduce their intake of saturated fats (see Chapter 22).

NURITIONAL SUPPORT FOR PATIENTS WITH RENAL DISEASE

A range of specialist products are available for use with patients with renal disease who require nutritional support. Patients requiring this are usually managed by a dietitian specialising in the treatment of renal disease.

KIDNEY STONES

70% of the kidney stones occurring in the UK contain calcium and in about 80% of them no underlying cause can be identified (Thomas 2001). Dietary risk factors

have been identified which increase the likelihood of developing kidney stones. These are:

- low fluid intake
- excessive vitamin D intake
- high oxalate intake
- high protein intake.

Dietary treatment for preventing recurrence of calcium stones

- Increase fluid intake.
- Avoid oxalate-rich foods—tea, all nuts, chocolate, rhubarb, beetroot and spinach.
- Avoid high dietary intake of protein.
- Avoid high dietary intake of sodium.
- Reduce intake of sucrose and refined carbohydrates.
- Restrict intake of calcium.

Goldfarb (1988) has shown that the effectiveness of calcium restriction is not certain and calcium-intake restriction depends on local policy.

Other forms of kidney stones are not usually treated with diet.

REFERENCES

Bennett S E, Robinson C, Walls J 1990 Is peritonitis a major factor in protein status in CAPD? EDTNA ERCA Journal 8: 15–17
Bergstrom J 1995 Nutrition and mortality in haemodialysis. Journal of the American Society of Nephrology 61: 329–341
Bower J 1989 Cooking for restricted potassium diets in dietary treatment of renal patients. Journal of Human Nutrition and Dietetics 2(1): 1, 31–38
Goldfarb S 1988 Dietary factors in the pathogenesis and prophylaxis of calcium nephrolithiasis. Kidney International 34: 544–555
Hadfield C 1992 Nutritional adequacy of a low protein diet. Journal of Renal Nutrition 2(3) (Suppl 1): 37–41
Lee H A 1980 Nutritional support in renal and hepatic failure. In: practical nutritional support. Pitman Medical, London: 275–282

Ikrizler T A, Hakim R M 1996 Nutrition in end-stage renal disease. Kidney International 50: 343–357
Mason P D, Pusey C D 1994 Glometulonephritis: diagnosis and treatment. British Medical Journal 309: 1557–1563
Oldrizzo L, Rugiu C, Maschio G 1989 The optimal protein intake in patients with early chronic renal failure. In: Oldrizzo L, Maschio G, Rugiu C et al (eds) The progressive nature of renal failure: myths and facts. Kager, Basel: 203–208
Thomas B (ed) 2001 Manual of dietetic practice, 3rd Edn. Blackwell Science, Oxford
Walker R, 1997 Recent advances: general management of end stage renal disease. British Medical Journal 315: 1429–1432

FURTHER READING

Allman M A 1990 Factors affecting the nutritional status of patients with chronic renal failure undergoing haemodialysis. Journal of Human Nutrition and Dietetics 3: 225–232
Blumenkrantz M J, Gahl J M, Kopple J D et al 1981 Protein losses during peritoneal dialysis. Kidney International 19: 593–602
Klahr S, Levey A S, Beck G J et al 1994 The effect of dietary protein restriction and blood pressure control on the

progression of chronic renal disease. New England Journal of Medicine 330: 877–884
Pender F T 1988 A study of dietary practices of chronic renal failure patients treated by haemodialysis at home. Journal of Human Nutrition and Dietetics 1: 15–21
Thomas B (ed.) 1994 Manual of dietetic practice, 2nd Edn. Blackwell Scientific Publications, Oxford
Vennegor M 1982 Enjoying food on a renal diet. Oxford University Press, Oxford

27

Diet in diabetes mellitus

LEARNING OBJECTIVES

After studying this chapter you should be able to:

- explain the causes and consequences of the different types of diabetes mellitus
- discuss how the microvascular and macrovascular complications of diabetes mellitus can be prevented
- describe the dietary modifications required for the treatment of diabetes mellitus for children and adults of all ages.

UNDERSTANDING DIABETES

The presence of sugar in the urine of people with diabetes mellitus has been known since the time of the ancient Greeks. However, it was not until early in the 19th century that the sugar was identified as glucose by the French chemist, Chevraul. Later in that century the link between the pancreas and diabetes was established and then the understanding and treatment of diabetes was revolutionised by the discovery of insulin by Banting and Best in the 1920s.

In the past, diabetes was primarily thought of as a disorder of carbohydrate metabolism, partly because of the ease with which the presence of glucose can be measured in the urine and blood. It is actually a complex metabolic disease in which lipid, protein and carbohydrate metabolism is disordered.

Diabetes mellitus occurs when the insulin activity is insufficient for normal metabolism. This can either be due to an insulin deficiency or inadequate insulin function. The islet cells of the pancreas produce the hormones insulin and glucagon, both of which are involved in the regulation of the blood glucose concentration.

Insulin is secreted in response to an increase in the blood glucose. Then, as the blood glucose level falls, so does the amount of insulin produced. Insulin has three major sites of action: muscle, liver and adipose tissue. It has a large number of actions at these sites, the most important of which are listed below.

The effects of insulin

Effects of insulin on muscle

- Increases glucose entry into the muscle cells.
- Increases protein synthesis.
- Increases glycogen synthesis.
- Decreases protein breakdown.

Effects of insulin on liver

- Increases protein synthesis.
- Increases lipid synthesis.
- Increases glycogen synthesis.
- Decreases the production of glucose from amino acids.

Effects of insulin on adipose tissue

- Increases glucose entry into the fat cells.
- Increases lipid synthesis.

From these lists, it is easy to see how a lack of insulin leads not only to disordered carbohydrate metabolism, but also to disordered protein and fat metabolism.

It has been estimated that the incidence of diabetes in the white UK population is 1%. The incidence increases with age and in the population aged over 75 years it may be as high as 10% (BDA 1988).

Normal control of blood glucose

The amount of glucose in the blood depends on the balance between the amounts entering and leaving it.

Glucose entering the blood comes from three sources:

1. *Carbohydrate-containing foods*. Once digested and absorbed, these are the body's most important glucose source.
2. *Glycogen*. This is stored in the muscle and liver and is broken down to release glucose.
3. Some amino acids are broken down by the liver to produce *glucose*. This use of protein to produce energy is particularly important during starvation and when the body's energy requirement is increased, for example after injury. If insufficient carbohydrate is provided in the diet, dietary protein will be metabolised to produce energy.

Insulin is not needed for any of the above processes to occur. However, once glucose has entered the bloodstream, insulin is needed to enable glucose to leave the blood and enter the tissues.

In the non-diabetic person, glucose leaving the circulation is used in two ways:

1. *As an immediate energy source* for all tissues.
2. *As a stored form of energy* as glycogen in liver and muscle, and as fat in the adipose tissue. These stores are utilised when the amount of energy provided by glucose in the circulation is inadequate.

Symptoms of diabetes mellitus

Glycosuria due to a high level of blood glucose is accompanied by an increased loss of water and electrolytes. This osmotic diuresis leads to increased thirst, dehydration, electrolyte disturbances and weight loss. To compensate for the unavailability of glucose as an energy source, the body increases the rates at which glycogen and fat stores are broken down to release energy sources, and produces glucose from the breakdown of body protein. This increased breakdown of fat from adipose tissue leads to the production of acetoacetic acid, β-hydroxybutyric acid and acetone, which are toxic, at a rate greater than the rate at which they can be metabolised.

If left untreated, these metabolic disturbances will proceed to dehydration, ketoacidosis and diabetic coma.

Both microvascular and macrovascular degenerative changes occur in diabetes:

- Microvascular changes cause diabetic retinopathy; minute aneurysms occur in retinal vessels which can haemorrhage resulting in visual loss.
- Changes in the glomerular capillaries of the kidneys reduce kidney function.
- Macrovascular degeneration involves the development of atherosclerosis, causing cardiovascular disease and peripheral vascular disease.
- Diabetic neuropathy affects all parts of the nervous system, except the brain, causing pain, muscular cramps and tingling sensations.

It has been generally assumed that the incidence of diabetic complications is less when the blood glucose is kept within the normal range. However, as there was no conclusive evidence for this, some diabetics felt that a higher level of blood glucose, associated with a more relaxed approach to their diabetic control, gave them a better quality of life.

Conclusive evidence of a link between reduction in incidence of diabetic complications and good diabetic control has been found as a result of a 10-year study by the US National Committee on Diabetes (NIDDKD 1993). The study compared a group of patients who received intensive treatment aimed at keeping their HbA1C at 6.05% with a group who aimed to keep their HbA1C below 13.1%. The group with an HbA1C of 6.05%, within the normal range, showed reduced risks of both retinopathy and neuropathy.

TYPE 1 AND TYPE 2 DIABETES

Patients with diabetes are normally diagnosed as having Type 1 insulin-dependent diabetes mellitus (IDDM) or Type 2 non-insulin-dependent diabetes mellitus (NIDDM). Both forms have similar symptoms but they differ in their speed of onset and their mode of treatment. See Table 27.1.

Type 1 occurs when the β cells of the pancreas fail to produce any (or very little) insulin. This is the most severe form of the condition and is always treated with insulin. It is usually diagnosed in the under-40 years age-group, often in childhood or adolescence, develops suddenly, and is fatal if not treated.

Type 2 occurs when, although the β cells are producing insulin, it is in an ineffective form or a reduced quantity. The group of patients with this type of diabetes are not routinely treated with insulin, although it may be used as treatment for a short time following diagnosis or during surgery or treatment of an infection. Some non-insulin-dependent diabetics do eventually require insulin routinely as part of their treatment.

Type 2 occurs in middle and later life and can present with the same symptoms as Type 1 although the rate of onset is not as rapid and the rate of weight loss generally less. Harris et al (1992) have shown that it is usual for people with Type 2 diabetes to have had it for many years before diagnosis. This supports the case for routine screening for diabetes mellitus so that complications can be reduced.

Epidemiological studies show that the incidence of Type 2 varies greatly within populations, the incidence increasing with increasing age. In the UK the incidence of Type 2 is four times as great in the Asian population as the white population (Mather & Keen 1985). The challenge this presents and the way in which the cultural and language problems can be overcome to provide a good service to the patient are discussed on page 277.

The blood glucose responses to an oral glucose tolerance test

A diagnosis of diabetes is made from a fasting plasma glucose level of 7 mmol/l or above (Expert Committee WHO 1999) or a random venous plasma glucose level of 11.1 mmol/l. An oral glucose tolerance test may be performed to confirm this diagnosis.

A standard glucose tolerance test now consists of 75 g glucose in 250 ml. The diagnosis of diabetes is made if the 2-hour plasma glucose concentration is 11.1 mmol/l or greater. The blood glucose responses of a non-diabetic and a diabetic can be seen in Figure 27.1.

The normal fasting blood glucose range is 3 to 5 mmol/l, which rises to a maximum of 8 mmol/l within the first hour after swallowing the glucose. The rise in blood glucose is modified by the action of insulin produced in response to the increase in blood glucose. By the end of $2\frac{1}{2}$ hours, the blood glucose has returned to the fasting value.

In the diabetic, the lack of insulin will mean that glucose cannot leave the circulation unless it is excreted via the kidneys. In the kidney, glucose passes freely into the glomerular filtrate but is normally reabsorbed before it leaves the renal tubule, thus preventing the loss of glucose in the urine. When the blood glucose rises above the renal threshold (about 10 mmol/l), the kidney can no longer resorb all the glucose and some is lost in the urine.

As a consequence of this, the blood glucose rises to a higher peak and the return to the fasting value takes longer. The fasting level in diabetics is higher than in non-diabetics.

Table 27.1 Types of diabetes mellitus

	Age of onset	Treatment
Type 1 Insulin-dependent (IDDM)	Usually under 40 years, can occur at any age but most often diagnosed in children and young people	Insulin and diet
Type 2 Non-insulin-dependent (NIDDM)	Usually over 40 years, sometimes referred to as maturity or late-onset diabetes	Diet alone Diet and oral hypoglycaemic drugs Diet and insulin

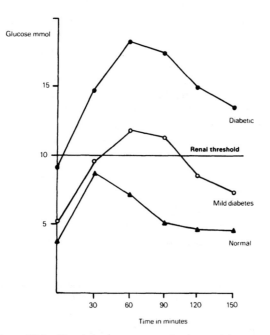

Figure 27.1 Blood glucose response to glucose tolerance test.

GENERAL PRINCIPLES OF DIETARY TREATMENT OF DIABETES

Dietary modification is a major part of treatment for all people who have diabetes. 40% of whom are treated by diet alone. The aims of dietary treatment are listed in Box 27.1.

All people with diabetes need dietary advice and they can be divided into three groups:

1. *Overweight and obese.* 80% of patients who are diagnosed as having Type 2 diabetes are overweight or obese at diagnosis. These patients need to be advised

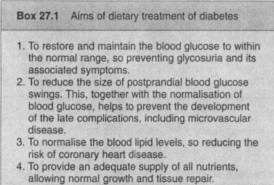

Box 27.1 Aims of dietary treatment of diabetes

1. To restore and maintain the blood glucose to within the normal range, so preventing glycosuria and its associated symptoms.
2. To reduce the size of postprandial blood glucose swings. This, together with the normalisation of blood glucose, helps to prevent the development of the late complications, including microvascular disease.
3. To normalise the blood lipid levels, so reducing the risk of coronary heart disease.
4. To provide an adequate supply of all nutrients, allowing normal growth and tissue repair.
5. To restore and maintain normal body-weight.

on how to lose weight and how to maintain their appropriate body-weight while eating a diet which is nutritionally adequate. Whether they require insulin injections, oral hypoglycaemic agents or no treatment, weight loss is of key importance in achieving optimal diabetic control.

2. *Those who do not require insulin injections or oral hypoglycaemic agents and are of normal weight.* This group need dietary advice to achieve and maintain their optimum body-weight and ensure good overall nutrition, as well as efficient use of the insulin that their bodies produce.

3. *Those who require insulin injections.* In addition to ensuring good overall nutrition and maintenance of body-weight, this group require dietary advice to ensure that the timing of their meals and the carbohydrate content are matched to their injected insulin.

Recommendations for nutrient contents of diabetic diets

For centuries, diets for diabetics have been surrounded by controversy and confusion. Before the discovery of insulin, when diet was the only treatment for diabetes, success was claimed for a variety of obscure diets. These included diets based on rice and on rancid meat. The current recommendations for diabetic diets (BDA 1992a) are summarised in Table 27.2.

These recommendations are important because they state that the principle of rigid carbohydrate restriction is no longer appropriate for the treatment of diabetes. A diet containing a higher amount of starchy foods rich in NSP (non-starch polysaccharides; dietary fibre) with a restricted fat content is now considered to be the appropriate form of treatment.

Energy

Identifying the correct energy intake for a person with diabetes is the cornerstone of good dietary advice. It is only if this is correct that the appropriate weight can be achieved and maintained and a diet with the correct amount of carbohydrate, protein and fat prescribed. If the patient's weight is stable at his/her correct weight, i.e. a body mass index (BMI) of around 22, then it can be assumed that his/her current energy intake is correct and it may be possible to estimate this from a dietary history.

If the person does not have a BMI of around 22, or his/her weight is not stable, then it will be necessary to estimate his/her energy requirement from his/her BMR (basal metabolic rate).

Table 27.2 Recommendations for diabetic diets: the dietary advice given to diabetics in the UK is based on these recommendations

Nutrient	Recommendations
Energy	Aim to maintain a BMI of 22
Carbohydrate	Should provide 50–55% of total energy
	Should consist of starchy high-fibre foods
	30 g dietary fibre per day (measured by Southgate analysis)
	Up to 25 g of sucrose or fructose per day could be included in the diet
Total fat	Should provide 30–35% of energy
	Saturated fat should provide no more than 10% of energy
	Polyunsaturated fat should never exceed 10% of energy
	Monounsaturated fatty acids should provide 10–15% of energy
Protein	Should provide 10–15% of total energy
Salt	Normotensive <6 g/day, Hypertensive <3 g/day

If the diet prescribed has too high an energy content, then the diabetic will gain weight. However, it is possible that the energy content of the prescribed diet is too low. Then it will:

- be difficult for the patient to keep to
- cause loss of lean body mass
- increase the risk of hypoglycaemia.

Carbohydrate

Most of the carbohydrate in the diet should come from foods which have their carbohydrates as polysaccharides (starch) and are also rich in NSP, such as fruit, vegetables and cereals, rather than refined carbohydrate.

A diet containing 50 to 55% of energy as carbohydrate, particularly as starchy high-fibre foods, can be bulky and difficult to get used to. The actual amount of carbohydrate in the diet will need to be decided on to suit the individual and it may be necessary to increase it from 45 to 50% over a period of time.

All carbohydrate-containing foods do not have the same effect on blood glucose levels. For example, 50 g of carbohydrate contained in a portion of fruit juice will have a far greater glycaemic effect than 50 g of carbohydrate contained in a portion of beans. The glycaemic effect of a food is determined by many factors including its physical form, chemical structure and fat, protein, sugar and NSP content. Carbohydrate-containing foods have been classified according to to their glycaemic effects in a glycaemic index. The glycaemic index compares the glycaemic effect of the portion of a particular food containing 50 g carbohydrate with the glycaemic response to 50 g carbohydrate either as glucose or white bread. Those foods with a low glycaemic index include pulses, pasta, raw fruit and milk. Those with a high glycaemic index include bread and fruit juices. There are practical difficulties in constructing diets based solely on low glycaemic index foods. However, Jarvi et al (1999) and Lafrance et al (1998) have shown improved glycaemic control in patients on a low glycaemic index diet and patients using insulin need to be aware that not all carbohydrates will have the same effect on their blood sugar levels.

The importance of NSP (dietary fibre) in the diabetic diet

The use of dietary fibre supplements as a treatment for diabetes has already been discussed in Chapter 8. Unrefined starchy foods are beneficial in the diets of diabetics for three reasons:

- Like the rest of the population, diabetics need NSP in their diet for healthy functioning of the gastro-intestinal tract.
- The carbohydrate that is contained in NSP-rich foods, particularly foods like pulses, which contain the viscous types of fibre, is absorbed slowly (Jenkins et al 1984). When carbohydrate is absorbed slowly from the gut, there is a correspondingly lower, more gentle rise in the blood glucose.
- The unrefined fibre-rich forms of foods are more bulky and so take longer to eat than their unrefined counterparts.

For the obese diabetic whose total energy intake is restricted, the extra bulk and feeling of satiety after eating the unrefined food is of particular value.

The dietary reference value for adults is 18 g/day NSP (DoH 1991) and individuals should not consume more than 32 g/day. As current recommendations are for NSP rather than dietary fibre, diabetics should aim to include in excess of 18 g/day NSP in their diet.

Sucrose

The British Diabetic Association (1990) now advises that the diet of a diabetic can contain up to 25 g per day of sucrose or fructose if it is already low in fat and high in starchy high-fibre foods. If sucrose is included in the diet, it should not be substituted for polysaccharide starch and should be included in meals. The inclusion of sucrose can make the diet more acceptable for some people and prevent the need for special diabetic products.

Fructose has no advantage over sucrose as a sweetener. This is because it causes a rise in blood glucose. Fructose also causes plasma triglycerides to rise when eaten in large quantities.

Fat

Diabetics should try to keep the proportion of their total energy intake that is provided by fat in the range of 30 to 35%.

The British Diabetic Association (1992a) recommends that energy intake from fat is provided as:

- 10 to 15% from monounsaturates
- 10% from polyunsaturates
- 10% from saturates.

These recommendations are broadly in line with those for the rest of the population (see Chapter 14). The reduction of fat intake is particularly important because of the increased risk of cardiovascular disease (CVD) in diabetics. The risk of coronary heart disease (CHD) and stroke in diabetics is at least twice that of the normal population and even higher in younger diabetics (DoH 1994, Fuller et al 1983).

Fat intake can be reduced by the following dietary changes:

1. Avoid fried and fatty foods.
2. Change to skimmed or semi-skimmed milk.
3. Spread margarine/butter on bread thinly or change to a low-fat spread.
4. Eat low-fat or half-fat cheese instead of full-fat cheese.
5. Cut off all visible fat from meat before cooking.
6. Avoid manufactured meat products such as pâtés and sausages.
7. Reduce intake of foods containing 'hidden fat', such as pastry and biscuits.

Current research links an increased intake of oily fish to a reduced frequency of heart disease in the general population and the general population has been recommended to eat more fish (DoH 1994). As diabetics are at an increased risk of heart disease, they should be encouraged to include oily fish in their diets.

Protein

This is an important nutrient. However, the diet of most people contains more than an adequate amount. Diabetics should be encouraged to have pulses in their diets instead of meat sometimes because, as well as being a valuable source of NSP, they are a protein source which contains no saturated fat, unlike meat.

As nephropathy is a complication for patients with diabetes and dietary protein intake influences renal function, studies suggest that it is wise to ensure that patients with diabetes have a protein intake that is at the lower end of the normal range (EASD 2000).

Special products and artificial sweeteners

Low-calorie sugar-free products increase the variety of the diabetic diet.

Special diabetic products are expensive and an unnecessary inclusion for diets (BDA 1992b).

Low-calorie sugar-free products

- Fruit tinned in water or unsweetened fruit juice
- Low-calorie soups
- Sugar-free fruit squashes and carbonated drinks.

All diabetics, including the overweight, will find these useful. However, not all low-sugar products are low-calorie. The calorie content of the fruits and soups is not negligible and must be considered, particularly if the patient is trying to lose weight.

Special diabetic products

These are luxury items and include cakes, biscuits, sweets, chocolates and preserves. They are sucrose-free and the alternative sweetening agents used are fructose and sorbitol. They are high in calories, often containing more calories than the ordinary products, and therefore are unsuitable for the overweight. It is better to include a small portion of a reduced-sugar product, for example reduced-sugar jam or marmalade in the diet, rather than the diabetic product. Diabetic lager has a lower carbohydrate content than ordinary lager but the carbohydrate is replaced with alcohol, making the lager higher in calories and more intoxicating.

The sweeteners used as alternatives to sucrose in the UK are saccharin, aspartame, sorbitol and fructose. Saccharin and aspartame are both calorie-free sweeteners, so are suitable for use by all diabetics, including those who are overweight. Fructose and sorbitol have the same calorie content as other sugars.

Saccharin is the most widely available artificial sweetener. It is derived from toluene and is 300 to 500 times as sweet as sucrose. It can be added to drinks and cooked food, but if it is added to food before it is cooked, it gives the food a metallic taste. The British Diabetic Association advises that no more than 14 saccharin tablets should be taken per day (BDA 1992a).

Aspartame is an artificial sweetener which is a dipeptide of aspartic acid and phenylalanine. It is approximately 200 times as sweet as sucrose. Aspartame is now widely used by the food industry as a sweetener in reduced-sugar products.

Sorbitol is a powdered sweetener which is used in the manufacture of cakes, biscuits and sweets for diabetics. When eaten in large amounts, sorbitol causes diarrhoea and abdominal pain, so should be restricted to 15 g per day. If artificial sweeteners are used, the British Diabetic Association recommends the use of a variety rather than just one type (BDA 1992a).

Alcohol

It is not necessary for people with diabetes to exclude alcohol from their diet unless it is specifically advised by their doctor. Diabetics should always discuss with their doctor whether or not they should drink alcohol. People who are prescribed the oral hypoglycaemic drug chlorpropamide may need to avoid alcohol because it causes flushing in some people.

Diabetics need to be aware that:

1. *Alcohol has a hypoglycaemic effect*—so it should never be drunk on an empty stomach. This hypoglycaemic effect can last several hours, so food should be taken with or after the drink.
2. *Alcoholic drinks contain calories*—so people who are trying to lose weight should exclude alcohol from their diet when possible. Regular drinking can cause weight gain.
3. *Beers and wines contain carbohydrate*—the carbohydrate contents should not be exchanged for those of food.
4. *Low-carbohydrate beers and lagers should be avoided*— they are high in calories and alcohol.

The British Diabetic Association (1992a), now known as Diabetes UK, recommends that men should drink no more than 3 units of alcohol a day and women 2 units (1 unit = $\frac{1}{2}$ pint ordinary beer or 1 glass of wine or 1 measure of spirits).

DIETS FOR DIABETES

For ease of classification, the type of dietary advice given is divided into three types. There are no hard-and-fast rules as to which diet is specific to a particular type of diabetes. Whether the diet is based on one or more of these types of advice depends on the severity of the diabetes, type of treatment, personality, age, weight and lifestyle of the diabetic.

The three types are:

* weight reduction followed by sugar-free weight maintenance
* sugar-free
* a measured-carbohydrate (exchange) diet.

Weight-reducing diet

It has been shown that weight loss will improve the life-expectancy of obese non-insulin-dependent diabetics (Lean et al 1990). These patients need encouragement, persuasion and practical help to ensure that weight is lost and the new weight maintained.

A diet should be prescribed which has an energy content calculated to allow for a weight loss of 500 to 700 g (1–1$\frac{1}{2}$ lb) per week. It has been shown that weight loss in an obese diabetic promotes a decrease in insulin resistance. This helps the blood glucose level to return to the normal range.

The energy requirement of an obese diabetic should be estimated using the basal metabolic rate (BMR). It is counterproductive to prescribe too strict a diet as it is difficult for the diabetic to keep to, so reducing the success of weight loss. In order for the diet to be easily managed it should not impose unnecessary restrictions. However, the guidelines in Box 27.2 need to be imposed.

It is important that the diabetic understands that meals should not be missed. Initially, overweight diabetics are well motivated and keen to lose weight. However, this motivation can be lost if:

* the diet is difficult to keep to
* weight loss is too slow
* the target weight seems unattainable.

Initial enthusiasm must be capitalised upon and encouraged by regular weight checks. Some diabetics benefit from the support and pressures of a slimming

---

Box 27.2 Guidelines for the diabetic on a weight-reducing diet

- Eat regular meals.
- Eat starchy foods instead of sugary foods.
- Eat less fat.
- Do not eat sugary foods.
- Eat more vegetables and fruit.

---

group but not all diets provided by commercial slimming organisations are suitable for diabetics, so it may be more beneficial for a practice nurse to organise a group specifically for people with diabetes.

Sugar-free diets

This type of diet is used for diabetics who do not need insulin injections and do not need to lose weight. It is based on three principles:

1. *Encourage healthy eating*
2. *Avoid sugar and sugary foods* such as:
   — all types of sugar
   — honey, jam and marmalade
   — sweets and chocolates
   — jam, chocolate and cream biscuits, cakes and puddings
   — fruit tinned in syrup
   — fruit squashes and fizzy drinks that contain sugar.
3. *Eat regular meals* which should contain carbohydrate in the form of starch, for example bread, potato, rice or chapattis, and these meals must be regularly spaced throughout the day.

The actual amount of carbohydrate allowed for each meal depends on the total energy requirement of the individual. Providing the carbohydrate as starch and distributing it evenly throughout the day will achieve the best match between carbohydrate intake and the available insulin produced by the patient. Box 27.3 gives an example of a day's meals on a sugar-free diet.

The carbohydrate exchange system

This system was designed to provide a method of regulating the dietary carbohydrate intake precisely and has been used both for those diabetics who are treated with insulin injections, and those on high doses of hypoglycaemic agents. A diet based on this system is more complicated for the diabetic to manage, but has the advantage of providing a diet which is more flexible and varied than the sugar-free type.

The weighed-portion carbohydrate exchange system is being used less now for newly diagnosed diabetics and is being replaced with a household measure type. This is because the diets currently prescribed have a more generous carbohydrate allowance and because of the differing glycaemic effects of different foods (Jenkins et al 1980).

The diet, as well as conforming to the nutritional guidelines published by Diabetes UK (see p. 268), must provide sufficient carbohydrate to cover periods of peak insulin activity and peak physical activity, so preventing hypoglycaemia. An understanding of this balance is a key to good blood sugar control and a diabetic's understanding of this point must be ensured by all those educating the diabetic.

The diet prescription will be calculated to provide the correct energy content to maintain the normal body-weight. The actual distribution of the food throughout the day depends on the individual's insulin regimen.

Weighing foods is not necessary, nor is strict calculation of the actual carbohydrate content of each meal, but best control is achieved if approximately the same amount of carbohydrate is eaten at approximately the same time, unless extra is required to cover extra exercise.

The weighed-portion exchange system needs to be understood by health care professionals working with diabetics because it is the system with which many diabetics are familiar and those diabetics who are used to it may not wish to change. It can also be a useful teaching aid as it helps in identifying those foods which have a high carbohydrate content.

In this country it is conventional for a carbohydrate exchange to be the amount of food which, on chemical analysis, contains 10 g of carbohydrate. A list of these carbohydrate exchanges has been produced by Diabetes UK. To avoid confusion all diabetics and dietitians should use this standard list. Box 27.4 lists portions of foods measured in household measures which contain 10 g carbohydrate; this information should be used in conjunction with the guide to foods which can be included in the diabetic diet (Table 27.3). The interchange of exchanges in the diet enables the diabetic to include a variety of foods in a meal and still keep the carbohydrate content constant.

An example of a day's meals using the 10 g exchange system can be seen in Box 27.5.

The number of carbohydrate exchanges a diabetic is allowed in a day depends on two factors:

- the total energy requirement

Box 27.3 Example of a day's meals on a sugar-free diet

Mrs Smith is a 69-year-old widow whose diabetes was diagnosed 3 years ago when she went to her GP because she was feeling unusually tired. Her diabetes is mild and controlled by a sugar-free diet alone. She weighs 59 kg, her height is 1.6 m, and her BMI is 23, so she is at her correct weight. Her energy requirement is estimated as 1600 kcal.

Breakfast

Bowl of high-fibre cereal such as bran flakes or porridge with semi-skimmed milk
One slice of wholemeal toast* thinly spread with reduced-sugar marmalade†
Tea, no sugar

Mid-morning

Coffee, no sugar
Piece of fruit if wanted

Lunch

Lean meat or fish
Portion of any vegetable or salad

Three potatoes, preferably boiled, or baked in skins
Fruit tinned in juice with sugar-free custard‡

Mid-afternoon
Tea, no sugar
One plain biscuit

Evening meal

Four slices wholemeal bread
Lean meat, fish, egg or cheese as sandwich filling
Salad
Portion of fruit such as an apple

During evening

Cup of semi-skimmed milk
One piece of fruit or slice of bread

*All bread/toast is spread thinly with either margarine high in polyunsaturates or a low-fat spread.
†A small amount of reduced- or low-sugar marmalade is allowed instead of diabetic marmalade.
‡Other puddings sometimes eaten are sugar-free milk puddings and diet yoghurts.

- the percentage of the total energy requirement that is to be provided by carbohydrate.

The total energy requirement is decided after the diabetic's current diet has been assessed or, more accurately, after his or her estimated energy requirement (EER) has been calculated. This depends on height, weight and age. A discussion of occupation and leisure activities will be needed to establish physical activity level (PAL). It is usual to aim for 55% of the total energy to be provided by carbohydrate, but this cannot always be achieved.

This individual prescription of a diet means that there will be a wide variation in the number of carbohydrate exchanges allowed. For example, an overweight diabetic may only be allowed 14 (140 g carbohydrate) a day while an 'ideal weight' diabetic may be allowed 30 (300 g carbohydrate) a day. Of course, both of these diabetics have different total energy requirements. It is important that both patients and carers understand that although the same principles apply there is no definitive, universal diabetic diet. Otherwise, confusion will arise as 'diabetic diets' are compared.

The way in which the carbohydrate exchanges are distributed throughout the day depends on the insulin regime. The aim is to balance insulin activity with food and so prevent both hypo- and hyperglycaemia.

If treatment is with mixtures of insulins or fast-acting insulin, then most of the carbohydrate should be eaten at the times of peak insulin activity. The use of the new (pen-type) injections for insulin has allowed insulin-dependent diabetics far more flexibility and freedom in when and what they eat.

Diabetics who are treated with slow-acting insulin or oral hypoglycaemic agents need to have their carbohydrate allocated evenly throughout the day.

Blood glucose monitoring

Frequent blood glucose monitoring is an essential component of blood sugar control and the patient should aim to maintain their blood glucose levels at 4 to 7 mmol/l.

MEDICATION FOR DIABETES MELLITUS

People with diabetes who are unable to maintain their blood glucose within the normal range by modifying their diet, and weight loss if overweight, require medication. Medication should be used in addition to achievement of ideal weight and dietary modification and not instead of them. Insulin has a metabolic effect, so unnecessarily large doses will cause weight gain. It is usual to use oral hypoglycaemic agents for Type 2 diabetes and injections of insulin for Type 1.

Box 27.4 Portions of carbohydrate-containing foods which contain approximately 10 g carbohydrate

One medium slice bread
One saucer-sized thin chapatti
Five tablespoons breakfast cereal
One Weetabix
Two crackers or crispbreads
One level tablespoon cooked rice or pasta
One small potato (50 g, egg-sized)
One small glass fruit juice
One apple, orange, pear, small bunch of grapes, small banana
One glass milk
One diet yoghurt
One small scoop ice-cream

Oral hypoglycaemic agents

Two types of oral hypoglycaemic agents are used—sulphonylureas and biguanides. Neither type should be used for pregnant women. For further information see the British National Formulary (BMA & RPS).

Sulphonylureas

This group is usually used for Type 2 with normal body-weight and acts by stimulating the β cells of the pancreas to produce more insulin, so maximising an individual's endogenous insulin production. They also act by increasing the sensitivity of peripheral tissues to insulin.

Table 27.3 A Guide to foods which can be included in the diet of a diabetic

	Choose these	Eat occasionally	Try to avoid
Starchy foods	Bread, preferably wholemeal, potatoes, rice, chapattis, pasta, whole grain breakfast cereals, porridge oats	Chips, roast potatoes, potato crisps, fried rice	Sugar-coated breakfast cereals
	Plain biscuits, crackers, muffins, crumpets, tea cakes	Scones, plain cake	Iced cakes and biscuits, croissants, cream biscuits
Fruit and vegetables	Fresh, frozen and tinned vegetables Herbs, spices	Fried vegetables	
	Fresh, frozen and tinned fruit (tinned in juice) Cooked, dried or tinned beans, lentils and dahl)	Avocado pears	Fruit tinned in syrup
Meat/fish	Lean meat (fat and poultry skin removed before cooking), all types of white and oily fish	Fried fish, sausages, pâté, meat pie	
Eggs		Limit egg yolks to two per week	
Dairy products	Skimmed and semi-skimmed milk, low-fat cottage cheeses, lower-fat cheeses—Edam, Camembert, low-fat Cheddar Fat-free yoghurt Fat-free fromage frais	Products containing cream, full-fat cheeses, full-fat yoghurt, condensed milk, evaporated milk	
Fats/oils	Wherever possible use a monounsaturated oil for cooking—olive/rapeseed—use as little as possible. Use a low-fat spread for bread, etc. or spread butter/margarine thinly	Lard, suet	
Confectionery and desserts	Sugar-free jelly, milk puddings and custards, diet yoghurts, diet fromage frais	Pastry, sugar-free crumble	Chocolate, sugar, honey, mincemeat, syrup, sweets, packet desserts, sweetened puddings, ordinary yoghurt and fromage frais
Miscellaneous	Tea, coffee, sugar-free squashes, sugar-free fizzy drinks, artificial sweeteners, Worcestershire sauce, tomato juice, soya sauce	Jam, marmalade— small amounts spread on bread, mayonnaise, salad cream, fruit juice	Sweetened drinks, ordinary squashes, fizzy drinks, Lucozade, Ribena (except when ill)

Box 27.5 An example of a day's meals using the 10 g exchange system

Sample diet for female aged 22 years, weight 57.6 kg, height 160 cm, BMI 22. BMR estimated as 1342.7 kcal: from this the EER is calculated as 2094 kcal. Carbohydrate is to provide 55% of total calories. Therefore diet should contain 270 g carbohydrate.

An example of a day's meals for two different insulin regimes is set out below:

Insulin regime	Inject Intermediate mixed with short-acting	Approximate carbohydrate content of meal (g)	Inject Intermediate and short-acting	Approximate carbohydrate content of meal (g)
Breakfast	Three slices toast* Two Weetabix or bowl of unsweetened cereal small glass fruit juice milk for cereal†	70	Three slices toast* Two Weetabix or bowl of unsweetened cereal small glass fruit juice milk for cereal†	70
Mid-morning	One piece of fruit	10	One piece of fruit *Inject short-acting*	10
Lunch	Four slices bread as sandwiches with lean meat, fish, egg or cheese filling One piece of fruit One diet yoghurt	60	Six slices bread as sandwiches with lean meat, fish, egg or cheese filling One piece of fruit One diet yoghurt	80
Mid-afternoon	One piece of fruit *Inject intermediate mixed with short-acting*	10	One piece of fruit *Inject short-acting*	10
Evening	Six potatoes or Six tablespoons boiled rice vegetables meat‡, fish, egg or pulse dish One piece of fruit One biscuit	90	Six potatoes or Six tablespoons boiled rice vegetables meat‡, fish, egg or pulse dish Two pieces of fruit	80
Bedtime	Two slices bread	20	One slice bread	10
Daily milk		10		10
TOTAL		270		270

*As in sugar-free diet, bread is spread with low-fat spread or a thin layer of polyunsaturated margarine.
†Milk should be skimmed or semi-skimmed.
‡Meat should be lean to ensure restriction of the saturated fat content of the diet.

Three different sulphonylureas are commonly used, each having a slightly different duration of activity.

1. *Tolbutamide*. This form has the shortest duration of activity, about 6 hours. This means it has to be taken two to three times a day, which can be a disadvantage.

However, because of its shorter duration of action, it is less likely to cause hypoglycaemia and so is valuable in the treatment of elderly diabetics.

2. *Glibenclamide* has a longer duration of action—approximately 12 hours. A large single dose can cause hypoglycaemia.

3. *Chlorpropamide* has activity of longer duration—up to 24 hours. Chlorpropamide can produce hypoglycaemia. This usually occurs during the night or when the usual dietary routine has been interrupted. The drug should not be used if renal function is impaired as the drug will not be excreted by the kidneys and so will accumulate. If renal failure is present, the sulphonylureas, gliquidone (duration of action 3 hours) and longer-acting gliclazide (duration 12 hours) are preferred as they are inactivated by metabolism in the liver.

Hypoglycaemia can also occur if other drugs—alcohol, sulphonamides, methyldopa and aspirin—are being used concurrently with oral hypoglycaemics.

Biguanides

Biguanides are used less often than the sulphonylureas. They are used to treat non-insulin-dependent diabetics who are overweight. Metformin is the only biguanide oral hypoglycaemic agent commonly used. It has a shorter duration of action than the sulphonylureas—approximately 2 hours. It can cause side-effects of nausea and anorexia. These effects can be minimised by taking it with food. Biguanides also reduce vitamin B_{12} absorption and so can be a cause of vitamin B_{12} deficiency. If used, biguanides are usually used in conjunction with a sulphonylurea to obtain optimal glycaemic control.

Insulin

Insulin is a polypeptide hormone used for treatment of ketoacidosis, non-ketotic hyperglycaemia and when blood glucose cannot be controlled by diet, weight reduction and oral hyperglycaemic agents. As it is a protein it is inactivated by gastrointestinal hormones and therefore cannot be given orally. It is given by injection, the normal injection sites being upper arms, thighs, buttocks and abdomen.

The choice of the type of insulin to be used in treatment should be made after consideration of the diabetic's preferred lifestyle, usual meal pattern, daily exercise, work pattern and hobbies. The insulins used can be divided into three broad categories and are summarised in Table 27.4.

Doses are small initially, to prevent hypoglycaemia developing, and are then gradually increased. It is usual to start insulin treatment with twice-daily injections of an intermediate-acting insulin to which injections of soluble insulin can be added to improve control. The final insulin regime and doses of insulin are determined on an individual basis in relation to individual lifestyle and blood glucose monitoring.

Four different insulin regimes are commonly used:

1. Short-acting mixed with intermediate-acting insulins injected twice daily, before breakfast and before the evening meal.
2. Short-acting mixed with intermediate-acting before breakfast, short-acting before the evening meal, and intermediate-acting at bedtime.
3. Short-acting three times a day before meals, and intermediate-acting at bedtime.
4. Short-acting mixed with intermediate-acting before breakfast only.

Obviously, the insulin regime intended for a retired person whose life follows a settled routine will not be suitable for the more erratic lifestyle of a shift worker or student.

Table 27.4 Onset and duration of action of insulins

	Onset of action*	Duration of action
Short-acting • Soluble • Rapid acting—analogues of human insulin which act rapidly and for a shorter time than soluble insulin	30 minutes after injection	Up to 8 hours
Intermediate-acting • Isophane (a suspension of insulin with Protamine), often used as a component of ready mixed combinations of long and shorter acting Insulins	1–2 hours after Injection	18–26 hours
Long-acting • Insulin zinc suspensions (often used to provide a background level of insulin to which small doses of soluble insulin are injected throughout the day)	1–2 hours after injection	24–36 hours
Mixture of short-acting and intermediate-acting	30 minutes after injection	16–24 hours

* The times for onset of action and duration do show individual variation in rates of absorption and variation depending on the injection site.

Ideally, the diet and eating habits of the diabetic should be assessed prior to prescription of the insulin regime, so that a combination of diet and insulin therapy maintains the best possible glycaemic control for each individual patient and his or her chosen lifestyle.

There are many different types of insulin and the British National Formulary (BMA & RPS) should be consulted for up-to-date information about current insulins.

It is increasingly likely that diabetics will be treated with a multi-injection regime; that is they will inject a long-acting insulin either at bedtime only or twice daily and, in addition to this, injections of a fast-acting insulin will be given before meals. As doses can easily be changed, this allows more flexibility as to when and what to eat. The pen injector system is a convenient way of managing this.

DIABETES AND PREGNANCY

Gestational diabetes

Most western women experience a deterioration in glucose tolerance during pregnancy. The metabolic changes which occur during pregnancy are accompanied by a reduction in sensitivity to insulin. This reduction in sensitivity to insulin can be up to 40% (Kuhl 1991). The pancreas in most pregnant women is able to produce extra insulin to compensate for this with only 2 to 3% of all pregnant women developing gestational diabetes. There is considerable variation in this figure between populations, with the incidence of gestational diabetes in the UK being eight times greater in women of Asian origin.

It is usual for women to be screened for glycosuria at routine antenatal appointments. If glycosuria is detected, then the presence of gestational diabetes is confirmed by a glucose tolerance test. The symptoms of gestational diabetes are the same as for Type 1 and Type 2, in addition to which there is an increased risk of perinatal mortality and postpartum hypoglycaemia. Maternal hyperglycaemia enhances the insulin produced by the foetus. The result of this is that the baby is likely to be larger.

Dietary treatment of gestational diabetes mellitus

The dietary treatment is based on similar principles to the sugar-free diet:

- Substitute unrefined starchy carbohydrate for refined starchy carbohydrate in the diet.

- Exclude sugar and sugary foods.
- Eat regular meals and snacks.
- Try to eat fewer fatty foods.

The increased nutritional requirements of pregnancy must be met, in particular the need for calcium. This is achieved by including 1 pint of semi-skimmed or skimmed milk a day in the diet.

Weight gain needs to be monitored carefully to ensure that enough of the bulky unrefined carbohydrate foods such as wholemeal bread, high-fibre breakfast cereals, potatoes and fruit are being eaten to provide sufficient energy. If the energy content of the diet is to be maintained, the calorie-dense, high-sugar, high-fat foods such as biscuits, cakes and sweets must be replaced by other foods. Between-meals snacks must be encouraged to provide the required energy. It is likely in the later stages of pregnancy that the woman will be eating three small meals and two to three substantial snacks. Sandwiches, fresh fruit and unsweetened breakfast cereals with milk (semi-skimmed or skimmed) are all useful snacks.

If the patient is obese, then the weight gain can be controlled by restricting fat intake, not by reducing carbohydrate intake. It is not appropriate to encourage weight loss at this stage, although the patient should be offered help to lose weight after the pregnancy. Patients should be encouraged to measure their own blood glucose levels and keep accurate records, so that the best possible glycaemic control can be achieved. Some patients with gestational diabetes eventually need insulin. This need for insulin injections stops after delivery. The same dietary advice applies as before insulin treatment, but the advice not to miss meals or snacks needs reinforcing and the eating of a snack before bedtime becomes more important; the pregnant woman should be advised to carry some fast-acting carbohydrate such as glucose tablets in case of hypoglycaemia.

Pregnancy and pre-existing diabetes

The diabetic control of women who intend becoming pregnant should ideally be reviewed before conception. Insulin treatment, exercise and diet should all be reviewed to ensure the best possible diabetic control before conception and during pregnancy. Good diabetic control is associated with a reduced incidence of stillbirths and congential abnormalities. The best way to provide this service to diabetic women is to provide a specialist diabetic antenatal clinic, where insulin and diet, along with blood glucose results, can be regularly reviewed at antenatal appointments.

Breast-feeding

Diabetic women should be encouraged to breast-feed as there is no reason why they should not succeed if they are given sufficient support.

They need to monitor their blood glucose levels regularly, as their energy requirement will increase and so they will need an extra 40 to 50 g carbohydrate per day to compensate for this. The diabetic who is breast-feeding should:

- Always eat before feeding.
- Drink sufficient fluid, 2 to 3 pints/day.
- Have an extra snack at bedtime.
- Have a snack and drink nearby while feeding. This is particularly important if the baby is a slow feeder. Not only will hypoglycaemia cause problems for the mother, it will reduce the milk supply.

DIABETES IN CHILDHOOD

For greater detail see Magrath et al (1993) and Shaw & Lawson (2001).

Most diabetics whose diabetes is diagnosed in childhood require insulin injections. Diabetes is a life-long condition and the incidence of its complications is reduced by good glycaemic control. These factors need to be considered at all stages when helping diabetics and their families come to terms with the condition and the management of it. Infants and young children are best served by being treated at a specialist centre, where the specific needs of children with diabetes and their carers are met and expertise can be developed. Wherever possible in the UK, newly diagnosed diabetics are stabilised and taught how to inject their insulin at home without a hospital admission. This means that the routine of insulin and diet can be tailored to fit in with the child and his or her life and not established in the artificial environment and routine of a hospital.

Nutritional needs of diabetic children

1. Requirements for vitamins, minerals, energy and protein are the same as for non-diabetic children.
2. Like non-diabetic children, they have food fads and periods of food refusal and may try to use food to manipulate their carers.
3. All children show tremendous day-to-day variations in energy expenditure. For example, a

10-year-old boy might spend all of a wet day watching the television with very little exercise and then play football all the next day.

The process of dietary education cannot and does not need to be completed within the first few days of diagnosis. However, there are some key points that need to be understood by the child and carers as a basis for further education:

- Eat regular meals; you may need to eat between-meal snacks.
- You need to eat some breakfast.
- You do not have to eat new, unusual foods.
- Do not be hungry; if you are, ask for bread, potatoes, fruit or breakfast cereal.
- Do not have sweets, sugary drinks or lots of fruit juice (your dietitian will explain when you can have these).
- Carry some glucose sweets with you.

Once the basic information has been assimilated, the process of education which will enable carers of children with diabetes to be given the advice and confidence to manage their children's diet in the range of different settings that are normal in the life of a child, for example a birthday party, football match, minor infection or period of 'faddy eating', can be started.

Summary of points which require special consideration for children with diabetes

Infancy

- The help of a specialist paediatric dietitian will be needed as diabetes is very rare in infancy.
- Infants with diabetes can be breast- or infant-formula-fed.

Under 5 years

- Children are unable to eat large quantities of unrefined starchy foods and are best managed with regular small meals and snacks.
- The consumption of starchy foods should be encouraged, but as these foods can be filling to eat and low in energy content, the diet should be reviewed regularly to check that it is providing sufficient energy.
- It is normal for children to go through periods of food refusal. This is a very difficult period for carers of diabetic children because of their anxiety about

the risk of hypoglycaemia. In these situations, hypoglycaemia will stimulate the appetite and foods which are not disliked but not seen as rewards, like sandwiches, breakfast cereals and milk or fruit, should be given.

- Children need to get into the routine of having sweets and chocolates before exercise or in small portions as part of a meal. It is very helpful if the whole family adopt this routine. Perhaps the introduction of a special place for storing sweets received as presents, prizes or at parties can be introduced.

School children

- For children who were diagnosed at a younger age this is a period when the diet is relatively easy to manage, as the child's eating patterns are restricted by the routine imposed by school.
- All children want to conform with their peers and every attempt should be made to ensure that the child does not feel too different. Diabetic children should be encouraged to have school meals with their friends, if school meals are provided. Liaison between school catering staff, school nurse and dietitian should ensure that the meals are satisfactory.
- Explanation of the diet to teachers and friends of the child and their parents should ensure that the child is not excluded from birthday parties, tea at friends' homes or sessions at school which include the preparation, tasting and discussion of food.
- Extra carbohydrate is essential before activity, particularly swimming, and should be in an easily eaten, rapidly absorbable form. Sweets, chocolates and biscuits are suitable for this.
- All staff caring for the child must be able to recognise the symptoms of hypoglycaemia. The school nurse has a key role in ensuring that they do and that they know how to act.

Adolescence

- It is normal for children of this age to have unconventional meals and eating habits and to want to conform to the diet that their friends eat. This makes dietary compliance difficult.
- Growth spurts can make good diabetic control difficult to achieve and changes in the insulin regime and diet will be necessary.
- If diabetes was diagnosed at a younger age, it should be possible to build on previous dietary habits so that a healthy diet is established for adulthood. For a newly diagnosed diabetic, there may need to be a

compromise between the carers and the health advisers who want the best possible glycaemic control and the teenager who wants to be like his friends. The principles of regular meals containing starchy foods and avoiding very sugary foods, except prior to exercise, must be encouraged. Changing over to the use of a 'pen' for multiple insulin injections may achieve better control when lifestyle is unpredictable.

- Children must be confident enough and well enough informed to manage their own diet. The resources produced by Diabetes UK are valuable teaching aids in helping the child to achieve this.

DIETARY ADVICE FOR THE ASIAN DIABETIC

There is a higher incidence of diabetes in the Asian population (Simmons et al 1991, Cruickshank et al 1991). Asians from the Indian sub-continent living in the UK are four times more likely than the indigenous population to develop Type 2 (Mather & Keen 1985). Therefore, dietary advice must be tailored to meet their needs and fit in with their culture and lifestyle (Govindji 1991) and build on their existing beliefs (Greenhaugh et al 1998).

The key to a good diet for this population is to reinforce their good traditional eating habits.

The traditional diet for this group of the population is high in unrefined carbohydrate and NSP and low in fat and refined sugars (see Chapter 18). It is the high-fat, high-sugar snack foods which have been incorporated into the diet which need restricting to improve the diet and so improve glycaemic control.

Dietary advice should be:

1. *Increase the NSP and carbohydrate intake by encouraging the consumption of:* wholemeal chapattis, rice, brown rice, wholemeal bread, high-fibre breakfast cereals, dahls, vegetables and fruit.

2. *Reduce the fat intake by:*

- reducing the amount of ghee, oil or spreading fat used
- avoiding fried snacks such as samosas and bahjis
- eating boiled rice instead of fried rice
- using a low-fat milk
- removing visible fat from meat before cooking.

3. *Reduce the intake of sugar by:*

- eating small portions of sweetmeats on special occasions only

- using artificial sweeteners
- drinking low-calorie drinks.

It is important that the health care professional understands the cultural and religious constraints imposed on the Asian diabetic. Particular care should be taken to ensure diet sheets include portions of familiar foods such as chapatti, dahl and vegetables traditionally eaten. There are a wide range of teaching aids available to overcome these problems, particularly the problems which occur if the patient cannot speak or read English.

Of particular use is a video produced by Diabetes UK called *Looking after Yourself* which is available in Bengali, Punjabi, Urdu and Gujerati. They also produce diet leaflets in these languages.

EXERCISE

Physical exercise has been shown to increase insulin sensitivity (Horton 1986) and should be encouraged alongside weight reduction for the treatment of Type 2 diabetes. Exercise also plays an important part in preventing CVD. Regular exercise is beneficial in lowering blood pressure and lowering blood lipids.

Exercise increases the utilisation of glucose, and extra carbohydrate is required to cover this. The amount and timing of the exercise in relation to the last meal influence the increased carbohydrate requirement. For example, increasing the amount of carbohydrate eaten at lunch time may be sufficient to sustain normoglycaemia during a period of walking, whereas a sugary snack such as a bar of chocolate may be more appropriate before a game of football or a swim.

During exercise the entry of glucose into muscle increases. This increase also occurs in the absence of insulin. As a result of this, the blood glucose concentration drops. To compensate for this drop and prevent hypoglycaemia, diabetics need extra carbohydrate (10–20 g) before exercise. It is important that extra carbohydrate is taken, as delayed hypoglycaemia can develop hours after strenuous activity.

It is not necessary to subtract this carbohydrate from the next meal's allowance—it is an addition needed for the additional exercise. This allowance makes dietary management of children easier, as they are allowed extra carbohydrate as confectionery before swimming or games sessions. Diabetics should be recommended to check their blood sugar level prior to starting an endurance event and ensure that they are able to consume extra carbohydrate at regular intervals, so preventing hypoglycaemia from developing.

HYPOGLYCAEMIA

Hypoglycaemia can occur in both diabetics who are treated by insulin and diabetics who are treated by long-acting oral hypoglycaemic drugs. An increased risk of hypoglycaemia is one of the potential consequences of improved diabetic control. For some elderly people it is appropriate to encourage them to maintain pre-prandial blood glucose levels of 5 to 9 mmol/l to reduce their risk of hypoglycaemia. The symptoms of hypoglycaemia vary with the individual, as does the blood sugar level at which they develop. It is usual for them to develop when the level falls to 2.8 to 3.3 mmol/l. Symptoms include hunger, weakness, tremor, apprehension, sweating and confusion. Hypoglycaemia can be very distressing and self-monitoring of blood glucose is a useful tool in preventing it. The causes of a low blood sugar include:

- increased energy expenditure such as extra or unexpected activity
- delayed or missed meal
- lack of carbohydrate at a meal
- mismeasurement of the insulin dose
- stress
- emotional trauma
- alcohol
- gastrointestinal disorder which causes anorexia, vomiting or diarrhoea
- weight loss reducing insulin resistance and so making insulin more effective
- renal failure
- hot weather, during which insulin is absorbed more rapidly.

The diabetic is usually aware of the symptoms of hypoglycaemia. When they are experienced, three sugar lumps or glucose tablets (= 15 g carbohydrate) should be taken.

This quick-acting carbohydrate should be followed by a snack containing a slower-acting carbohydrate such as sandwiches or fruit. This snack is additional to the next meal and is intended to prevent the blood glucose from dropping again before the next meal.

People with Type 1 need to carry some form of rapidly absorbed carbohydrate, such as glucose tablets or sugar lumps, with them in case of hypoglycaemia. They should also carry some form of diabetic identification.

Patients in hospital should be allowed to keep their own supply of rapidly absorbed carbohydrate, so that they can manage hypoglycaemic events themselves (BDA 1994).

If symptoms routinely occur at the same time, both the diet and the insulin regime should be reviewed.

DIET IN ILLNESS

During illness, energy requirements increase as a response to the metabolic stress, more glucose is released from body stores and the blood glucose level rises. Therefore, it is important to monitor blood glucose and to continue taking medication. It may be necessary for the insulin dose to be increased to prevent ketoacidosis.

People with diabetes need to be taught that if they are ill they need to:

- continue medication
- drink plenty of fluid
- test blood at least 4-hourly
- if vomiting or illness continues or the patient is concerned, call the doctor.

It may be that during a period of illness a person with non-insulin-dependent diabetes will require insulin for a short time.

It is important that during periods of illness the usual insulin dose is maintained. If, because of illness,

---

Box 27.6 Carbohydrate exchanges suitable for diet in illness

50 ml Lucozade
Two heaped teaspoons drinking chocolate powder
One tablespoon undiluted Ribena
One small glass orange juice (100 ml)
One cup thick soup
200 ml milk
Two level teaspoons glucose powder or sugar
One small scoop ice-cream

---

appetite is lost and the usual diet cannot be eaten, then other carbohydrate-containing foods such as milk drinks, fruit juice, soups and ice-creams can be eaten instead—see Box 27.6 for portion sizes.

THE COST OF THE DIABETIC DIET

Diabetics should not need to spend more on food when they are on a diet unless their previous diet was particularly poor or unusual. Those who find the diet expensive are usually the diabetics who are buying expensive diabetic products or large amounts of fresh fruit and vegetables out of season (see Chapter 14 on healthy eating on a budget).

REFERENCES

British Diabetic Association (BDA) 1988 Diabetes in the United Kingdom. British Diabetic Association, London
British Diabetic Association (BDA) Nutrition Sub-Committee 1990 Sucrose and fructose in the diabetic diet. Diabetic Medicine 7: 764–769
British Diabetic Association (BDA) Nutrition Sub-Committee 1992a Dietary recommendations for people with diabetes: an update for the 1990s. Diabetic Medicine 9: 189–202
British Diabetic Association (BDA) Nutrition Sub-Committee 1992b Discussion paper on the role of 'diabetic' foods. Diabetic Medicine 9: 300–306
British Diabetic Association (BDA) 1994 Diabetes: what care to expect in hospital. British Diabetic Association, London
British Medical Association (BMA) and Royal Pharmaceutical Society of Great Britain (RPS) British National Formulary. BMA and RPS, London (Published March and September each year)
Cruickshank J K, Cooper J, Burnett M, MacDuff J, Drubra U 1991 Ethnic differences in fasting plasma C-peptide and insulin in relation to glucose tolerance and blood pressure. Lancet 338: 842–847
Department of Health (DoH) 1991 Dietary reference values for food energy and nutrients for the United Kingdom. Report of the Panel on Dietary Reference Values of the Committee on Medical Aspects of Food Policy (COMA) (Report on Health and Social Subjects 41). HMSO, London

Department of Health (DoH) 1994 Nutritional aspects of cardiovascular disease. Report of the Cardiovascular Review Group of the Committee on Medical Aspects of Food Policy (COMA) (Report on Health and Social Subjects 46). HMSO, London
European Association for the Study of Diabetes (EASD) 2000 Diabetes and Nutrition Study Group. Recommendations for the nutritional management of patients with diabetes mellitus. European Journal of Clinical Nutrition 54: 353–355
Expert Committee on the Diagnosis and Classification of Diabetes Mellitus 1999 Committee report. Diabetes Care 22 (Supp 1): S5–S19
Fuller J H, Shipley M J, Rose G, Jarrett R J, Keen H 1983 Mortality from coronary heart disease and stroke in relation to degree of glycaemia: the Whitehall study. British Medical Journal 287: 267–270
Govindji A 1991 Dietary advice for the Asian diabetic. Practical Diabetes 8(5): 202–203
Greenhaugh T, Helman C, Chowdhury A M 1998 Health beliefs and folk models of diabetes in British Bangladeshis: a qualitative study. British Medical Journal 316: 978–983
Harris M I, Klein R, Welborn T A, Kuniman M W 1992 Onset of NIDDM occurs at least 5–7 years before clinical diagnosis. Diabetes Care 15(7): 815–819

Horton E S 1986 Exercise and physical training: effects on insulin sensitivity and glucose metabolism. Diabetes Metabolic Review 2: 1–17

Jarvi A E, Karlstrom B E, Granfeldt Y E, Bjorck I E, Asp N G, Vessby B O 1999 Improved glycaemic control and lipid profile and normalised fibrinolytic activity on a low glycaemic index diet in type 2 diabetic patients. Diabetes Care 22(1): 10–18

Jenkins D J A, Wolever T M S, Taylor R H et al 1980 Rate of digestion of foods and postprandial glycaemia in normal and diabetic subjects. British Medical Journal 2: 14–17

Jenkins D J A, Wolever T M S, Jenkins A L, Josse R G, Wong G S 1984 The glycaemic response to carbohydrate foods. Lancet 2: 388–391

Kuhl C 1991 Insulin secretion and insulin resistance in pregnancy and GDM. Implications for diagnosis and management. Diabetes 40 (Suppl 2): 18–24

Lafrance L, Rabasa-Lhoret R, Poisson D, Ducros F, Chiasson J L 1998 Effects of different glycaemic index foods and dietary fibre intake on glycaemic control in Type 1 diabetic patients on intensive insulin therapy. Diabetic Medicine 15(11): 972–978

Lean M E J, Powrie J K, Anderson A S, Garthwaite P H 1990 Obesity, weight loss and prognosis in Type 2 diabetes. Diabetic Medicine 7: 228–233

Magrath G, Hartland B V and the Nutrition Sub-Committee of the British Diabetic Association's Professional Advisory Committee 1993 Dietary recommendations for children and adolescents with diabetes: an implementation paper. Journal of Human Nutrition and Dietetics 6: 491–507

Mather H M, Keen H 1985 The Southall diabetes survey: prevalence of known diabetes in Asians and Europeans. British Medical Journal 291: 1081–1084

National Institute of Diabetes, Digestive and Kidney Diseases (NIDDKD) 1993 Diabetes control and complications trial. New England Journal of Medicine 329(14): 977–986

Shaw M, Lawson V (eds) (for the Paediatric Group of the British Dietetic Association) 2001 Clinical paediatric dietetics, 2nd Edn. Blackwell Science, Oxford

Simmons D, Williams D R R, Powell M J 1991 The Coventry Diabetes Study: prevalence of diabetes and impaired glucose tolerance in Europids and Asians. Quarterly Journal of Medicine, New Series 81(296): 1021–1030

FURTHER READING

American Diabetes Association 2001a Position Statement. Tests of glycemia in diabetes. Diabetes Care 24 (Suppl 1)

American Diabetes Association 2001b Position Statement. Nutrition recommendations and principles for people with diabetes mellitus. Diabetes Care 24 (Suppl 1)

Amos A F, McCarty D J, Zimmet P 1997 The rising global burden of diabetes and its complications: estimates and projections to the year 2010. Diabetic Medicine 14 (Suppl 5): S1–S85

British Diabetic Association (BDA) Nutrition Sub-Committee 1991 Dietary recommendations for people with diabetes: an update for the 1990s. Journal of Human Nutrition and Dietetics 4: 393–412

Day J L 1998 Living with diabetes. The British Diabetic Association guide for those treated with insulin. John Wiley & Sons, Chichester

Day J L 1998 Living with diabetes. The British Diabetic Association guide for those treated with diet and tablets. John Wiley & Sons, Chichester

Frost G, Wilding J, Beecham J 1994 Dietary advice based on the glycaemic index improves dietary profile and

metabolic control in type 2 diabetic patients. Diabetic Medicine 11

Krentz A J 2000 Churchill's Pocketbook of Diabetes. Churchill Livingstone, Edinburgh

Laing S P, Swerdlow A J, Slater S D et al 1999 The British Diabetic Association Cohort Study I: All-cause mortality in patients with insulin-treated diabetes mellitus. Diabetic Medicine 16: 459–465

MacKinnan M 1998 Providing diabetes care in general practice. A practical guide for the Primary Care Team, 3rd Edn. Class Publishing, London

Mandrup-Poulsen T 1998 Diabetes. British Medical Journal 316: 1221–1225

Vermeulen A, Turnbull W H 2000 Feasibility of the G I guide to increase knowledge about the glycaemic index in practice. Journal of Human Nutrition 13: 397–405

Viberti G C, Marshall S, Beech R et al 1996 Report on renal disease in diabetes. Diabetic Medicine 13 (9 Suppl 4): S6–S12

USEFUL ADDRESSES

Diabetes UK (NB Formerly The British Diabetic Association)
10 Queen Anne Street
London W1G 9LH
Tel: 020 7323 1531
Website: www.diabetes.org.uk

Patients with diabetes should be encouraged to join the
Association as its local branch meetings provide a link
between diabetics. The literature published by the
Association includes a wide range of leaflets, booklets,
videos and a bi-monthly magazine, *Balance* (also available
on cassette), which give practical advice about a wide
variety of topics.

28

Diet in some disorders encountered in paediatrics

See also Chapter 15, 'Diet in Infancy, Childhood and Adolescence'; Chapter 16, 'Diet and Dental Disease'; 'Coeliac Disease' in Chapter 24, 'Diet in Disorders of the Gastrointestinal Tract'; Chapter 27, 'Diet in Diabetes Mellitus'

LEARNING OBJECTIVES

After studying this chapter you should be able to:

- describe the causes and treatment of failure to thrive
- describe the practical difficulties encountered by parents and carers when providing therapeutic diets for children
- explain the dietary treatment of cystic fibrosis
- outline the scientific rationales for diets used for the treatment of paediatric metabolic disorders
- describe the causes, symptoms and treatment of food allergies and intolerances.

The imposition of dietary restrictions or modifications on any individual requires careful monitoring to ensure that optimal nutrition is maintained. This is especially important for infants and children, as adequate nutrition is essential for their normal growth and development as well as the maintenance of good health.

Having a child on a special diet imposes many restrictions and strains on the family. For example, treats like an ice-cream at the seaside, or a visit to a friend's home for tea, can require careful planning. It is important that everybody involved in a child's care understands the diet. This includes relatives, child minders, nurses, health visitors and teachers.

This chapter is not intended to give detailed explanations of all the dietary modifications used in paediatric practice, particularly in specialist units, but rather to explain those diets most usually encountered in clinical practice by health workers. This will enable them to understand the reason for the diet and enable them to support parents and carers of children whose diets require specific modifications. Sources of information on diets not mentioned in this chapter are included in the list of further reading.

MONITORING OF GROWTH

Accurate records of weight and height and comparison with standards are the only way in which a child's growth can be monitored accurately. These weights and heights should be plotted on the correct centile charts (Tanner et al 1966). These charts are available from the Child Growth Foundation (see useful addresses at the end of this chapter). There are different charts for males and females and special charts for preterm infants (Gairdner & Pearson 1983). By a comparison of the points plotted on the chart it can be seen whether the infant/child's growth is proceeding in the expected way. Standards exist for weight-for-height-for-age, weight-for-height, weight-for-height velocity, head circumference and mid-arm circumference.

Weight. Infants should be weighed nude and children should be weighed in their vest and pants.

Height. Children under the age of 3 years should be measured lying supine on a flat surface using a sliding board which is brought into contact with the child's heels. Children over this age should be measured standing upright with bare feet.

When plotted, the heights and weights should not differ from each other by more than two major centiles. It is usual to measure the head circumference of children aged under 2 years. The stunting of growth and failure of the head circumference to increase correctly indicate chronic malnutrition. If a child is only marginally malnourished, even though the child is underweight, normal growth can still occur. In this situation a diet history will give valuable information as to the child's normal diet and eating habits and give guidance as to the likelihood of any specific nutrient deficiencies being present.

FEEDING THE LOW-BIRTH-WEIGHT (LBW) BABY

The choice of feed for a LBW baby is complex and should be reviewed regularly by a specialist paediatric dietitian who will modify the feed's composition as the infant progresses. The following three factors influence the choice of feed:

- Gestational age—babies born preterm have immature kidneys, liver and gastrointestinal systems. Nutrients must be provided in a form that can be metabolised by these immature systems.
- Actual weight—the actual weight of the child in relation to his or her gestational age will show whether the child has suffered intrauterine growth retardation (IUGR). These children will have a higher energy and protein requirement than those who have not suffered IUGR, so that they can 'catch up' on this growth.
- Any medical condition the infant has.

These babies all have higher nutrient requirements than babies whose birth-weight is normal. Their requirements for fluid, energy and protein are summarised in Table 28.1.

Table 28.1 Nutritional requirements of normal-birth-weight (NBW) and low-birth-weight (LBW) babies aged 0–3 months (ESPGAN 1987, from DoH 1991 with permission)

Nutrient	Quantity/kg body weight/day	
	NBW	LBW
Fluid	150 ml	150–200 ml
Energy	100–115 kcal	130 kcal
Protein	2.1 g	3–4 g

Mode of feeding

Babies born prior to 26 weeks gestational age will require parenteral nutrition in specialist units, as their gut is not mature enough for enteral feeding. After 26 weeks, enteral feeding can be started as this will aid gut maturation. At this stage, suckling is not properly developed so tube feeding is necessary until at least 34 weeks.

Frequency of feeds

It is usual for feeds to be given 1- to 2-hourly until the baby's weight has reached 1.5 to 1.8 kg.

Choice of feed for the preterm baby

Energy

Infants' needs are variable and are increased by:

- *Prematurity.* Preterm infants have a higher surface area to body-weight ratio, so have an increased requirement.
- *Intrauterine growth retardation (IUGR).* Infants whose growth has been retarded before birth need to grow

to correct this; they thus have higher energy requirements than those who are the correct weight for gestational age.

- *Metabolic state.* Stress, infection and surgery all increase energy requirements.

Energy intake should be calculated using expected weight rather than actual weight. Otherwise there will not be sufficient energy for catch-up growth.

If the decision is made to fortify a feed with an energy source, the energy:protein ratio needs to be considered to check that it is still within the acceptable range.

Fluid

Low-birth-weight infants have a fluid requirement that is higher than infants whose birth-weight is normal, but the intake of some infants may need to be restricted because of renal, cardiac or respiratory problems.

Protein

Protein requirement is higher than for term babies of normal weight. The amino acids cysteine, glycine and taurine, which are not normally essential, are essential for the preterm baby and are included in infant formulae. Care must be taken to ensure protein requirements are not exceeded, as immature organ systems are unable to cope.

Choice of carbohydrate

Intestinal disaccharidase enzymes such as lactase are not present in the gut until the 24th week of gestation and these levels vary, some infants tolerating lactose better than others. If lactose is not tolerated, infant formula and breast-milk cannot be used and a lactose-free formula should be used. Most infants tolerate the use of glucose polymers, which are often added to increase energy content of feed. If these are not tolerated, then a fat supplement may be used instead to increase the energy content of the feed.

Fats

In preterm infants the enzyme systems necessary for the conversion of the essential fatty acids linoleic and alphalinolenic to arachidonic and decosahexanoic acids, which are important for prostaglandin and phospholipid development, are lacking (Koletzko et al 1989) and these essential fatty acids, which are important for brain development, must be included in the formulation (ESPGAN 1991). Fat digestion of preterm infants is impaired, so medium-chain triglycerides may be used.

Vitamins and minerals

Preterm infants have a low store of minerals (iron, copper, zinc, calcium, magnesium and phosphorus) and therefore have increased requirements to ensure that stores are adequate.

The feed options available are:

1. totally breast-fed
2. breast-feeding plus low-birth-weight formula
3. breast-feeding plus use of a breast-milk fortifier
4. low-birth-weight formula
5. standard formula
6. specialist formula.

Infants fed breast-milk require extra vitamin A. Infants fed pooled breast-milk which has been heat treated will also require vitamin C, thiamin and folate.

Wherever possible breast-milk should be included in the infant's diet, as it exerts a favourable effect on the neurodevelopment of infants born preterm (Lucas et al 1994). Mothers of preterm infants produce a breast-milk which is different in composition from that of mothers of term babies, and breast-feeding should be encouraged. However, it is unlikely that the optimum amount of energy will be supplied and it seems that currently the best way to feed preterm babies is a combination of both human breast-milk and a low-birth-weight infant formula or fortified breast-milk.

Term LBW babies

These babies have been exposed to some intrauterine growth retardation and weigh less than the 10th centile for post-conception age. They are born with smaller glycogen and lower body-fat stores than their better-nourished counterparts. This means that they are more susceptible to hypoglycaemia if allowed to go for periods without food, so may need to be woken for regular feeds.

Weaning the preterm baby

The preterm baby is very demanding and it is not surprising that parents are eager to reduce the frequency of feeding by the introduction of solid foods. Parents need to understand the difference between birth age and post-conceptional age and be supported so that they do not introduce solids at an inappropriately early age.

When deciding when to wean the preterm baby, the degree of prematurity, chronological age, developmental level and rate of growth of the baby all need to be considered. The introduction of solids should be postponed until the infant weighs more than 5 kg, has lost the extrusion reflex and is able to eat from a spoon (DoH 1994).

FAILURE TO THRIVE (FTT)

Failure to thrive exists when infants and young children do not achieve their expected rate of growth. This can easily be identified by serial measurements of growth, height and, in children under 2 years old, head circumference, plotted longitudinally on centile charts. A decline in rate of weight gain is the first sign of FTT. This is followed by decline in gain in length and finally in reduced increase in head circumference. Infants whose weight is persistently more than two major centiles below their height centile show FTT. Stunting of growth and head circumference occurs in prolonged and severe FTT and can be associated with a reduction in mental ability.

The incidence of FTT is varied and is greatest in inner city areas (Moy et al 1990). It is always caused by under-nutrition. However, the causes of this under-nutrition are varied and are discussed by Skuse (1992). FTT identified in infants is likely to be due to physiological causes which will respond to the appropriate medical treatment and appropriate feeding, for example:

- neurological problems
  — poor swallowing/sucking
  — oral hypersensitivity
- reflux
- cystic fibrosis
- coeliac disease
- lactose intolerance.

However, it may also be caused by inadequate feeding and an accurate dietary assessment plays an important part in the diagnosis and treatment of FTT. Iron-deficiency anaemia can result in poor appetite leading to poor weight gain.

In older infants and toddlers the previously listed causes may still be important, but in many cases no organic cause is identified and the problems are due to a combination of behavioural and social problems. Many older infants and toddlers are fussy eaters and go through periods of food refusal. This does not always result in FTT but in some situations the problems are particularly acute or the carer is unable to resolve them and FTT develops.

Causes of FTT in older infants and toddlers

Poor parenting skills

- Carers may be unaware of their child's nutritional needs so feed an inappropriate diet.
- Some carers are unhappy about allowing children to experiment with food and learn to feed themselves because it is too messy.

Health workers can help carers to understand why their child is failing to thrive and help them to overcome the problems.

Family diet

- If the family diet includes frequent snacks and drinks, such as biscuits, crisps and fruit squashes, the child will not be hungry at meal times. The snacks and drinks usually have a high fat and sugar content and low vitamin and mineral contents.
- Children whose diets contain a lot of less energy-dense foods (fruit and vegetables) at the expense of other more energy-dense foods (bread, cereals, potatoes, rice and protein foods) will not have a sufficient energy intake. This can result in FTT (Clark & Cockburn 1988).

Delayed weaning

A diet of infant formula alone does not provide sufficient energy or nutrients beyond 6 months-of-age. If a large volume is consumed beyond this age, this will reduce the appetite for more energy-dense foods.

Child's temperament

Some children are slow eaters and do not enjoy eating, while others are not prepared to concentrate for long enough to finish a meal or are conservative, not wanting to try new tastes or textures.

Carers need to be helped to accept their child's limitations and be prepared to spend time encouraging their child to eat and enjoy food, and be confident in their own ability to help their child.

Poverty

Poverty can result in difficulty in obtaining and preparing an adequate diet for all members of the family. It can also mean that the children's diet relies heavily on snack foods which reduce the appetite for other foods.

Treatment of FTT

If the cause of FTT is identified as malabsorption or poor dietary intake due to a medical condition, this can be overcome by reviewing the child's current diet and then either fortifying the child's diet or providing nutrients in forms that can be absorbed, for example changing to a lactose-free infant formula. However, in many situations no specific medical cause is identified and the best approach is treatment by a team which includes a speech and language therapist, a health visitor, a paediatrician, a social worker, a clinical psychologist and a dietitian.

There are two aims for the treatment of FTT:

1. Improve the child's nutritional status to ensure normal growth and development.
2. Maintain the improved nutritional status.

If the cause of FTT is behavioural, then a third aim is to enable parents and carers to manage their child's behaviour.

Strategies for overcoming food refusal

- *Provide regular meals and snacks.* This means that the child does not go for long periods without food, so becoming too bad tempered to eat, and also helps carers say 'no' to between meal snacks of sweets and biscuits which reduce appetite for meals.
- *Include nutrient-dense foods in all meals.* Foods like fruit and vegetables, although full of vitamins and minerals, are poor sources of energy and protein, so meals should also include a starchy food such as bread, potato or breakfast cereal and a protein food.
- *Never force the child to eat.*
- *Set a time-limit for meals.* 20 minutes is appropriate unless the child is a very slow eater. Once this has been reached, the meal is cleared away and nothing else is eaten until the next official snack/meal time.
- *Try to make meal times shared, pleasant occasions.* Carers and their children should look forward to, rather than dread, meals and meals should become social events. Many fussy eaters eat well on picnics or at friends' houses and try foods as part of a school meal that they would not eat at home.
- *Praise.* Children respond well to praise and any improvement in their dietary habits should be acknowledged and praised by their carers.

A study by Wright et al (1998) showed that structured health visitor intervention within the community dietetic, paediatric and social work interventions, if required, resulted in better long-term weight and height gain than conventional hospital-based management of FTT.

CYSTIC FIBROSIS

This is an inherited disorder which is estimated to have an incidence of 1 in 2500 live births (BPA 1988); it is usually diagnosed in early childhood. The symptoms are FTT and recurrent respiratory infections. Its diagnosis is confirmed by a sweat test when the sweat is found to have an abnormally high sodium content.

The exocrine glands of the body produce abnormally thick, viscid secretions. All of these exocrine glands are affected but most of the clinical problems are due to involvement of those glands in the lungs and pancreas. The frequent and severe chest infections result from the congestion of the lungs and cause permanent lung damage. Before improved treatment with antibiotics, mucolytic agents and physiotherapy, these were a common cause of death.

Pancreatic exocrine insufficiency is present in 90% of cases of cystic fibrosis and, for these individuals, normal digestion and absorption of fat cannot occur and pancreatic enzyme supplements are essential. The abnormal secretions produced by the pancreas block the ducts, eventually causing fibrosis of the gland. The incidence of diabetes mellitus is much higher than that in the normal population and increases with age. Cystic fibrosis is a cause of malnutrition and FTT and is a well-documented cause of short stature (Gaskin et al 1990). The causes of malnutrition are summarised in Table 28.2.

Recent studies show that aggressive nutritional intervention is essential to ensure and maintain proper growth and development (Corey et al 1988). Not only does improving nutritional status enhance growth, but it has also been shown to improve depressed immunological systems and increase respiratory muscle strength, which are both important in preserving lung function. Dietary treatment must ensure a high intake of all nutrients. The calorie intake should never be less than the estimated average requirement (EAR) of a noncystic child of similar age and activity and it is usual to aim for 120 to 150% of the EAR. This is difficult to achieve, especially during periods of infection, which are accompanied by loss of appetite. The high calorie intake is usually achieved by a high-fat, high-sugar diet which includes frequent snacks as well as regular meals (see example of a day's meals in Box 28.1).

Table 28.2   Summary of causes of malnutrition in cystic fibrosis

Cause	Treatment
Malabsorption of protein, fat and fat-soluble vitamins due to pancreatic insufficiency	Routine use of pancreatic supplements Daily supplements of the fat-soluble vitamins A, D, E, K Ensure energy and protein content of diet adequate to compensate for losses

Increased requirement of energy due to:
    energy lost in stools
    malabsorption
    energy cost of expectorating sputum
    energy cost of chronic infections
	Increase dietary intake of energy-dense, high-sugar, high-fat foods
	Use of energy supplements such as Maxijul

Reduced dietary intake due to:
    loss of appetite during periods of infection
    vomiting associated with coughing
    meal-time anxiety, created by loss of appetite and
    knowledge that dietary intake is essential to maintain
    good health
	Provision of small high-energy meals
	Use of dietary supplements
	Enteral feeding

Box 28.1   Examples of a day's meals for a child with cystic fibrosis

Breakfast

Cereal with full-cream milk and sugar
Toast, butter and jam
Fruit juice and energy supplement*

Mid-morning

Packet of crisps
Squash and energy supplement*

Lunchtime

Cheese sandwich
Chocolate biscuit
Fruit yoghurt (full-fat)
Piece of fruit
Drink containing energy supplement*

Mid-afternoon

Glass of milk
Two biscuits

Evening meal

Meat or fish (fried or grilled)
Chips or mashed potato with butter or margarine added
Vegetables
Fruit pie and custard

Bedtime

Milk drink
Toast, butter and jam

*Energy supplement—it is usual to use a glucose polymer such as Maxijul (see Chapter 23).

Enteral feeding

During periods of infection it may be impossible to achieve an adequate intake and it is likely that there will be periods when enteral feeding will be necessary, either to prevent further weight loss or aid regaining of weight that has been lost.

Feeding may be overnight for short periods, for example the fortnight while individuals are in hospital for intravenous antibiotic treatment for lung infections, or long-term for some people. It is usual to use standard polymeric feeds (see Chapter 23). For children weighing less than 20 kg, a specialist paediatric enteral feed should be used. Nasogastric, jejunostomy or gastrostomy tubes can all be used. The use of a gastrostomy button is gaining in popularity for long-term feeding. The overnight feeding regime should stop at least 1 hour before the morning physiotherapy session.

Pancreatic enzyme supplements are necessary for the digestion and absorption of the feed. They can be either added to the feed or taken before and during tube-feeding. The actual practice depends on the routine practice of specific units. Overnight enteral feeding does result in a reduction of daytime nutrient intake. However, long-term studies of patients who have been enterally fed have shown that even so there is an increase in total energy intake which is beneficial (Ramsey et al 1992).

A diet for a child with cystic fibrosis can be particularly difficult for other people to understand, as it contradicts the basics of healthy eating. Children are encouraged to increase the energy content by eating fatty foods and foods which have been fried, and include sugar and sugary foods in their diet. The reason for this is that fats and sugar are concentrated sources of energy and, without adequate energy, the child will not grow properly and will be less resistant to infections. As the dietary intake of sucrose is likely to be high, special care must be taken with dental care and, wherever possible, foods containing sucrose should be included as part of a meal rather than as a between-meal snack.

Pancreatic enzyme supplements

Pancreatic enzyme supplements are available in powder, tablet or capsule forms. Most UK centres use enteric-coated microspheres which are administered as granules or gelatine capsules. They need to be taken with each meal and snack. Individuals' requirements for pancreatic enzyme supplements vary and depend on the severity of their condition (Owen et al 1991). The optimal dose for an individual controls the frequency of bowel movements to an acceptable level and prevents abdominal discomfort.

It is usual for infants to be given their enzyme supplement before their feed. Enteric-coated granules are mixed with expressed breast-milk, infant formula or puréed fruit and given from a spoon.

Dietary supplements

These should be used routinely when nutrient intake is poor, perhaps due to a respiratory infection, when growth is inadequate and when nutrient requirements are increased. They should be used in addition to food rather than in place of it.

The glucose polymer energy supplements can easily be routinely added to drinks without the child feeling difficult or awkward. Nutritional supplements, if needed, should be given as sip-feeds after meals and at bedtime, rather than between or before meals when they will reduce the child's meal-time appetite.

PHENYLKETONURIA (PKU)

PKU is a recessively inherited condition, with an incidence in the UK of 1 in 10 000 live births. The enzyme phenylalanine hydroxylase is lacking and so the conversion of the amino acid phenylalanine to tyrosine is impaired. Phenylalanine is an essential amino acid and is present in most protein-containing foods. Approximately 5% of dietary protein is phenylalanine.

Failure of conversion of the phenylalanine in the diet to tyrosine results in an accumulation of abnormal phenylalanine breakdown products known as phenyl ketones. Failure to treat PKU means that these accu-

mulated products cause progressive brain damage and intellectual impairment. Early diagnosis and treatment of the condition is essential to prevent intellectual impairment.

In the UK all infants are screened for PKU by the Guthrie test between 6 and 10 days after birth (Guthrie & Susi 1963). Infants with PKU have normal blood phenylalanine levels at birth, the raised levels only developing following the introduction of breast- or formula-milk feeds.

Aims of dietary treatment of PKU

This section outlines the principles of treatment. If more detailed recommendations are required, Shaw & Lawson (2001) should be consulted.

Phenylalanine is an essential amino acid, so it cannot be totally excluded from the diet. There are four aims of dietary treatment of PKU:

- reduction of dietary intake of phenylalanine to a level which ensures that the plasma phenylalanine level is within the normal range (120–360 μmol/l)
- supplementation of the diet with tyrosine, as sufficient quantities are not produced by the conversion of phenylalanine
- provision of adequate intakes of all other nutrients to ensure optimal growth
- enabling the child and family to continue to enjoy their food.

Regular monitoring of the blood phenylalanine levels is used to assess the success of the diet and as a basis for modifying its phenylalanine content, the frequency of monitoring depending on the child's age and state of health. It is usual for blood levels to be measured once-a-week until the age of 4 years, as this is the time of most rapid growth and when dietary intake can be unpredictable, for example during weaning and toddler tantrums. After the age of 4 years, growth is less rapid and eating habits better established.

Feeding infants with PKU

Many mothers have already established breast-feeding when the positive result of a Guthrie test is confirmed. They will need to stop breast-feeding their infants for a short period of time, so that the infant can be fed a prescribed phenylalanine-free substitute until the infant's raised plasma phenylalanine level has dropped. During this time the mother should maintain her lactation by expressing her milk. The infant can then be stabilised on a regime of a measured amount of the phenylalanine-free formula before five or six of the breast-feeds, combined with demand breast-feeding. The volume of formula given depends on the plasma levels of phenylalanine.

Infants who are not breast-fed are fed measured quantities of phenylalanine-free formula and ordinary infant-formula milk.

Feeding children with PKU

The diet for a child with PKU has four components:

1. *Phenylalanine-free protein supplement which contains tyrosine.* The phenylalanine-free infant formula is replaced by a phenylalanine-free protein substitute at weaning. This can be mixed to a paste and given from a spoon. For older children, other forms are available which can be taken as a flavoured drink.

2. *Phenylalanine-containing foods.* As the child is weaned, measured portions of foods which contain small amounts of protein are substituted for the infant formula and breast-feeds and become the basis around which meals are built. These measured portions of food are known as PKU exchanges and some examples are given in Box 28.2. The allowance of ordinary food is normally very small and 4 exchanges a day is the usual average for a 4-year-old.

3. *Free foods.* These are foods which do not contain protein—see Box 28.3. They are an important part of all meals and only by ensuring an adequate intake of these and special protein-free products will the diet contain enough energy.

4. *Vitamin and mineral supplements.* These are needed for children with PKU because of their very restricted diets, the actual type and amount depends on the diet of the individual child and the protein supplement used.

Monitoring of phenylalanine levels

It cannot be assumed that both raised and abnormally low phenylalanine levels are due to poor dietary compliance, as this is not always the case. Other causes of

Box 28.2 Food portions that supply approximately 50 mg phenylalanine (1 PKU exchange)	
Ordinary bread	15 g
Biscuits	15 g
Cornflakes	15 g
Rice Krispies	15 g
Milk	30 ml
Potato, boiled	80 g
Potato chips	30 g

Box 28.3 These items may be taken in unrestricted amounts by a child with PKU
Sugar
Clear boiled sweets
Syrup
Honey
Jam and marmalade
Butter and margarine
Lard
Vegetable cooking fats and oils
Tea and coffee
Fizzy drinks and squashes (not diet drinks)
Flavouring essences (not artificial sweeteners)
Spices and condiments
Cornflour and custard powder
Sago, arrowroot and tapioca

raised blood phenylalanine that should be considered, other than dietary non-compliance, are catabolism of body protein due to inadequate dietary energy intake or increased energy requirement due to infection or surgery. Low levels may occur during growth spurts or recovery from injury.

Other disorders of amino acid metabolism occur, but very infrequently. In some conditions, it may be necessary to control the intake of more than one amino acid; for example in maple syrup urine disease, the intakes of valine, leucine and isoleucine are all restricted. These three amino acids are also essential amino acids and cannot be completely excluded from the diet.

CARBOHYDRATE INTOLERANCE
Disaccharidase deficiency

This section deals with a particular aspect of the malabsorption syndrome. See also Chapter 24. It is a condition which is sometimes seen in infancy, when it causes diarrhoea with bulky or frothy acid stools and FTT. Normally, carbohydrate digestion proceeds as shown in Figure 28.1, the simple sugars (monosaccharides) being finally absorbed into the body.

A common cause of carbohydrate intolerance is insufficient activity of one or more of the disaccharide-splitting enzymes. This results in the presence in the bowel of abnormally large amounts of the sugar which cannot be digested. The enzyme deficiency may be due to temporary immaturity of the gut for a period following birth or may be secondary to disease of the bowel such as in coeliac disease or gastroenteritis. Carbohydrate intolerance due to an inborn defect of carbohydrate-digesting enzymes occurs, although more rarely.

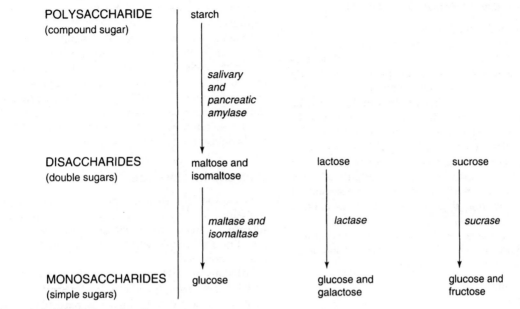

Figure 28.1 Carbohydrate digestion.

Treatment of malabsorption is dietary and consists of identifying the cause of the malabsorption and the sugar that is being malabsorbed (see Table 28.3). This malabsorbed sugar is then excluded from the diet and replaced with an alternative energy source, so ensuring that the diet is still nutritionally adequate.

Lactose intolerance

This condition is usually transitory, developing when the intestinal mucosa is damaged, for example by gastroenteritis or in coeliac disease. Congenital alactasia does exist but is very rare.

Diet for infants with lactose intolerance

The milk of all mammals contains lactose and cannot be used (this includes breast-milk); neither can infant-formula milks. Specialised lactose-free infant formulae are available. These include:

- SMA LF (SMA Nutrition)
- AL 110 (Nestle)
- Enfamil Lactofree (Mead Johnson)
- Glactomin Formula 17 (Scientific Hospital Supplies).

Suitable weaning foods are milk-free baby rice and puréed fruits and vegetables. If commercially prepared weaning foods are used, their contents should be studied carefully to ensure that they do not contain milk or milk products. As weaning progresses, other suitable foods from the list of foods suitable for lactose-intolerant children can be included.

Table 28.3 Carbohydrates which need to be excluded from the diet in carbohydrate intolerance

Condition	Carbohydrate(s) not tolerated	Tolerance of small amounts of some carbohydrate(s)
Congenital alactasia	Lactose	No
Secondary lactase deficiency	Lactose	Maybe
Sucrase–isomaltase deficiency	Sucrose	Maybe
Hereditary fructose intolerance	Fructose Sucrose Sorbitol	No

Lactose-free diet for toddlers and older children

As all milk and milk products are excluded from the diet, an alternative substitute must be included to ensure an adequate calcium intake. If the child was accustomed to, and enjoyed, milk prior to developing the intolerance he or she may be unwilling to drink the substitute as it tastes different. This problem can be overcome by flavouring the milk or using it in cooking, for making custard and sauces. Some children are able to tolerate the traces of lactose that remain in the following cheeses—reduced-fat Cheddar, Edam and Gouda. However, many will need an additional calcium supplement prescribed for them, as the amount of milk substitute that they consume does not contain sufficient of this mineral.

Lists of lactose-free products are available and it is not only those foods which contain milk that should be avoided but also those containing:

- skimmed milk powder
- milk solids
- non-fat milk solids
- whey and whey products.

Foods to avoid. Some examples of foods to avoid, or about which details should be sought as to the ingredients used in their manufacture and preparation are:

- milk, cheese, ice-cream, butter and margarine
- bought breads, biscuits, cakes and pastries, unless known to be free from milk
- prepared cake and pudding mixes
- proprietary infant foods
- breakfast cereals
- canned or packet soups and sauces
- confectionery.

Foods permitted are:

- bread—check with manufacturer that it is milk-free
- unmixed starchy foods such as flour, cornflour, rice, semolina, oatmeal, sago and tapioca
- vegetable oils and cooking fats
- milk-free margarine and low-fat spreads
- fresh meat, fish and eggs
- fresh, frozen or dried vegetables, or vegetables canned in brine
- fresh, frozen, canned or dried fruit
- fruit juices
- jam, marmalade, honey and syrup
- tea, coffee made from coffee grounds, soft drinks.

Where proprietary foods are concerned, lactose-free varieties are frequently available. Most manufacturers will supply information about the lactose content if requested.

The degree of intolerance will depend on the degree of damage to the intestinal villus and the child's normal milk intake. For example, a child with secondary lactose intolerance following gastroenteritis may be able to tolerate the small amount of milk present in milk-containing foods such as biscuits. In practice this child does not need to select a diet of totally milk-free foods but cannot tolerate milk drinks.

Sucrose intolerance

This is due to deficiency of the enzyme sucrase-isomaltase and is rare. It is identified either once sucrose is introduced into the diet during weaning or sometimes in babies whose feeds are fortified with glucose polymers.

The daily sucrose intake of children and adults is variable and symptoms can be intermittent, only occurring when sucrose intake is particularly high, making the diagnosis of sucrose intolerance difficult.

Children find the exclusion of all sucrose-containing foods (such as sweets, biscuits and cakes) from their diet very difficult and may decide to tolerate their diarrhoea rather than exclude sucrose. If this decision is made, the child's growth must be monitored to ensure that the resulting malabsorption is not so great as to cause malnutrition which inhibits growth.

Sucrose is present in many manufactured savoury products. Glucose and honey can be used in most situations to replace sucrose and some low-sucrose products are available.

Fructose intolerance

This is a hereditary disorder caused by deficiency of the enzyme fructose-1-phosphate aldolase B which is found in the liver and kidney as well as the small intestine.

The dietary treatment is lifelong and is the strict exclusion of all foods containing fructose, sucrose and sorbitol. This is because:

- sucrose is digested to glucose and fructose
- sorbitol is converted to fructose in the liver.

If fructose is not excluded from the diet, liver and kidney damage can be caused. This condition is usually diagnosed once fructose-containing foods are introduced at weaning. The symptoms include poor feeding, FTT, vomiting and abdominal distension.

Fructose occurs naturally in:

- fruits
- some vegetables such as sweetcorn and root vegetables
- honey.

These foods should be excluded from the diet, as should all foods which contain sucrose.

A fructose-free diet is likely to require supplementation with vitamin C and folate, as they are provided by fruit and vegetables in the diet. An adequate intake of cereal fibre should be encouraged to compensate for the lack of fruit and vegetable fibre.

GALACTOSAEMIA

Galactosaemia is an inherited disorder of galactose metabolism. The simple sugar galactose is converted to glucose in the body as a result of a series of chemical reactions, each of which requires the presence of a specific enzyme. There are three forms of this disorder; in the most commonly occurring form the enzyme galactose-1-phosphate uridyl transferase is deficient. This causes an accumulation in the tissues of galactose and intermediate conversion products, galactose-1-phosphate, galactitol and galactonic acid. These cause damage to the brain, liver and kidneys, and to the lens of the eye causing cataracts. Symptoms develop during the first few days or weeks of life and include vomiting, refusal of food, loss of weight, FTT and jaundice.

Diet

The major dietary source of galactose is lactose present in milk and products containing milk, which is digested to glucose and galactose. In galactosaemia, milk and its products must be excluded from the diet. This diet must be continued for life and kept to strictly. There are long-term complications of galactosaemia (Schweitzer et al 1993) which include learning disability, growth retardation and speech abnormalities.

As well as foods containing lactose, two other groups of foods are excluded from the diet. These are:

- foods rich in nucleoproteins, such as offal and eggs
- foods containing galactosides—pulses, soya protein, chocolate and nuts.

There is no consensus on this but it is usual to exclude them for at least the first 2 years of life. A specialist infant formula such as Infasoy (Cow & Gate), Wysoy (SMA Nutrition), Glactomin Formula 17 (Scientific Hospital Supplies) or Farley's Soya Formula (Farley/

Heinz) must be used in infancy and the infant cannot be breast-fed.

Weaning

Following the introduction of weaning, care should be taken to exclude any foods likely to contain traces of milk, egg and soya. These will be in many manufactured foods and only the most recent information about a product's ingredients should be referred to, as recipes and formulations for manufactured foods are frequently changed.

FOOD INTOLERANCES (INCLUDING FOOD ALLERGY)

There is great interest in both the scientific and popular press about the causes of food intolerance and the conditions with which it might be associated. The term 'food intolerance' is defined as: 'any non-psychological, undesirable reaction to a specific food or ingredient' (ESPGAN 1992).

Five distinct categories of food intolerance exist including food allergy:

1. *Toxic.* The food acts as a toxic agent. For example:
   a. infected food causing gastrointestinal symptoms as in food poisoning
   b. food acting as a gastric irritant.
2. *Metabolic.* The food or specific nutrient contained in it cannot be digested or metabolised normally because of an enzyme deficiency, e.g. lactase deficiency and as in PKU (see above).
3. *Pharmacological.* Many substances which occur naturally in foods have a pharmacological effect. Individuals differ in their susceptibility to these substances and the amount needed to cause an undesirable reaction, e.g. the stimulants methylxanthines, caffeine and theobromine which occur in coffee, tea, cocoa, chocolate and cola drinks. The vasoactive amines—tyramine, which occurs in fermented products (e.g. cheese and red wine), and phenylethylamine, found in cocoa and chocolate—often trigger a migraine attack. Some foods stimulate a non-allergic production of histamine or prostaglandins. The symptoms caused are similar to those of a true food allergy but the immune system is not involved. Foods which can cause this type of reaction include red wine, eggs, strawberries, shellfish, tomatoes, citrus fruits and alcohol.
4. *Idiosyncratic.* This is a difficult category of intolerance to identify, as any food can cause an idiosyncratic food intolerance in a susceptible person. The person

responds to ingestion of this food with reproducible symptoms when challenged with the food (given a small portion of the food disguised so that they do not know whether or not they are eating the food) but no reason for the response can be identified.

5. *Food allergy.* When a true food allergy exists there is an immune response to the presence of the food. For some individuals the food may not have to be eaten. They are so sensitive that symptoms can develop rapidly once the food has entered the mouth or touched the lips. Some of the components of the food, usually proteins, are identified as harmful and antibodies are manufactured to protect against this harmful antigenic food, thus causing the allergic reaction. As the structure of proteins is changed by heating, some individuals, although allergic to the raw food, find they can tolerate the cooked food, but this is not always the case.

Food-induced anaphylaxis. This is a potentially life-threatening allergic response which occurs usually in infants and children when the food to which they are allergic is eaten. The symptoms of red itchy weals on the skin, oedema and circulatory collapse develop quickly after a very small amount of the food has been eaten. It is assumed that the individual has become sensitised to that food by the transmission of the antigen from the mother, either in breast-milk or in utero. Because of the severity of the reaction it is essential that the cause is identified immediately and excluded from the diet (Brostoff & Hawk 1991). Examples of foods which can cause this response are nuts and eggs. Peanut allergy is a particular cause of concern in the UK where it affects 1.3% of the general population (Hourihane et al 1996).

Symptoms of food intolerance

The symptoms caused by a food intolerance show individual variation in both nature and severity depending on the nature of the intolerance and the susceptibility to the food of an individual, but are specific and reproducible in an individual with a food intolerance. An example is the variation in response to red wine; the alcohol present can act as a gastric irritant causing gastritis and nausea in some individuals, while for another group the tyramine may trigger migraine, and a further group of the population are unaffected.

Symptoms of food intolerance include:

- asthma, hayfever, rhinitis
- diarrhoea, constipation, abdominal distension, vomiting, FTT

- headaches, lethargy, behavioural changes, attention deficit disorder and hyperactivity
- skin rashes, urticaria, eczema.

The foods most commonly implicated in causing a food intolerance are milk, soya, eggs, wheat and nuts. The symptoms can develop rapidly or slowly following a period of consumption of that food, e.g. milk intolerance can develop as soon as milk is introduced into the weaning diet or gradually as the milk intake increases.

Prevention of food allergy

The highest incidence of food allergy is during the first year of life. For those infants who are at risk of developing a food allergy because there is a family history of food allergy, gluten enteropathy or allergic asthma, the Committee on Medical Aspects of Food Policy (COMA) panel (DoH 1994) recommended that the following steps should be taken:

1. Breast-feeding should be encouraged for 4 to 6 months, preferably longer.
2. Early weaning should be discouraged.
3. Foods regarded as potentially allergenic should be avoided until 6 months. These include cow's milk, gluten, eggs, soya proteins, wheat and citrus fruits.

Breast-feeding has been shown to be preventive against food allergy and, in infants at high risk of developing an allergy, if the mother excludes the potential allergen from her diet this is also beneficial (Chandra et al 1989). However, if the mother is advised to do this, she will need expert help to ensure that her diet is adequate. The most likely food that will be excluded from her diet is milk and an alternative calcium source is essential.

Identification of the food intolerance

Diet history

In many cases an accurate diet history is sufficient to identify the cause of a food intolerance. This is relatively easy when the range of foods eaten is limited and the onset of symptoms is rapid. However, when the diet includes a wide range of foods and ingredients and the symptoms of the food intolerance develop slowly, a dietary history may not be as useful in identifying the cause. An accurate record of everything eaten and drunk and a record of symptoms will still be of help in identifying potential causes of the intolerance, which can then be further investigated by dietary exclusion.

Dietary exclusion

Once potential causes of the food intolerance are suspected, they are excluded from the diet totally for a period of up to 3 weeks to see if symptoms disappear or reduce. For example, a child who develops atopic eczema at weaning might be tried on a milk-free diet and if the condition improved only slightly might then be tried on an egg- and milk-free diet.

In some cases when multiple allergies are suspected or the actual allergy is difficult to identify, the infant will be fed a hydrolysed protein formula which is hypoallergenic, such as Nutramigen (Mead Johnson) or Pregestimil (Mead Johnson), or the child/adult will be kept on a very limited diet which is constructed from foods known to be unlikely to cause an intolerance and then slowly other foods are introduced into the diet.

The reintroduction of foods has to be done slowly to ensure that each food is tolerated before the next food is introduced. Foods are usually introduced in their simplest forms. For example, wheat would be introduced before bread, as bread also contains yeast and sometimes soya flour. The actual order in which foods are reintroduced depends on the individual's preference, unit policy and suspected causes of intolerance. The dietetic management of exclusion diets and a programme of reintroduction of foods is beyond the scope of this book and the section on diagnosis of food allergy and intolerance in Shaw & Lawson (2001) should be consulted.

Conditions which may be associated with food allergy

FTT

Cow's milk protein intolerance can result in gastrointestinal symptoms and FTT. In this situation an infant soya formula should not be used because the infant may also become sensitive to soya protein (Milla 1991). Infant formulas which are semi-elemental, that is they contain protein which has already been hydrolysed, such as Pregestimil (Mead Johnson), Pepti Junior (Cow & Gate) and Nutramigen (Mead Johnson) should be used. A paediatric dietitian should be part of the team caring for the child, to ensure that the nutrient intake is adequate and to provide information and guide the carers through the weaning period so that the infant's diet can become as varied as possible. Milk-free weaning foods will be necessary for weaning (see p. 292).

Atopic eczema

All children with atopic eczema do not need to go on a restricted diet. The condition of most children with eczema will improve with conventional topical treatment and will not require any dietary modification (Atherton 1988).

In those situations where the symptoms are severe and food intolerance is suspected the following foods have been implicated: milk, egg and additives. While the exclusion of additives and eggs from the diet does not pose any potential nutritional risk, a nutritionally adequate substitute for milk must be included in the diet if milk is to be excluded. Hydrolysed protein infant formula should be used in this situation.

Attention deficit disorder and hyperactivity (ADDH)

Children with ADDH need identifying and specialist help as their difficulty in concentration, irritability and recklessness can lead to antisocial behaviour and poor academic achievement. However, food intolerance is not always the cause and behavioural treatment is more successful than dietary exclusion in many situations.

The diet tried for the treatment of this condition is the exclusion of additives and preservatives. The additives and preservatives which should be avoided are:

- E102–155 artificial colours
- E210–219 benzoate preservatives
- E220–224 sulphur dioxide preservatives
- E249–252 nitrite preservatives.

It would appear that for a minority of children their behaviour is related to their diet (Kaplan et al 1989) and for them a properly supervised dietary exclusion regime, which identifies the food or foods that the child is intolerant of, is essential.

Use of alternative mammalian milks

Goats' and sheep's milk are not suitable alternatives for infant formula or breast-milk. They can be used for infants aged over 1 year as long as the milks are microbiologically safe. However, they do not have the same nutritional composition as cows' milk:

- goats' milk contains less iron, vitamin A, vitamin D and folate than cows' milk
- sheep's milk contains less iron, vitamin D and folate than cows' milk.

Children drinking these milks need the nutritional content of their diet assessed and vitamin and iron supplements may be necessary.

Nut-free diet

Some children respond to the introduction of nuts into their diet with an anaphylactic reaction. This is an extreme life-threatening response and means that a lifelong nut-free diet must be followed.

Foods which should be avoided are:

- peanuts, nuts, nut products
- groundnut oil, arachis oil
- vegetable oil
- all nut oils.

Nut products and nut oils are not always easily identified in the contents list of manufactured foods and it is easy for foods to become contaminated with traces of groundnut oil or nuts if a range of products are manufactured in the same unit. The advice must be given that if in doubt, avoid the food.

REFERENCES

Atherton D J 1988 Diet and atopic eczema. Clinical Allergy 18: 215–228

British Paediatric Association (BPA) Working Party on Cystic Fibrosis 1988 Cystic fibrosis in the United Kingdom 1977–1985: an improving picture. British Medical Journal 297: 1599–1602

Brostoff J, Hawk L J 1991 Food allergy in children. European Journal of Clinical Nutrition 45 (Suppl 1): 11–15

Chandra R K, Puri S, Hamed A 1989 Influence of maternal diet during lactation and use of formula feeds on development of atopic eczema in high risk infants. British Medical Journal 299: 228–230

Clark B, Cockburn F 1988 Fat, fibre and the under-fives. Nursing Times 84: 59–64

Corey M, McLaughlin F J, Williams M, Levison H 1988 A comparison of survival, growth and pulmonary function in patients with cystic fibrosis in Boston and Toronto. Journal of Clinical Epidemiology 41: 583–591

Department of Health (DoH) 1991 Dietary reference values for food energy and nutrients for the United Kingdom. Report of the Panel on Dietary Reference Values of the Committee on Medical Aspects of Food Policy (COMA) (Report on Health and Social Subjects 41). HMSO, London

Department of Health (DoH) 1994 Weaning and the weaning diet. Report of the Working Group on the Weaning Diet of the Committee on Medical Aspects of Food Policy (COMA) (Report on Health and Social Subjects 45). HMSO, London

European Society of Paediatric Gastroenterology and Nutrition (ESPGAN) 1987 Committee on Nutrition of the Preterm Infant. Nutrition and feeding of preterm infants. Acta Paediatrica Scandinavica (Suppl 336)

European Society of Paediatric Gastroenterology and Nutrition (ESPGAN) 1991 Committee Report. Comment on the content and composition of lipids in infant formulas. Acta Paediatrica Scandinavica 80: 887–896

European Society for Paediatric Gastroenterology and Nutrition (ESPGAN) 1992 Working Group for the Diagnostic Criteria for Food Allergy. Diagnostic criteria for food allergy with predominantly intestinal symptoms.

Journal of Pediatric Gastroenterology and Nutrition 14: 108–112

Gairdner D, Pearson J 1983 Growth and development records preterm–2 years. Castlemead Publications, Ware, Hertfordshire

Gaskin K J, Walters D L, Baur L A, Soutter V L, Gruca M A 1990 Nutritional status, growth and development in children undergoing intensive treatment for cystic fibrosis. Acta Paediatrica Scandinavica 366 (Suppl): 106–110

Guthrie R, Susi A 1963 A simple phenylalanine method for detecting phenylketonuria in large populations of new-born infants. Paediatrics 32: 338–343

Hourihane J O'B, Dean T P, Warner J O 1996 Peanut allergy in relation to heredity, maternal diet and other atopic diseases: results of a questionnaire survey, skin prick testing and food challenges. British Medical Journal 313: 518–521

Kaplan B J, McNicol J, Conte R A, Moghadam H K 1989 Dietary replacement in preschool-aged hyperactive boys. Pediatrics 83: 7–17

Koletzko B, Schmidt E, Bremer H J, Haug M, Harzer G 1989 Effects of dietary long-chain polyunsaturated fatty acids on the essential fatty acid status of premature infants. European Journal of Paediatrics 148: 669–675

Lucas A, Morley R, Coles J J, Gore S M 1994 A randomised multicentre study of human milk versus formula and later development in infants. Archives of Disease in Childhood 70: F141–146

Milla P J 1991 The clinical use of protein hydrolysates and soya formulae. European Journal of Clinical Nutrition 45 (Suppl 1): 23–28

Moy R J D, Smallman S, Booth I W 1990 Malnutrition in a UK children's hospital. Journal of Human Nutrition and Dietetics 3(2): 93–100

Owen G, Peters T J, Dawson S, Goodchild MC 1991 Pancreatic enzyme supplement dosage in cystic fibrosis. Lancet 338: 1153

Ramsey B W, Farrell P M, Penchar P 1992 Nutritional assessment and management in cystic fibrosis: a consensus report. American Journal of Clinical Nutrition 55: 108–116

Schweitzer S, Shin Y, Jacobs C, Brodehl J 1993 Long-term outcome in 134 patients with galactosaemia. European Journal of Pediatrics 152: 36–43

Shaw M, Lawson V (eds) (for the Paediatric Group of the British Dietetic Association) 2001 Clinical paediatric dietetics, 2nd Edn. Blackwell Science, Oxford

Skuse D 1992 Failure to thrive: current perspectives. Current Paediatrics: 105–110

Tanner J M, Whitehouse R H, Takaishi M 1966 Standards from birth to maturity for height, weight, height velocity and weight velocity for British children in 1965. Archives of Disease in Childhood 41: Part I: 454–471; Part II: 613–635

Wright C M, Callum J, Birks E, Jarvis S 1998 Effect of community based management in failure to thrive: randomised control trail. British Medical Journal 317: 571–574

FURTHER READING

British Dietetic Association 1990 Policy statement: food allergy and intolerance. BDA, Birmingham

Chandra R K 1997 Food hypersensitivity and allergic disease: a selective review. American Journal of Clinical Nutrition 66: 526–529

Kay A B 1998 Clinical review. ABC of allergies: good allergy practice. British Medical Journal 316: 535–537

McHenry P M, Williams H C, Bingham E A 1995 Fortnightly review: management of atopic eczema. British Medical Journal 310: 843–847

Ministry of Agriculture, Fisheries and Food (MAFF) 1992 Foodsense No. 2: About food additives (Guide from the Food Safety Directorate PB0552). MAFF, London

Ministry of Agriculture, Fisheries and Food (MAFF) 1992 Foodsense No. 3: Understanding food labels (Guide from the Food Safety Directorate PB0553). MAFF, London

Ministry of Agriculture, Fisheries and Food (MAFF) 1994 Foodsense: Food allergy and other unpleasant reactions to food (Guide from the Food Safety Directorate PB1696). MAFF, London

Robertson A F, Bhatia J 1993 Feeding premature infants. Clinical Paediatrics 32: 36–44

Smith I 1993 Recommendations on the dietary management of phenylketonuria. Archives of Disease in Childhood 68: 426–427

Taitz L S, Wardley B L 1990 Handbook of child nutrition. Oxford University Press, Oxford

Truswell A S 1999 Food Sensitivity. In: Truswell A S (ed) ABC of nutrition, 3rd Edn. British Medical Journal, London: 96–100

USEFUL ADDRESSES

British Allergy Foundation
St. Bartholomew's Hospital
W. Smithfield
London EC1A 7BE

Child Growth Foundation
2 Mayfield Avenue
London W4 1PW

Cystic Fibrosis Trust
11 London Road
Bromley
Kent BR1 1BY
Tel: 0208 464 7211
Website: www.cftrust.org.uk

Galactosaemia Support Group
31 Cotysmore Road
Sutton Coldfield
West Midlands

National Eczema Society
163 Evershold Street
London NW1 1BU
Tel: 0207 388 4097

National Society for Phenylketonuria (NSPKU)
7 Southfield Close
Willen
Milton Keynes
Bucks. MK15 9LL

29

Diet in HIV infection

LEARNING OBJECTIVES

After studying this chapter you should be able to:

- explain the scientific basis for the nutritional and dietary therapy used in the treatment of human immunodeficiency virus (HIV)/acquired immunodeficiency syndrome (AIDS)
- provide practical dietary advice to improve the nutritional status of a person with HIV/AIDS.

THE IMPORTANCE OF GOOD NUTRITION IN HIV INFECTION

Nutritional advice is an important part of the care of all HIV-positive people at all stages of their disease, to:

- maintain optimal nutritional status
- prevent food-and water-borne infections
- optimise drug therapy
- treat and prevent gastrointestinal symptoms such as anorexia, nausea, vomiting and diarrhoea
- help fight infection
- enable clients to make decisions about the appropriateness and safety of alternative diets and dietary supplements.

Good nutrition not only improves quality of life and prevents weight loss, it prevents further weakening of the immune system and appears to extend the life-expectancy of the patient (Kotler 1989).

Nutrition following diagnosis

Following diagnosis, patients should undergo a full nutritional assessment to identify potential causes of malnutrition and identify effective strategies for their prevention and treatment. They can be provided with help and advice on how they can achieve an adequate diet within the constraints imposed by their own particular social and financial circumstances.

In addition the following issues should also be considered:

1. the feasibility of restoring nutritional status
2. the prognosis and desire for wellbeing of the client
3. the medical treatment plan
4. the health care setting in which the nutrition care will be provided (American Dietetic Association 2000).

Doing this will ensure that the opinions and requests of the patient are incorporated into the dietary advice wherever possible, and this will encourage the patient to keep to the diet advised and feel that he or she has some control over the situation. Peck & Johnson (1990) have shown that there is psychological benefit in nutritional advice which empowers individuals to maintain control over their own health.

Provision of a good diet is not always easy, as clients may have limited access to facilities for food storage and preparation. They may be totally dependent on government benefits or may have the type of lifestyle which excludes the eating of regular meals. Dietary advice given must therefore be tailored to individual requirements and may include advice on the use of convenience foods and budgeting.

Treatment with alternative diets. The range of complementary and alternative therapies used has been surveyed by Calabrese et al (1998). Clients should be enabled to make informed decisions about the usefulness for them of nutrition-related therapies. It is understandable that, while there is no cure for AIDS, patients may try alternative diets and therapies (Gowen et al 1993), however, the risks that accompany the use of some of them must be explained. Restricted diets can provide inadequate supplies of some nutrients and excessive amounts of others and the justification for some diets may be based on inaccurate information. It must be remembered that too much of a nutrient can be as harmful as too little.

HIV infection and body-weight

Ysseldyke (1991) has shown that severe weight loss is common in the later stages of HIV disease, and Summerbell (1994) has suggested that those with HIV may prolong their survival by aiming at maintaining their BMI within the range of 25 to 30. Ideally, nutritional advice should be given soon after the diagnosis that a person is HIV-positive. This advice should explain the basics of good nutrition and how to maximise intake of nutrients from food which will also enable individuals to make informed judgements about the potential benefits or risks of any alternative therapies they may wish to try.

Sore mouth and throat. Many patients experience this condition, which is caused by infection with *Candida* or herpes simplex, and by lesions of Kaposi's sarcoma in the mouth and throat.

These symptoms can be reduced by:

- avoiding spicy, salty or acidic foods
- eating soft foods
- stimulating salivary production by sucking boiled sweets or chewing gum
- thickening liquids with products like Instant Carobel or Thixo D for those patients who find liquids difficult to swallow
- eating an anti-candida diet (Crook 1985).

The anti-candida diet excludes all yeast-containing foods (bread, vinegar, wine) and foods rich in refined carbohydrates (sugar, sweets, confectionary and preserves). It is proposed that by excluding these foods the gut no longer provides a suitable environment for candida growth. However, there is as yet no conclusive evidence to show that this diet is effective.

Malabsorption and diarrhoea. These are experienced by 30 to 50% of patients with AIDS. If untreated, this leads to rapid loss of fluid and electrolytes resulting in metabolic disturbances. There are several causes including:

- *Cryptosporidium* infection
- emotional stress
- food poisoning (Kotler 1989)
- cytomegalovirus-induced enteritis and colitis.

HIV-positive individuals should be given information on safe food handling in their initial nutritional consultation, to ensure that they minimise their risk of bacterial food poisoning.

- They should also know how to calculate BMI and the importance of maintaining body-weight. This is particularly important in individuals who decide to adopt vigorous exercise plans which will increase their energy expenditure, or change their diet, e.g. become vegetarian, which may decrease their intake of energy-dense foods and some nutrients.

Nutrition and AIDS

At later stages, when the patient develops AIDS, the dietitian's and carer's skills are needed to ensure an adequate dietary intake, in spite of a range of clinical symptoms which include sore mouth, anorexia, vomiting and diarrhoea. These symptoms may appear independently or together and result from the many opportunistic infections that develop due to reduced immunity and also as the side-effects of treatment. Unless advice is given, the symptoms can prevent an adequate nutrient intake for long periods of time and will be accompanied by rapid weight loss. Nutritional support using supplements is an important part of treatment and should be used to help prevent weight loss when oral intake is reduced or energy requirements increased, and to help regain the weight lost during an acute infection.

Anorexia, nausea and vomiting. These result from depression, anxiety, opportunistic infections, tiredness and the side-effects of certain drugs and chemotherapy.

Reduction of these symptoms can be achieved by:

- eating small, frequent meals
- drinking 30 to 60 minutes before eating and not with meals
- eating dry foods, such as toast and plain biscuits
- avoiding greasy foods
- avoiding spicy, aromatic meals; cold meals which have no smell are often better tolerated
- resting in an upright position after meals. *Salmonella* and *Listeria* infections are far more common and serious in individuals whose immune function is reduced.

When the diarrhoea is not severe, it usually responds to antidiarrhoeal agents; a diet low in fruit and vegetable fibre may also be helpful. The use of sip-feeds which contain extra fibre, such as Entera Fibreplus (Fresenius Kabi Ltd) and Resource Fibre (Novartis Consumer Health) are beneficial for some people. The use of milk-free sip-feeds such as Provide Xtra (Fresenius Kabi Ltd) and Fortijuice (Nutricia Clinical Care) is beneficial for those people who develop lactose intolerance and need a milk-free diet.

In the most severe cases of malabsorption an elemental feed, which contains nutrients which do not need digesting, is used. The fat in this type of feed is provided as medium-chain triglycerides and the protein as hydrolysed amino acids. Because these feeds are unpalatable, it is usual for them to be fed enterally. When the gut function is severely impaired, total parenteral nutrition (TPN) may be the only way of maintaining adequate nutrition.

Meal timing and drug therapy

The interactions that occur between foods and drugs can include reduced drug-absorption, reduced nutrient-absorption, nutrient depletion and gastrointestinal side-effects. Anti-retroviral drugs show considerable variation in the best timing for drug therapy, some needing to be taken with food, others without, so the appropriate manufacturer's recommendations should be consulted.

As drug treatment becomes more complex and more successful, dietary treatment for HIV and AIDS is changing. Pharmaceutical interventions can result in fat accumulation, and increased lipid levels. These will need addressing to reduce the risk of developing diabetes, cardiovascular disease and obesity.

Breast-feeding and HIV infection

See Chapter 15 on infant feeding.

REFERENCES

American Dietetic Association 2000 Nutrition intervention in the care of persons with human immunodeficiency virus infection—position of the American Dietetic Association and Dietitians of Canada. Journal of the American Dietetic Association 100: 708–717

Calabrese C, Wenner C A, Reeves C, Turet P, Standish L J 1998 Treatment of human immunodeficiency virus-positive patients with complementary and alternative medicine: a survey of practitioners. Journal of Alternative Complementary Medicine 4: 281–287

Crook W G 1985 The yeast connection: a medical breakthrough. Professional Books/Future Health, Jackson TN

Gowen S L, Erskine D, McAskill R 1993 An assessment of the usage of non-prescribed medication by HIV-positive patients. Hospital Pharmacy Practice: 77–90

Kotler D P 1989 Diarrhoea in AIDS: diagnosis and management. Medical Times 177(3): 101–108

Peck K, Johnson S 1990 The role of nutrition in HIV infection. Journal of Human Nutrition and Dietetics 3: 145–157

Summerbell C 1994 Appetite and nutrition in relation to human immunodeficiency virus (HIV) infection and acquired immunodeficiency syndrome (AIDS). Proceedings of the Nutrition Society 53: 139–150

Ysseldkye L L 1991 Nutritional complications and incidence of malnutrition among AIDS patients. Journal of the American Dietetic Association 91: 217–218

FURTHER READING

British Dietetic Association 1995 Nutrition intervention in human immunodeficiency virus infection—position paper. British Dietetic Association, Birmingham

Fields-Gardner C, Thomson C A, Rhodes S S 1997 A clinicians guide to nutrition in HIV and AIDS. American Dietetic Association, Chicago

Macallan D C, Noble C, Baldwin C, Foskett M, McManus T, Griffin G 1993 Prospective analysis of patterns of weight change in stage IV human immunodeficiency virus infection. American Journal of Clinical Nutrition 58: 417–424

30

Diet in the treatment of multiple sclerosis

LEARNING OBJECTIVE

After studying this chapter you should be able to:

- provide appropriate dietary advice for a person with multiple sclerosis, that will improve their nutritional status and general wellbeing.

DIET AND MULTIPLE SCLEROSIS

Multiple sclerosis is a chronic degenerative disease in which patches of the myelin sheath surrounding the neurone axons are destroyed. The result of this is that the nerve impulses can no longer be transmitted along the nerve. The progression of this condition is unpredictable and it shows periods of remission and relapse, with most patients surviving for more than 20 years after the initial onset of the disease.

Many different dietary treatments have been tried for this condition but none have been shown to be consistently beneficial. An individual's nutritional status needs to be assessed regularly throughout the course of the disease and particular attention paid to:

1. *Fluid intake*. Patients with urinary incontinence may reduce their fluid intake—this should be discouraged as it can lead to both urinary tract infections and constipation.

2. *Non-starch polysaccharide (NSP) intake*. Increasing the intake of NSP will help to prevent constipation, this should be as fruit, vegetables and wholegrain cereal products.

3. *Body-weight*. Weight gain caused by the reduced energy expenditure resulting from reduced mobility will further reduce mobility. If the increase is due to 'comfort eating' because of isolation or depression, the gain in weight may cause further depression and low self-esteem. Treatment with steroids can also result in weight gain. If steroid-induced diabetes develops, it is treated with a diabetic diet (see Chapter 27).

4. *Weight loss.* As the condition progresses it may be difficult for patients to shop and prepare meals for themselves. Muscular weakness may make chewing and swallowing difficult. These problems can be overcome with supportive care and the use of nutritional supplements (see Chapter 23).

Weight loss should be prevented for two reasons:

- It reduces resistance to infection and relapses are more likely to occur following an infection.
- As mobility is reduced, the likelihood of pressure sores developing is greater. Good nutrition is important in their prevention.

People with multiple sclerosis use a range of alternative therapies including special diets (Winterholler et al 1997).

Diets which may be tried by people with multiple sclerosis include:

Exclusion diets. Particular foods or groups of foods are excluded because individuals consider themselves to be allergic to them. This type of dietary manipulation can be harmful, leading to malnutrition, particularly if large numbers of foods are avoided and if all energy-dense foods are eliminated.

Gluten-free diet. (see Chapter 24) There is no conclusive evidence that this diet is beneficial, although many multiple sclerosis sufferers claim their condition is helped by it. Gluten-free products are not prescribable for people with multiple sclerosis, so this can be an expensive diet to keep to, as bread, biscuits, flour, pasta and some breakfast cereals contain gluten, as do many manufactured products.

Action and Research for Multiple Sclerosis (ARMS) diet. This diet is low in saturated fat and high in essential fatty acids, which are necessary for the myelination of nerves.

Dietary supplements. Many people with multiple sclerosis take dietary supplements rich in essential fatty acids, such as evening primrose, starflower and wheatgerm oils. There is no definitive evidence that these are beneficial in the long term. While dietary supplements are not necessary for those people who are able to eat a diet that is nutritionally adequate, they should be considered to ensure the best possible nutritional status and to prevent malnutrition.

Malnutrition does occur in people with multiple sclerosis. A study by Timmerman & Stuifbergin (1999) showed that 10% of women with multiple sclerosis had an inadequate intake of NSP, vitamin E, calcium and zinc.

REFERENCES

Timmerman G M, Stuifbergin A K 1999 Eating patterns in women with multiple sclerosis. Journal of Neuroscience Nursing 31(3): 152–158
Winterholler M, Erbguth F, Neundorfer B 1997 The use of alternative medicine by multiple sclerosis patients (German). Fortschritte der Neurologie-psychiatrie 65 (12): 555–561

FURTHER READING

Mayer M 1999 Essential fatty acids and related molecular and cellular mechanisms in multiple sclerosis: new looks at old concepts. Folia Biologica 45(4): 133–141

USEFUL ADDRESSES

The Multiple Sclerosis Society
372 Edgeware Road
London NW2 6ND

Tel: 0808 8008 000
Website: www.mssociety.org.uk

31

Diet and arthritis

LEARNING OBJECTIVES

After studying this chapter you should be able to:

- discuss how dietary treatment can be used to reduce the severity of symptoms and improve the wellbeing of people with osteoarthritis and rheumatoid arthritis
- describe the dietary treatment of gout.

DIETARY TREATMENT OF ARTHRITIS

There are many unproven dietary remedies for both osteoarthritis and rheumatoid arthritis and, while there is little evidence to support their use, it is likely that patients with arthritis will wish to discuss the benefits of a special diet with those who care for them. Restricting the range of foods included in the diet can cause a dietary deficiency and, if any dietary changes are made, the diet must be assessed to ensure:

- optimal intake of all nutrients is maintained
- weight is maintained within the normal range.

Osteoarthritis

It is usual to advise people with osteoarthritis to try to maintain their body mass index (BMI) within the range of 20 to 25, as extra mechanical stress imposed on joints by obesity can result in further damage to the joints. Obesity also makes exercise more difficult and painful and reduces mobility. Some people find that supplementing their diets with fish oil is beneficial to them (Stammers et al 1989) and do this either by taking liquid fish oils or fish-oil capsules.

Rheumatoid arthritis

This condition is thought to be a disease of the autoimmune system. Not only is there swelling, inflammation and stiffness of the joints, but other symptoms associated with the condition are tiredness and loss of appetite. This can lead to weight loss and specific nutritional deficiencies, particularly iron-deficiency anaemia.

People with either osteoarthritis or rheumatoid arthritis are likely to encounter difficulties in shopping for, preparing and eating food and so should have their nutritional status monitored regularly, so that difficulties can be identified and resolved before they cause a decline in nutritional status.

Some of these difficulties can be overcome by using:

- *cups with special handles,* which are easier and safer to use and help maintain independence, dignity and adequate fluid intake
- *non-slip mats,* which stop plates from moving around on the table and are also useful for resting utensils on at the table, e.g. a mixing bowl
- *specially adapted kitchen utensils,* for example tin openers, spiked boards, jar openers and teapot stands, which all help to overcome some of the limitations imposed by stiff and swollen joints
- *large-handled cutlery,* which is easier to grip and use
- *high-sided dishes,* which are easier to eat from if only one hand can be used, as food can be pushed against the side.

GOUT

Gout can be a very painful condition and is characterised by recurrent episodes of acute joint inflammation, which is caused by raised plasma uric acid levels resulting in the deposition of sodium bicurate crystals in the cartilage of the joints. It is usually treated with the drug allopurinol, which reduces the serum uric acid by inhibiting renal tubular reabsorption of uric acid. Dietary treatment is used for those people who cannot be treated with drugs.

Dietary treatment for gout

1. *Achieve a BMI of 20 to 25.* A range of environmental and social factors are important in the causation of gout. It has been shown that the mean blood uric acid level is higher in overweight men than in men of normal weight (Phoon & Pincherle 1972) and that moderate weight loss is accompanied by a reduction in blood uric acid level (Nicholls & Scott 1972).

2. *Avoid fasting.* The weight loss to achieve an ideal body-weight must be slow and gradual and include regular meals. Plasma urate levels rise during starvation and increases can be measured after a 24-hour fast. The levels rise because the ketoacids produced as ketosis develops reduce the renal excretion of uric acid.

3. *Ensure adequate fluid intake.* A fluid intake of 1 to 2 litres should be aimed for, as this will dilute the urine and prevent the formation of kidney stones.

4. *Dietary purines.* These are contained in offal, such as liver, kidneys, brain and sweetmeats, meat extracts, oily fish and shellfish. However, these sources only contribute a small amount of the excess uric acid present in gout. Their restriction does not have a major impact on the blood uric acid level. However, their restriction will be beneficial for those people who cannot be treated with drugs.

REFERENCES

Nicholls A, Scott J T 1972 Effect of weight loss on plasma and urinary levels of uric acid. Lancet 2: 1223–1224
Phoon W H, Pincherle G 1972 Blood uric acids in executives. British Journal of Biological Medicine 29: 334–337

Stammers T, Sibbald B, Freeiling P 1989 Fish oil in osteoarthrosis (letter). Lancet: 503

FURTHER READING

Kershner R B, Lasswell A B 1992 Nutritional considerations in the management of arthritis in the home health patient. Journal of Home Health Care Practice 4(2) 23–33

USEFUL ADDRESSES

Arthritis Research Campaign (ARC)
Capeman House
St Mary's Court
St Mary's Gate
Chesterfield
Derbyshire S41 7TD
Tel: 01246 558033
Website: www.arc.org.uk

Arthritis Care
18 Stephenson Way
London NW1 2HD
Website: www.arthritiscare.org.uk

Appendices

Appendices

Weight

1000 micrograms (µg)	= 1 milligram (mg)
1000 milligrams	= 1 gram (g)
1000 grams	= 1 kilogram (kg)
28.35 grams (30 approx.)	= 1 ounce
1 kilogram	= 2.205 pounds (2.2 approx.)

Volume

1000 millilitres (ml)	= 1 litre (l)
28.4 millilitres (30 approx.)	= 1 fluid ounce (fl oz)
568 millilitres (550 approx.)	= 1 pint (p)
1 litre	= 1.76 pints (1¾ approx.)

1 teacup	=	150 ml	=	5 fluid ounces	Approximately
1 glass	=	225 ml	=	8 fluid ounces	

Energy

4.184 joules (4.2 approx.) = 1 calorie

Appendix 2 Reference nutrient intakes for vitamins. (Reproduced with permission from Department of Health 1991 Dietary reference values for food energy and nutrients for the United Kingdom. Report of the Panel on Dietary Reference Values of the Committee on Medical Aspects of Food Policy [COMA]. [Report on Health and Social Subjects 41] HMSO, London.)

Age	Thiamin	Riboflavin	Niacin (nicotinic acid equivalent)	Vitamin B6	Vitamin B12	Folate	Vitamin C	Vitamin A	Vitamin D
	mg/d	mg/d	mg/d	mg/d†	µg/d	µg/d	mg/d	µg/d	µg/d
0–3 months	0.2	0.4	3	0.2	0.3	50	25	350	8.5
4–6 months	0.2	0.4	3	0.2	0.3	50	25	350	8.5
7–9 months	0.2	0.4	4	0.3	0.4	50	25	350	7
10–12 months	0.3	0.4	5	0.4	0.4	50	25	350	7
1–3 years	0.5	0.6	8	0.7	0.5	70	30	400	7
4–6 years	0.7	0.8	11	0.9	0.8	100	30	400	–
7–10 years	0.7	1.0	12	1.0	1.0	150	30	500	–
Males									
11–14 years	0.9	1.2	15	1.2	1.2	200	35	600	–
15–18 years	1.1	1.3	18	1.5	1.5	200	40	700	–
19–50 years	1.0	1.3	17	1.4	1.5	200	40	700	–
50+ years	0.9	1.3	16	1.4	1.5	200	40	700	**
Females									
11–14 years	0.7	1.1	12	1.0	1.2	200	35	600	–
15–18 years	0.8	1.1	14	1.2	1.5	200	40	600	–
19–50 years	0.8	1.1	13	1.2	1.5	200	40	600	–
50+ years	0.8	1.1	12	1.2	1.5	200	40	600	**
Pregnancy	+0.1***	+0.3	*	*	*	+100	+10	+100	10
Lactation:									
0–4 months	+0.2	+0.5	+2	*	+0.5	+60	+30	+350	10
4+ months	+0.2	+0.5	+2	*	+0.5	+60	+30	+350	10

*No increment
**After age 65 the RNI is 10 mg/d for men and women
***For last trimester only
†Based on protein providing 14.7% of EAR for energy

Appendix 3 Estimated average requirements (EAR) for energy for children and adolescents, aged 0 to 18 years. (Reproduced with kind permission from HMSO, from Salmon J [for the Department of Health] 1991 Dietary reference values: a guide. HMSO, London.)

Age	EAR – MJ/d (kcal/d)	
	Boys	Girls
0–3 months	2.28 (545)	2.16 (515)
4–6 months	2.89 (690)	2.69 (645)
7–9 months	3.44 (825)	3.20 (765)
10–12 months	3.85 (920)	3.61 (865)
1–3 years	5.15 (1230)	4.86 (1165)
4–6 years	7.16 (1715)	6.46 (1545)
11–14 years	9.27 (2220)	7.92 (1845)
15–18 years	11.51 (2755)	8.83 (2110)

Appendix 4 Estimated average requirements (EARs) for energy (MJ/d) for groups of men and women at various ages, weights and activity levels. (Reproduced with kind permission from HMSO, from Salmon J [for the Department of Health] 1991 Dietary reference values: a guide, HMSO, London.)

Body Weight kg	BMR MJ/d	Physical activity level (PAL)								
		1.4	1.5	1.6	1.7	1.8	1.9	2.0	2.1	2.2
Men 19–29 years										
60	6.7	9.3	10.0	10.7	11.4	12.0	12.7	13.4	14.1	14.7
65	7.0	9.8	10.5	11.2	11.9	12.6	13.3	14.0	14.7	15.4
70	7.3	10.2	11.0	11.7	12.5	13.2	13.9	14.6	15.4	16.1
75	7.6	10.7	11.5	12.2	13.0	13.7	14.5	15.2	16.0	16.8
80	7.9	11.1	11.9	12.7	13.5	14.3	15.1	15.9	16.7	17.5
Men 30–59 years										
65	6.8	9.5	10.2	10.8	11.5	12.2	12.9	13.5	14.2	14.9
70	7.0	9.8	10.5	11.2	11.9	12.6	13.3	14.0	14.7	15.4
75	7.3	10.2	10.9	11.6	12.4	13.1	13.8	14.5	15.3	16.0
80	7.5	10.5	11.3	12.0	12.8	13.5	14.3	15.0	15.8	16.5
85	7.7	10.8	11.6	12.4	13.2	13.9	14.7	15.5	16.3	17.0
Women 18–29 years										
45	4.8	6.8	7.2	7.7	8.2	8.7	9.2	9.7	10.2	10.6
50	5.1	7.2	7.7	8.2	8.7	9.2	9.7	10.3	10.8	11.3
55	5.4	7.6	8.2	8.7	9.3	9.8	10.4	10.9	11.5	12.0
60	5.8	8.1	8.7	9.2	9.8	10.4	11.0	11.5	12.1	12.7
65	6.1	8.5	9.1	9.7	10.3	10.9	11.5	12.1	12.7	13.3
70	6.4	8.9	9.6	10.2	10.8	11.5	12.2	12.8	13.4	14.0
Women 30–59 years										
50	5.2	7.3	7.9	8.4	8.9	9.4	9.9	10.5	11.0	11.5
55	5.4	7.6	8.2	8.7	9.2	9.7	10.3	10.8	11.3	11.9
60	5.6	7.8	8.4	8.9	9.5	10.0	10.6	11.2	11.7	12.3
65	5.7	8.0	8.6	9.2	9.8	10.3	10.9	11.5	12.0	12.6
70	5.9	8.3	8.9	9.5	10.1	10.7	11.3	11.8	12.4	13.0

Appendix 5   Changes that would be needed in consumption of foods normally eaten during one week, to achieve the COMA nutrient target. The figures represent national averages, not recommendations for individuals. Food and drinks provided and eaten away from home would be additional to the amounts shown below. (Reproduced with permission from Department of Health 1994 Nutritional aspects of cardiovascular disease. Report of the Cardiovascular Review Group of the Committee on Medical Aspects of Food Policy [COMA]. [Report on Health and Social Subjects 46] HMSO, London.)

Food group	Average household food consumption 1992 (National Food Survey)		Illustrative example of average household food consumption meeting COMA recommendations		Comment
	g/person/ week*	Rough equivalent in terms of portions	g/person/ week*	Rough equivalent in terms of portions	
Milk	1960 (ml)	1 glass whole milk plus 1 glass semi skimmed milk each day	2140 (ml)	½ glass whole milk and 1¾ glasses semi skimmed milk each day	Continues trend to low fat milk.
Other milk and cream	260 (ml)	1 tablespoon cream each day	130 (ml)	½ tablespoon each day	Cheese consumption is currently steady
Cheese	115	filling for 2–3 sandwiches each week	60	filling for 1–2 sandwiches each week	
Carcase beef and lamb	210	2 portions each week	210	2 portions *lean* meat each week (trimmed off visible fat)	For carcase meat the amount is left unchanged but a switch to leaner meat assumed; for meat products the example shows reduced consumption with no change in fat content
Pork and poultry	300	3 portions each week	300	3 portions each week	
Other meat and meat products	440	7 portions each week	220	3½ portions each week (assumes 30% reduction in sodium content)	
Fish and fish products	140	1 portion white fish or fish products plus ½ portion oily fish	190	1 portion white fish or fish products plus 1 portion oily fish	In effect this means doubling the number of people eating sardines, salmon, etc in any week
Eggs	60	1 egg each week	60	1 egg each week	Assumes no change
Butter	40	spread for 3 slices bread each day	20	spread for 1½ slices bread each day	Continues switch to low-fat spreads and move from butter/margarine/lard to vegetable oils for cooking
Margarine	80		40		
Low and reduced fat spreads	50	spread for 1 slice bread each day	120	spread for 2½ slices bread each day	
Vegetable oils	50	4½ tablespoons each week	100	9 tablespoons each week	
Other fats	25	1½ tablespoons each week	10	¾ tablespoons each week	
Potatoes	900	1 small portion potatoes (2 egg sized potatoes) each day	1260	1 medium portion potatoes (3 egg sized potatoes) each day	
Potato products	170	each week either: 2 potato croquettes or 1 medium portion chips	80	each week either: 1 potato croquette or small portion chips	
Vegetables and products	1130	2–3 portions each day	1690	4 portions each day (assumes 30% reduction in sodium content of processed vegetables)	Assumes 50% increase in main categories; present trends are for fruit to increase (mainly juice) but potatoes and bread falling
Fruit and products	930	1½ pieces of fruit each day	1290	2 pieces fruit each day	
Bread	750	3 slices each day (of which 1½ slices wholemeal)	1130	4½ slices each day of which 1 slice wholemeal (assumes 30% reduction in sodium content)	

Buns, cakes and biscuits	290	3–4 biscuits each day	145	1–2 biscuits each day	Assumes 50% reduction, with no change from current composition
Breakfast cereals	130	1 bowl each day	130	1 bowl each day	Assumes no change
Other cereals	285	1 serving pasta or rice each day	285	1 serving pasta or rice each day	
Sugar and preserves	200	6 teaspoons sugar each day (or good spread for 2 slices bread)	190	5 teaspoons sugar each day (or thin spread for 2 slices bread)	Continues trends on sugar/preserves and move to low-calorie soft drinks.
Soft drinks (containing sugar)	720 (ml)	2 cans	360 (ml)	1 can each week plus any amount of sugar free drinks	Assumes small reduction in consumption of confectionery.
Chocolate confectionery	35	1 small bar each week	30	¾ small bar each week	Consumption of soft drinks and confectionery is probably heavily understated because
Sugar confectionery	15	3 boiled sweets each week	15	3 boiled sweets each week	much is bought for consumption away from home
All other foods	440	2 tablespoons pickle or dressing each day	440	2 tablespoons pickle or dressing each day	Assumes no change

*Unless otherwise stated

Appendix 6 A guide to foods for inclusion during weaning. (Reproduced with permission from Department of Health 1994 Weaning and the weaning diet. Report of the Working Group on the Weaning Diet of the Committee on Medical Aspects of Food Policy [COMA]. [Report on Health and Social Subjects 45] HMSO, London.)

	4–6 months	6–9 months	9–12 months	After 1 year	Extra information
Milk *Dairy products and substitutes*	**Minimum 600 ml breast or infant formula daily** Cow's milk products can be used in weaning after 4 months (*e.g. yoghurt, custard, cheese sauce*).	**500–600 ml breast milk, infant formula or follow-on formula daily** Also use any milk* to mix solids. Hard cheese (*e.g. Cheddar*) can be cubed or grated and used as 'finger food'.	**500–600 ml breast milk or infant milks daily** Also use any milk* to mix solids.	**Minimum 350 ml milk daily or 2 servings dairy product** (*e.g. yoghurt, cheese sauce*) Whole milk can be used as a drink and soft cheeses included after 1 year. Lower fat milks can be used in cooking, but not as main drink.	If milk drinks are rejected, use alternatives (*e.g. cheese*) and give water to drink. Discourage large volumes of milk after 1 year (i.e. more than 600 ml) as it will stop appetite for other foods. Discourage feeding from a bottle after 1 year.
The starchy foods	**Introduce after 4 months** Mix smooth cereal with milk: use low-fibre cereals (*e.g. rice based*). Mash or puree starchy vegetables.	**2–3 servings daily** Start to introduce some wholemeal bread and cereals. Foods can be a more solid 'lumpier' texture. Begin to give 'finger foods' (*e.g. toast*).	**3–4 servings daily** Encourage whole-meal products; discourage foods with added sugar (*biscuits, cakes, etc*). Starchy foods can be of normal adult texture.	**Minimum of 4 servings daily** At least one serving at each mealtime. Discourage high fat foods (*crisps, savoury snacks and pastry*).	Most baby and breakfast cereals are fortified with iron and B vitamins. Cereals and bread derived from whole-meals are a richer source of nutrients and fibre than refined cereals.
Vegetables and fruits	**Introduce after 4 months** Use soft-cooked vegetables and fruit as a smooth puree.	**2 servings daily** Raw soft fruit and vegetables (*e.g. banana, melon, tomato*) may be used as 'finger foods'. Cooked vegetables and fruit can be a coarser, mashed texture.	**3–4 servings daily** Encourage lightly-cooked or raw foods. Chopped or 'finger food' texture is suitable. Unsweetened orange juice with meals especially if diet is meat free.	**Minimum of 4 servings daily** Encourage unsweetened fruit if vegetables are rejected. Food can be adult texture though some fibrous foods may be difficult (*e.g. celery, radish*).	Vegetables may be prefered raw (*e.g. grated carrot, chopped tomato*) or may need to be disguised in soups, pies and stews. To improve iron absorption, give vitamin C (*fruits and vegetables*) with every meal.
Meat and meat alternatives	**Introduce after 4 months** Use soft-cooked meat/pulses. Add no salt or sugar or minimum quantities to food during or after cooking.	**1 serving daily** Soft-cooked minced or pureed meat/fish/pulses. Chopped hard-cooked egg can be used as 'finger food'.	**Minimum 1 serving daily from animal source or 2 from vegetable sources** In a vegetarian diet use a mixture of different vegetable and starchy foods (*macaroni cheese, dhal and rice*).	**Minimum 1 serving daily or 2 from vegetable sources** Encourage low-fat meat and oily fish (*sardine, herring, mackerel*). Liver paté can be used after 1 year.	Trim fat from meat Use little or no added fat when cooking foods which already contain fat, such as meat.

Appendix 6 (*cont.*)

	4–6 months	6–9 months	9–12 months	After 1 year	Extra information
Occasional foods	Choose low-sugar desserts; avoid high salt foods.	Encourage savoury foods rather than sweet ones. Fruit juices are not necessary—try to restrict to meal times or alternatively offer water/milk.	May use moderate amounts of butter, margarine. Small amounts of jam (if necessary) on bread. Try to limit salty foods.	Limit crisps and savoury snacks. Give bread, or fruit if hungry between meals. Do not add sugar to drink. Try to limit soft drinks to mealtimes.	Encourage a pattern of three main meals each day. Discourage frequent snacking on fatty or sugary foods.

*Includes breast milk, infant formula, follow-on formula and whole cow's milk.

Appendix 7 Recommendations for maintaining good nutritional status in elderly people. (Reproduced with permission from Department of Health 1992 The nutrition of elderly people. Report of the Working Group on the Nutrition of Elderly People of the Committee on Medical Aspects of Food Policy [COMA]. [Report on Health and Social Subjects 43] HMSO, London.)

1. The Working Group endorsed the recommendations for people aged over 50 years in the Government publication *Dietary Reference Values for Food Energy and Nutrients for the United Kingdom*.

2. Recommendations for dietary energy intakes of elderly people should tend to the generous, except for those who are obese.

3. Elderly people should derive their dietary intakes from a diet containing a variety of nutrient dense foods.

4. An active life style, with prompt resumption after episodes of intercurrent illness, is recommended as contributing in several ways to good health.

5. Steps should be taken to increase the awareness by health professionals of the importance of both overweight and underweight in elderly people.

6. For the majority of elderly people, the same recommendations concerning the dietary intake of non-milk extrinsic sugars apply as for the younger adult population.

7. Intakes of non-starch polysaccharides comparable to those recommended for the general population are advised for most elderly people. Foods with high phytate content, especially raw bran, should be avoided or used sparingly.

8. The statutory fortification of yellow fats other than butter with vitamin A and D should continue, and manufacturers are encouraged to fortify other fat spreads voluntarily.

9. Elderly people should be encouraged to increase their dietary intakes of vitamin C..

10. Adequate intakes of vitamin C need to be ensured for elderly people who are dependent on institutional catering.

11. Elderly people, in common with those of all ages, should be advised to eat more fresh vegetables, fruit, and whole grain cereals.

12. Elderly people should be encouraged to adopt diets which moderate their plasma cholesterol levels.

13. There should be encouragement of elderly people to consume oily fish and to maintain physical activity in order to reduce the risk of thrombosis.

14. The Working Group endorsed the WHO recommendation that 6 g/d sodium chloride would be a reasonable average intake for the elderly population in the UK, and recommends that the present average dietary salt intakes be reduced to meet this level.

15. The calcium intakes of elderly people in the UK should be monitored.

16. Doorstep deliveries of milk for elderly people should be maintained.

17. All elderly people should be encouraged to expose some skin to sunlight regularly during the months May to September.

18. If adequate exposure to sunlight is not possible, vitamin D supplementation should be considered especially during the winter and early spring.

19. Health professionals should be made aware of the impact of nutritional status on the development of and recovery from illness.

20. Health professionals should be made aware of the often inadequate food intake of elderly people in institutions.

21. Assessment of nutritional status should be a routine aspect of history taking and clinical examination when an elderly person is admitted to hospital.

Appendix 8 Body mass index chart. (Adapted from Garrow J.S. in *Obesity and Related Diseases* 1988, published by Churchill Livingstone, and Bray G.A. in *Human Obesity. Annals of the New York Academy of Sciences* 1989; 499. Reproduced with permission from Servier Laboratories Ltd.)

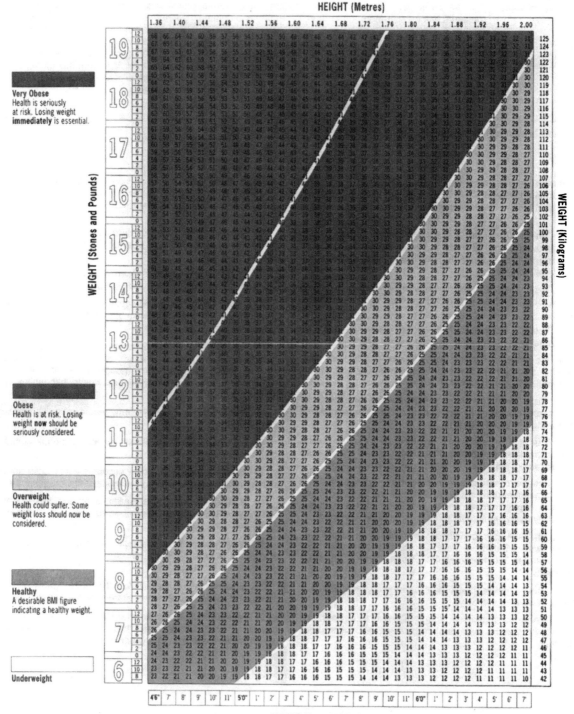

Appendix 9 Activity and injury factors for estimation of energy requirements. (Reproduced with permission from Long C L 1984 The energy and protein requirement of the critically ill patient. In: Wright R A, Heymsfield S (eds) Nutritional assessment. Blackwell Scientific, Boston.)

Basal energy Expenditure × activity factor × injury factor

Activity factors
Patients confined to bed	× 1.2
Patients out of bed	× 1.3

Injury factors
Minor surgery	× 1.20
Skeletal trauma	× 1.35
Major sepsis	× 1.60
Severe thermal burn	× 2.10

Appendix 10 Adult fluid and electrolyte requirements per kg actual body weight. (Based on Elwyn, D H 1980 Nutritional requirements of adult surgical patients. Critical Care Medicine 8: 9–20.)[a]

Change in basal metabolic rate	Water (ml/kg)	Sodium (mmol/kg)	Potassium (mmol/g nitrogen intake)[b]	Phosphate (mmol/day)
Normal (up to 25%)	30–35	1.0[c]	5.0	20
Intermediate (25–55%)	30–35	1.0	5.0	20–30
Hypercatabolic (45–100%)	30–35	1.0	7.0	50 (Max.)

[a]Pyrexia—for each 1°C above 37°C, give an additional 500–750 ml, water and 30 mmol Na^+.
[b]Potassium—give an additional 2 mmol/g nitrogen if serum $[K^+]$<3.5 mmol/litre and if refeeding severely malnourished patients.
[c]Minimum total daily intake.

Index

References to figures are indicated by 'f' and references to tables are indicated by 't' when they fall on a page not covered by the text reference.

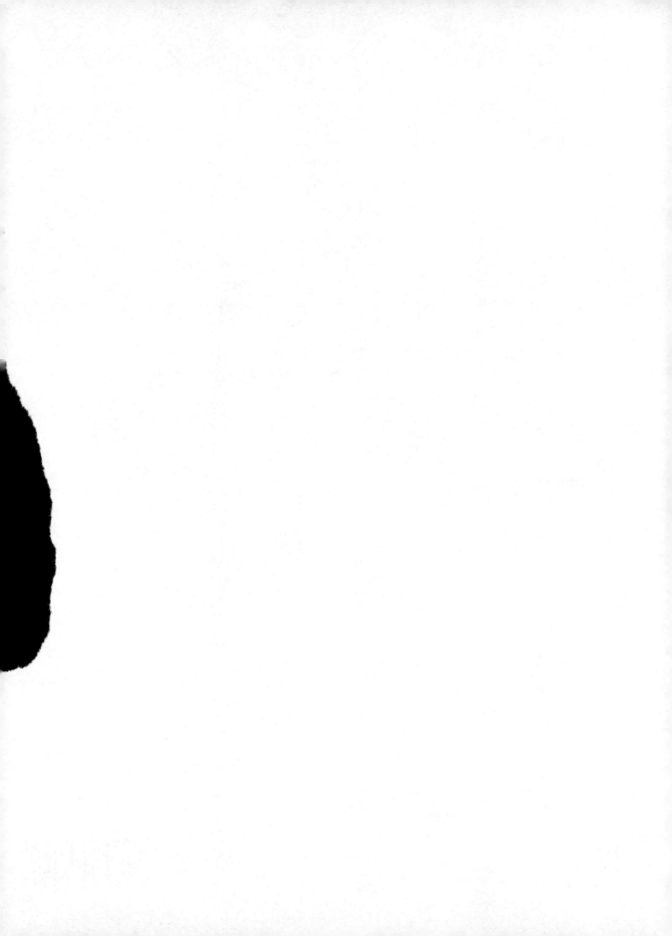

Lightning Source UK Ltd.
Milton Keynes UK
01 August 2010

157640UK00002B/1/P